THE KETO DIET FOR BEGINNERS

The Comprehensive Guide to Ketogenic Diet for Weight Loss, to Heal Your Body and Living Keto Lifestyle PLUS 100 Keto Recipes & 21-Day Meal Plan Program

TASHA RYAN

COPYRIGHTS

© Copyright NATASHA RYAN 2020 - All rights reserved.

The content contained within this book may not be reproduced, duplicated, or transmitted without direct written permission from the author or the publisher.

Under no circumstances will any blame or legal responsibility be held against the publisher, or author, for any damages, reparation, or monetary loss due to the information contained within this book. Either directly or indirectly. You are responsible for your own choices, actions, and results.

Legal Notice:

This book is copyright protected. This book is only for personal use. You cannot amend, distribute, sell, use, quote, or paraphrase any part, or the content within this book, without the consent of the author or publisher.

Disclaimer Notice:

Please note the information contained within this document is for educational and entertainment purposes only. All effort has been executed to present accurate, up to date, and reliable, complete information. No warranties of any kind are declared or implied. Readers acknowledge that the author is not engaging in the rendering of legal, financial, medical, or professional advice. The content within this book has been derived from various sources. Please consult a licensed professional before attempting any techniques outlined in this book.

By reading this document, the reader agrees that under no circumstances is the author responsible for any losses, direct or indirect, which are incurred as a result of the use of the information contained within this document, including, but not limited to, — errors, omissions, or inaccuracies.

DESCRIPTION

Are you planning to lose weight with a new diet regime? Would you like to heal your body while losing weight and change your lifestyle for the better? Have you heard of the ketogenic diet but want to learn more before you try it?

The ketogenic diet has taken the world by storm for some exceptionally good reasons that include a healthier lifestyle, delicious food, and, of course, that all-important weight loss that stays off. For millions of people, it has been their savior after years of trying and failing with other diets that simply didn't work.

Now, with this book, **The Keto Diet for Beginners: The Comprehensive Guide to Ketogenic Diet for Weight Loss, to Heal Your Body and Living Keto Lifestyle PLUS 100 Keto Recipes & 21-Day Meal Plan Program**, you can start on your own road to success with chapters that include:

- **Keto versus other diets**
- **The secret of ketosis and what it does to the body**
- **The benefits of the keto diet**
- **Safety advise while using the keto diet**
- **Side effects**
- **Avoiding common mistakes when starting out**
- **Keto catered for individuals**
- **How to follow the ketogenic diet on a budget**
- **And lots more...**

Even if you are someone who has yo-yo dieted for years and have all but given up, the ketogenic diet offers you something different that can really work and will see you lose weight quickly and easily once ketosis has been achieved. **The Keto Diet for Beginners** will talk you through each step of the process and provide you with the motivation to lose the weight you always wanted to.

TABLE OF CONTENTS

COPYRIGHTS	II
DESCRIPTION	III
TABLE OF CONTENTS	IV
INTRODUCTION	1
CHAPTER 1: ALL ABOUT KETO DIET	**2**
What Is The Keto Diet?	3
History Of The Keto Diet	8
Is Keto The Most Controversial Diet?	13
The Truth About Carbs And Fat Loss!	15
The Truth About Fat And Fat Facts	18
Myths about the Ketogenic Diet	22
Before Keto. Overview Of Various Diets	25
The Standard Ketogenic Diet (SKD)	27
The Cyclical Ketogenic Diet (CKD)	29
The Targeted Ketogenic Diet (TKD)	32
Keto VS Other Diets	40
What We Can And Can't Eat On The Ketogenic Diet	42
Food to Enjoy	50
Food to Avoid	51
Make Your Own Decision About Dieting	52
Conclusion	55
CHAPTER 2. KETO GENERAL BENEFITS	**56**
How The Body Adapts To The Ketogenic Diet — The Main Reason for Many of the Benefits	57
How The Ketogenic Diet Benefits Us All	59
Boosts Brain Function	59
Increases Energy	59
Help To Weight Loss	59
Decreases Inflammation and Pain	60

Increase Your Performance 60
Helps Build More Lean Muscles While Losing Fat 60
Improves Body Composition 60
Treating Epilepsy — The Origins Of The Ketogenic Diet 61
The Ketogenic Diet In Reversing Type 2 Diabetes 61
Controlling Type 1 Diabetes with the Ketogenic Diet 62
Improving Blood Pressure With the Ketogenic Diet 62
Booster Of The Digestive Health 63
The Power To Improve The Alzheimer's Disease 63
Parkinson's Disease Symptoms Reduced By Ketogenic Diet 64
Improve Cholesterol Levels And Reverse Heart Disease With The Ketogenic Diet 65
A Potential Treatment For Polycystic Ovary Syndrome And Infertility 65
Reverse Non-Alcoholic Fatty Liver Disease With The Ketogenic Diet 66
The Ketogenic Diet Helps Cancer Patients 67
Prevent And Reduce The Severity Of Migraines 67
Conclusion 69

CHAPTER 3. COMMON CONCERNS WITH A KETO DIET 70

Dawn Effect Of The Ketogenic Diet 71
Who Should Be Cautious With A Keto Diet? 72
How Safe Is The Keto Diet? 72
Is Keto Safe For Long-Term? 73
Is The Keto Diet Safe For You? 73
Are There Any Side-Effects Of This Diet? 74
Short-Term Side Effects 75
Long-Term Effects 75
What To Do About Keto Diet Side Effect 77
Other Cautions And How To Avoid Them 78
More About Keto Flu 79
The Simplest Cure For The Keto Flu 79
Conclusion 82

CHAPTER 4. ALL ABOUT KETOSIS 83
Short Introduction To Ketosis 84
What Is The Ketosis? 85
What Are Ketones? 87
Key Benefits Of Ketosis 88
Ketosis Health Effects 89
Ketosis Phases 89
Main Types Of Ketosis 90
Signs Of Ketosis 91
Ketones Measuring 92
How To Enter Ketosis? 94
Conclusion 95

CHAPTER 5. KEY PRINCIPLES OF THE KETO DIET 96
Fundamental Rules To Be On A Keto 97
Know What Side Effects to Expect 99
Use The Macro Calculator 101
Frequent Mistakes Of Beginners And How To Avoid Them 104
Possible Difficulties with Keto for beginners 107
Make a concrete nutrition plan 110
Keto Diet Plan Nutrition 111
Example Keto Diet Plan 114
How Many Meals Should Eat On The Keto Diet 115
Best Keto Products 116
How To Determine If A Product Is Keto-Friendly 122
Which Keto Products Are Right for You? 122
Conclusion 127

CHAPTER 6. KETO SPECIFIC 128
Keto For Women 129
Keto For Men 132
Keto For People Over 40/50/60 134
Keto For Sportsmen 138

Keto For Diabetes 141

Keto For Children 145

Conclusion 147

CHAPTER 7. KETO AND WEIGHT LOSS **148**

About Weight Loss With Keto 149

Low-Carbohydrate Diets Weight Loss 151

High-Protein Diets for Weight Loss 152

Foods You Can Eat on a Ketogenic Diet for Weight Loss 155

Using another approach: keto with intermitting fasting 160

Other information for weight loss with keto 162

Most Important Principles For Weight Loss 164

Conclusion 168

CHAPTER 8. KETO MISTAKES AND HOW TO AVOID THEM **169**

Fear of Eating Too Much Fat 170

Not Eating the RIGHT Fats 170

Not Drinking Enough Water 170

Not Consuming Enough Sodium 171

Too Much Dairy 171

Too Much Snacking 171

Having Cheat Meals 171

Not Sleeping Enough 172

Worrying Too Much About the Scale 172

Consuming Too Much Protein 172

Consuming More Carbs Than Recommended Levels 173

Not Being Patient 173

Eating Too Many Nuts 173

Eating Products that Are Labeled "Low-Carb" 173

Not Planning Your Meals 174

Not Getting Enough Exercise 174

Not Dealing with Stress 174

Conclusion 175

CHAPTER 9. KETO TIPS AND TRICKS 176

Keto On A Budget 177
Keto Grocery List On A Budget 178
Sample Meal Plan For Keto On A Budget 179
Essential Tips To Keto Lifestyle 181
Conclusion 187

CHAPTER 10. KETO MEAL PREP 188

What Is Meal Prepping? 189
How to Meal Prep in a Few Easy Steps? 189
Benefits Of Planning Meals 191
Must-Have Kitchen Essentials 192
Amazing Meal Prep Ideas 194
The Common Mistakes Made By Meal Prepping Beginners 195
Tips And Tricks For Making Meal Prep Easy 197
Measurements Conversion Tables 199
About Recipes 200

CHAPTER 11. KETO RECIPES and 21-day meal plan 202

21-DAY MEAL PLAN 203
Meal Plan. Week 1 203
Meal Plan. Week 2 204
Meal Plan. Week 3 205

Recipes Part 1 KETO SWEET BREAKFAST 206

Smooth Coconut Porridge 207
Keto Coconut Pancakes 208
Keto Cereal 209
Nut & Coconut Porridge 210
Sweet or Savory Breakfast Cookies 211
Cream Cheese Pancakes 212
Keto Pancake Bites 213
Keto Porridge 214

Peanut Butter Cupcakes 215

Coffee And Chia Pudding 216

Recipes Part 2 KETO BREAKFAST 217

Keto Mushroom Omelet 218

Baked Cheesy Egg Muffins 219

Vibrant Scrambled Eggs 220

Lettuce Sandwich 221

Beefy Baked Eggs 222

Keto Tuna Salad 223

Avocado And Egg Delight 224

Egg Salad 225

Classic Bacon And Eggs 226

Asparagus And Poached Eggs 227

Frittata With Spinach 228

Keto Bread 229

Sausage And Cheese Casserole 230

Salmon And Asparagus Frittata 231

Veggie Scramble 232

Scrambled Tofu 233

Tomato And Spinach Muffins 234

Keto Smoked Salmon And Egg Butter 235

Keto Egg Casserole 236

Breakfast Salad 237

Recipes Part 3 KETO SMOOTHIE 238

Spinach And Ginger Smoothie 239

Blueberry Smoothie 240

Keto Chocolate Smoothie 241

Turmeric Keto Smoothie 242

Avocado Smoothie 243

Coffee Smoothie 244

Spinach And Raspberry Smoothie 245

Chocolate Almond Smoothie ... 246
Avocado And Cucumber Smoothie ... 247
Raspberry And Yoghurt Smoothie ... 248

Recipes Part 4 KETO SALADS ... 249

Salmon, avocado, and arugula salad ... 250
Green Bean Salad ... 251
Salmon And Avocado Salad ... 252
Grilled Vegetable Salad ... 253
Chicken Salad ... 254
Cheesy Bacon Mushroom Salad ... 255
Cauliflower Salad ... 256
Strawberry Avocado Salad ... 257
Fun Cucumber Salad ... 258
Broccoli And Kale Salad ... 259

Recipes Part 5 KETO SOUP ... 260

Chicken Enchilada Soup ... 261
Zucchini Noodle Soup ... 262
Garlic Chicken Soup ... 263
Shrimp Chowder ... 264
White Chicken Chili Soup ... 265
Creamy Asparagus Soup ... 266
Mushroom Soup ... 267
Cauliflower Soup ... 268
Chicken Fajita Soup ... 269
Zucchini And Basil Soup ... 270

Recipes Part 6 KETO LUNCHES ... 271

Salmon Avocado Devilled Egg ... 272
Salmon With Pesto ... 273
Chicken Jalapeno Fritters ... 274
Prosciutto Mozzarella Balls ... 275

Green Beans And Bacon 276
Taco Pie 277
Chipotle Beef Chili 278
Keto Fried Chicken 279
Mexican Ground Beef With Veggies 280
Bread Rolls 281
Chicken Paprika Meatballs 282
Lamb Chops 283
Low-Carb Curry Chicken 284
Cheesy Beef Stuffed Peppers 285
Keto Cheesy Cauliflower 287
Keto Bread Sandwich 287
Tuna Steak 288
Salsa Chicken 289
Keto Pepperoni Pizza 290
Butter Chicken 291

Recipes Part 7 KETO DINNER 292

Skillet Lasagna 293
Garlic Butter Salmon 294
Chicken Caprese 295
Lamb Kofta 296
Garlic Chicken 297
Low-Carb Pasta 298
Butter Poached Shrimp 299
Mangolian Beef 300
Salmon With Spinach 301
Stuffed Avocado 302
Buttery Chicken With Broccoli 303
Cheese Stuffed Meatballs 304
Cabbage Casserole 305
Chicken Adobo 306
Keto Meatloaf 307

Roasted Pork Belly	308
Bacon Wrapped Chicken	309
Lamb With Kale	310
Cauliflower And Broccoli Casserole	311
Yakitori Chicken	312
REFERENCES	**313**
ABOUT AUTHOR	**314**

INTRODUCTION

Thank you for purchasing this book!

Living a keto lifestyle is possible for you, as long as you know about the diet and what you can and can't eat. The Ketogenic diet has revived the hope of individuals who are on the verge of giving up on their weight loss routine. This type of diet is unique. In a sense, it works on low carb diet composition. However, it does not put you in a starving mode because you will simply replace most carbs with fat, vitamins, and some proteins.

The main reason why you find it difficult to lose weight is that your body has been conditioned to rely on carbs for energy. Carbs can be hard to break down in the body system, and the fact that they slow down your metabolism simply means your weight loss will be ridiculously slow.

The Ketogenic weight loss diet works on a simple rule, and that is, to switch your body from carbohydrate-reliant to fat-burning mode. When your body enters into ketosis (the specific body condition with a keto diet), it uses up fat instead of carbs. That means your body will burn fat faster than when it is on carb-burning mode.

This book has comprehensive information about the ketogenic diet that will supercharge your weight loss journey.

Happy Reading!

CHAPTER 1.
ALL ABOUT KETO DIET

What Is The Keto Diet?

These days, it seems like everyone is talking about the ketogenic (in short, keto) diet — the very low-carbohydrate, moderate protein, high-fat eating plan that transforms your body into a fat-burning machine. Hollywood stars and professional athletes have publicly touted this diet's benefits: from losing weight, lowering blood sugar, fighting inflammation, reducing cancer risk, increasing energy, to slowing down aging. So is keto something that you should consider taking on? The following will explain what this diet is all about, the pros and cons, as well as the problems to look out for.

This chapter discusses some general ideas about ketogenic diets, as well as defining terms that may be helpful.

You must be aware that the body uses sugar (glucose) in the form of glycogen to function. The keto diet that is extremely restricted in sugar forces your body to use fat as fuel instead of sugar, since it does not get enough sugar (glucose). When the body does not get enough sugar (glucose) for fuel, the liver is forced to turn the available fat into ketones that are used by the body as fuel - hence the term ketogenic.

This diet is a high fat diet with moderate amounts of protein. Depending on your carb intake the body reaches a state of ketosis in less than a week and stays there. As fat is used instead of sugar for fuel in the body, the weight loss is dramatic without any supposed restriction of calories.

The keto diet is such that you should aim to get 60-75% of your daily calories from fat, 15-30% from protein, and only 5-10% from carbohydrates. This usually means that you can eat only 20-50 grams of carbs in a day. It depends on the type of keto diet, but we'll talk about that a little later.

So, in the most general terms, a ketogenic diet is any diet that causes ketone bodies to be produced by the liver, shifting the body's metabolism away from glucose and towards fat utilization. More specifically, a ketogenic diet is one that restricts carbohydrates below a certain level, inducing a series of adaptations to take place. Protein and fat intake are variable, depending on the goal of the dieter. However, the ultimate determinant of whether a diet is ketogenic or not is the presence (or absence) of carbohydrates.

The Keto In Other Words

Normally, the body uses glucose as the main source of fuel for energy. When you are on a keto diet and you are eating few carbs with only moderate amounts of protein (excess protein can be converted to carbs), your body switches its fuel supply to run mostly on fat. The liver produces ketones (a type of fatty acid) from fat. These ketones become a fuel source for the body, especially the brain which consumes plenty of energy and can run on either glucose or ketones.

When the body produces ketones, it enters a metabolic state called ketosis. Fasting is the easiest way to achieve ketosis. When you are fasting or eating very few carbs and only moderate amounts of protein, your body turns to burning stored fat for fuel. That is why people tend to lose more weight on the keto diet.

An Ideal Keto

An ideal ketogenic diet should consist of:

• 70-80% fat

• 20-25% protein

• 5-10% carbs.

Fuel Metabolism And The Ketogenic Diet

Under 'normal' dietary conditions, the body runs on a mix of carbohydrates, protein, and fat. When carbohydrates are removed from the diet, the body's small stores are quickly depleted. Consequently, the body is forced to find an alternative fuel to provide energy. One of these fuels is free fatty acids (FFA), which can be used by most tissues in the body. However, not all organs can use FFA. For example, the brain and nervous system are unable to use FFA for fuel; however, they can use ketone bodies.

Ketone bodies are a by-product of the incomplete breakdown of FFA in the liver. They serve as a non-carbohydrate, fat-derived fuel for tissues such as the brain. When ketone bodies are produced at accelerated rates, they accumulate in the bloodstream, causing a metabolic state called ketosis to develop. Simultaneously, there is a decrease in glucose utilization and production. Along with this, there is a decrease in the breakdown of protein to be used for energy, referred to as 'protein sparing'. Many individuals are drawn to ketogenic diets in an attempt to lose bodyfat while sparing the loss of lean body mass.

PERFECT
KETO BALANCE

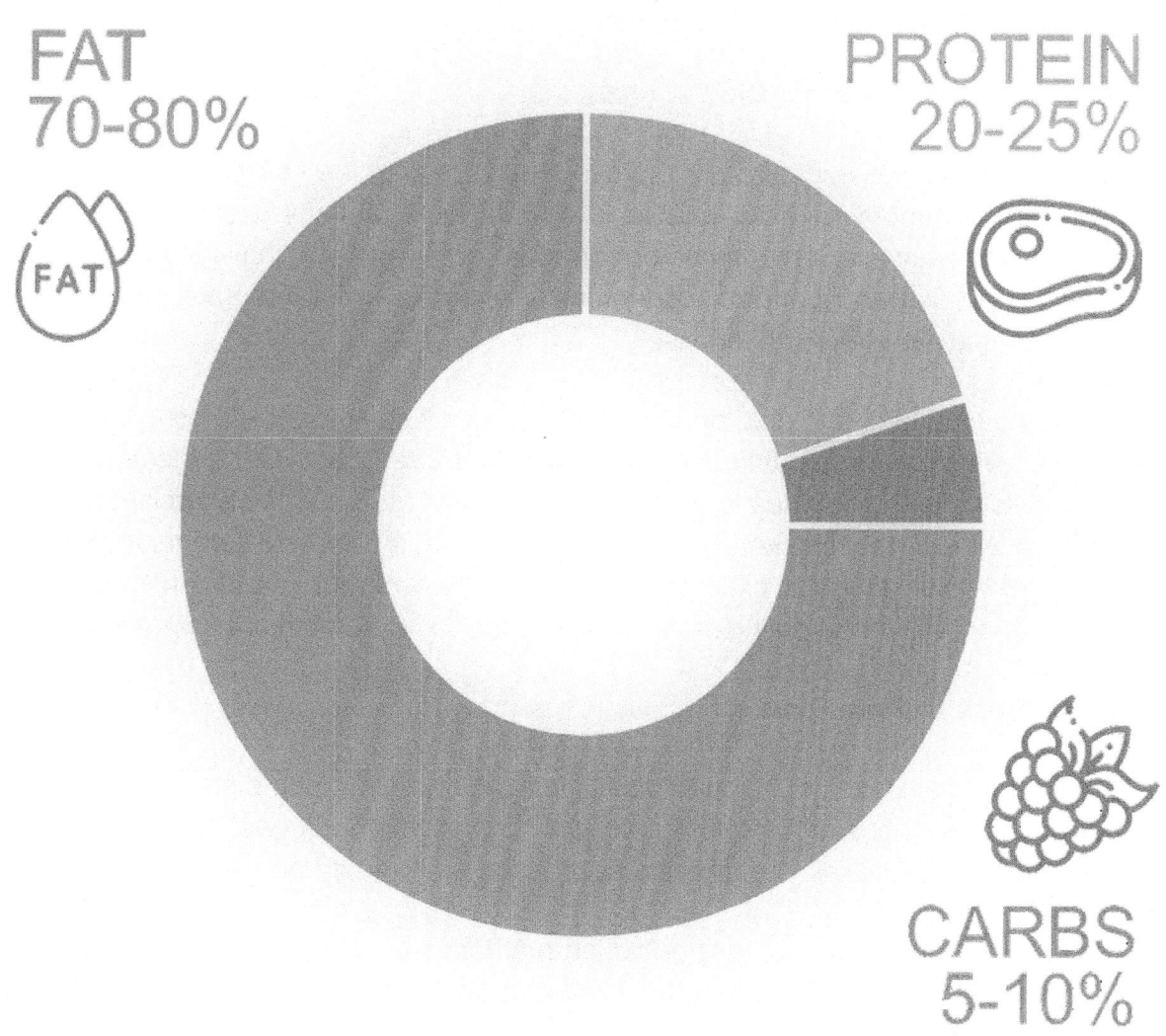

FAT
70-80%

PROTEIN
20-25%

CARBS
5-10%

Hormones And The Ketogenic Diet

Ketogenic diets cause the adaptations described above primarily by affecting the levels of two hormones: insulin and glucagon. Insulin is a storage hormone, responsible for moving nutrients out of the bloodstream and into target tissues. For example, insulin causes glucose to be stored in muscle as glycogen, and FFA to be stored in adipose tissue as triglycerides. Glucagon is a fuel-mobilizing hormone, stimulating the body to break down stored glycogen, especially in the liver, to provide glucose for the body.

When carbohydrates are removed from the diet, insulin levels decrease and glucagon levels increase. This causes an increase in FFA release from fat cells, and increased FFA burning in the liver. The accelerated FFA burning in the liver is what ultimately leads to the production of ketone bodies and the metabolic state of ketosis. In addition to insulin and glucagon, a number of other hormones are also affected, all of which help to shift fuel use away from carbohydrates and towards fat.

Exercise And The Ketogenic Diet

As with any fat-loss diet, exercise will improve the success of the ketogenic diet. However, a diet devoid of carbohydrates is unable to sustain high-intensity exercise performance although low-intensity exercise may be performed. For this reason, individuals who wish to use a ketogenic diet and perform high-intensity exercise must integrate carbohydrates without disrupting the effects of ketosis.

One main (the standard keto diet, or SKD) and two modified ketogenic diets are described in this book, which approach this issue from different directions. The targeted ketogenic diet (TKD) allows carbohydrates to be consumed immediately around exercise, to sustain performance without affecting ketosis. On the other hand, the cyclical ketogenic diet (CKD) alternates periods of ketogenic dieting with periods of high-carbohydrate consumption. The period of high-carbohydrate eating refills muscle glycogen to sustain exercise performance.

The Main Types Of Keto Diets

There are three main types of ketogenic diets in total. However, some are categorized into four classes, including a high-protein keto diet. But in this book, we'll consider three of them, and each of these takes a different approach to fat and carbohydrate intake.

After reading the book, you can decide which method is best for you. But remember that the most important thing when choosing is to understand your goals and your fitness level and lifestyle clearly.

The standard ketogenic diet [SKD]. It's the most common and recommended keto diet. Here, you stay in the range of 20-50 grams of net carbs per day. You should pay special attention to adequate protein intake and high fat intake.

Targeted Ketogenic Diet (TKD). This type will suit you if you are an active person. On a targeted keto diet, you can consume about 25-50 grams of net carbs before, during, or after exercise.

The cyclic ketogenic diet [CKD]. The best choice if a standard or targeted keto diet is difficult for you. It is also a great way to start keto. During CKD, you cycle through periods of a low-carb diet. For several days, you eat high-fat foods. This period is followed by a period of carbohydrate consumption (usually 1-2 days).

So, let's move on to the next questions. It will help us understand more about the keto diet. Also, I hope this helps to change some of your beliefs about dieting.

TYPES OF THE KETO DIET

STANDARD [SKD]

- 20-50g net carbs per day
- best for weight loss and start

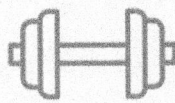

TARGETED [TKD]

- carbs 30 min. before and after exercise
- best for athletes and activity

CYCLICAL [CKD]

- high-fat low-carb diet 5-6 days
- couple days eating high-carb

History Of The Keto Diet

With discussing the theory and metabolic effects of the ketogenic diet, it is useful to briefly review the history and how it has evolved. There are two primary paths (and numerous sub-paths) that the ketogenic diet has followed since its inception: treatment of epilepsy and the treatment of obesity.

It should be understood that fasting (the complete abstinence of food) and ketogenic diets are metabolically very similar. The similarities between the two metabolic states (sometimes referred to as 'starvation ketosis' and 'dietary ketosis' respectively) have in part led to the development of the ketogenic diet over the years. The ketogenic diet attempts to mimic the metabolic effects of fasting while food is being consumed.

Cure For Epilepsy

The ketogenic diet has been used to treat a variety of clinical conditions, the most well-known of them is childhood epilepsy. Writings as early as the middle ages discuss the use of fasting as a treatment for seizures. The early 1900's saw the use of total fasting as a treatment for seizures in children. However, fasting cannot be sustained indefinitely and only controls seizures as long as the fast is continued.

Due to the problems with extended fasting, early nutrition researchers looked for a way to mimic starvation ketosis, while allowing food consumption. Research determined that a diet high in fat, low in carbohydrate, and providing the minimal protein needed to sustain growth could maintain starvation ketosis for long periods of time. This led to development of the original ketogenic diet for epilepsy in 1921 by Dr. Wilder. in many cases, he controlled pediatric epilepsy where drugs and other treatments had failed. The ketogenic diet as developed by Dr. Wilder is essentially identical to the diet being used in 1998 to treat childhood epilepsy.

The ketogenic diet fell into obscurity during the 30's, 40's, and 50's as new epilepsy drugs were discovered. The difficulty in administering the diet, especially in the face of easily prescribed drugs, caused it to all but disappear during this time. A few modified ketogenic diets, such as the Medium Chain Triglyceride (MCT) diet, which provided greater food variability were tried but they too fell into obscurity.

In 1994, the ketogenic diet as a treatment for epilepsy was essentially 'rediscovered' in the story of Charlie, a 2-year-old with seizures that could not be controlled with medications or other treatment, including brain surgery. Charlie's father found reference to the ketogenic diet in the literature and decided to seek more information, ending up at Johns Hopkins medical center.

Charlie's seizures were completely controlled as long as he was on the diet. The amazing success of the ketogenic diet where other treatments had failed led Charlie's father to create the Charlie Foundation. They have produced several videos, published the book "The Epilepsy Diet Treatment: An introduction to the ketogenic diet", and has sponsored conferences to train physicians and dietitians to implement the diet. Although the exact mechanisms of how the ketogenic diet works to control epilepsy are still unknown, the diet continues to gain acceptance as an alternative to drug therapy.

Other clinical conditions. Epilepsy is arguably the medical condition that has been treated the most with ketogenic diets. However, preliminary evidence suggests that the ketogenic diet may have other clinical uses including respiratory failure, certain types of pediatric cancer, and, possibly, head trauma. Interested readers can examine the studies cited, as this book focuses primarily on the use of the ketogenic diet for fat loss.

Cure For Obesity

Ketogenic diets have been used for weight loss for at least a century, making occasional appearances into the dieting mainstream. Complete starvation was studied frequently, including the seminal research of Hill, who fasted a subject for 60 days to examine the effects, which was summarized by Cahill. The effects of starvation made it initially attractive to treat morbid obesity as rapid weight/fat loss would occur. Other characteristics attributed to ketosis, such as appetite suppression and a sense of well being, made fasting even more attractive for weight loss. Extremely obese subjects have been fasting for periods up to one year given nothing more than water, vitamins, and minerals.

The major problem with complete starvation is a large loss of body protein, primarily from muscle tissue. Although protein losses decrease rapidly as starvation continues, up to one half of the total weight lost during a complete fast is muscle and water, a ratio which is unacceptable.

Alternative approach. In the early 70's, an alternative approach to starvation was developed, termed the Protein Sparing Modified Fast (PSMF). The PSMF provided high quality protein at levels that would prevent most of the muscle loss without disrupting the purported 'beneficial' effects of starvation ketosis, which included appetite suppression and an almost total reliance on bodyfat and ketones to fuel the body. It is still used to treat severe obesity but must be medically supervised.

At this time, other researchers were suggesting 'low-carbohydrate' diets as a treatment for obesity based on the simple fact that individuals tended to eat less calories (and hence lose weight/fat) when carbohydrates were restricted to 50 grams per day or less. There were many debates as to whether ketogenic diets caused weight loss through some peculiarity of metabolism, as suggested by early studies, or simply because people ate less.

Dr. Atkins Diet Revolution. The largest increase in public awareness of the ketogenic diet as a fat loss diet was due to "Dr. Atkins Diet Revolution" in the early 1970's. With millions of copies sold, it generated extreme interest, both good and bad, in the ketogenic diet. Contrary to the semi-starvation and very low calorie ketogenic diets which had come before it, Dr. Atkins suggested a diet limited only in carbohydrates but with unlimited protein and fat. He promoted it as a lifetime diet which would provide weight loss quickly, easily, and without hunger, all while allowing dieters to eat as much as they liked of protein and fat. He offered just enough research to make a convincing argument, but much of the research he cited suffered from methodological flaws.

For a variety of reasons, most likely related to the unsupported (and unsupportable) claims Atkins made, his diet was openly criticized by the American Medical Association and the ketogenic diet fell back into obscurity. Additionally, several deaths occurring in dieters following "The Last Chance Diet" - a 300 calorie-per-day liquid protein diet, which bears a superficial resemblance to the PSMF - caused more outcry against ketogenic diets.

From that time, the ketogenic diet (known by this time as the Atkins diet) all but disappeared from the mainstream of American dieting consciousness as a high carbohydrate, low-fat diet became the norm for health, exercise performance, and fat loss.

Recently, there has been a resurgence in low carbohydrate diets including "Dr. Atkins New Diet Revolution" and "Protein Power" by the Eades but these diets are aimed primarily at the typical American dieter, not athletes.

The Keto Diet And Athletes

Low carbohydrate diets were used quite often in the early years of bodybuilding (the fish and water diet). As with general fat loss, the use of low carbohydrate, ketogenic diets by athletes fell into disfavor as the emphasis shifted to carbohydrate based diets.

As they have reentered the diet arena in the 1990's, modified ketogenic diets have been introduced to athletes, primarily bodybuilders. These include so-called cyclical ketogenic diets (CKD's) such as "The Anabolic Diet" and "Bodyopus".

During the 1980's, Michael Zumpano and Daniel Duchaine introduced two of the earliest CKD's: 'The Rebound Diet' for muscle gain, and then a modified version called 'The Ultimate Diet' for fat loss. Neither gained much acceptance in the bodybuilding subculture. This was most likely due to difficulty in implementing the diets and the fact that a diet high in fat went against everything nutritionists advocated.

In the early 1990's, Dr. Mauro DiPasquale, a renowned expert on drug use in sports, introduced "The Anabolic Diet" (AD). This diet alternated periods of 5-6 days of low carbohydrate, moderate protein, moderate/high-fat eating with periods of 1-2 days of unlimited carbohydrate consumption. The major premise of the Anabolic Diet was that the low-carb week would cause a 'metabolic shift' to occur, forcing the body to use fat for fuel. The high-carb consumption on the weekends would refill muscle carbohydrate stores and cause growth. The carb-loading phase was necessary as ketogenic diets can not sustain high intensity exercise, such as weight training.

DiPasquale argued that his diet was both anti-catabolic (preventing muscle breakdown) as well as overtly anabolic (muscle building). His book suffered from a lack of appropriate references (using animal studies when human studies were available) and drawing incorrect conclusions. Moreover, his book left bodybuilders with more questions than it provided answers.

The Ketogenic Diet Nowadays

In the 1960s, people began using the keto diet for weight loss, but for the most part, the diet continued to toil in relative obscurity.

That started to change in the 1990s, with TV exposure about how the diet had cured two cases of epileptic children where pharmaceutical treatment had failed. The first case was aired in 1994 on NBC's Dateline, concerning the son of Hollywood producer Jim Abrahams. The second case appeared in 1997, in a true-to-life movie entitled First Do No Harm, starring Meryl Streep.

Nowadays, it seems everyone is already talking about the ketogenic diet. Many people prefer it to a standard diet. So, let's make our informed choice regarding this diet.

Is Keto The Most Controversial Diet?

We must all now be familiar with the term keto diet. Of all of the 'trendy' nourishment systems that move through our popular culture, none has caused as much interest or controversy. The diet that has caused a storm is continuing to acquire both dedicated followers and severe opponents both within and without the medical community.

The keto diet itself is only the most popular of an approach, usually called low-carb diets because of the primary interest in restricting consumption of carbohydrates. Since the entire spectrum of our food is drawn from proteins, fats, carbohydrates, or water, severe restriction of one group is seen by many as an arbitrary and, possibly, even dangerous step.

Most of the controversy surrounding low-carb approaches is not that they lie about weight loss (studies continue to show marked weight loss in many who use the diets) but the disturbing possibility that cutting the carbs out of your diet just isn't healthy.

The first and most obvious carbohydrate group (the one we rarely have much argument about reducing) is sugar. It is a catch-all term for a number of simple carbohydrates, including fructose (fruit sugar), galactose (milk sugar), sucrose (table sugar), and glucose (simple sugars such as blood sugar). Sugar consumption has been on the increase for decades and, despite the numerous campaigns against saturated fats, is certainly the biggest contributing factor to the increasing obesity epidemic.

Eating sugar causes a number of physiological effects in the body. The most striking of these is the sudden and marked increase in blood insulin. It is the hormone in our body responsible for 'taxiing' the food broken down in out stomach to the various parts of our body that require these substances, although it has numerous uses. First, and most importantly, when glucose levels rise in our blood, the process becomes extremely toxic. Left in our bloodstream without control elevated sugar levels would kill us quickly, so the powerful release of insulin helps keep our blood cleared of excess glucose. Unfortunately, insulin is a double-edged sword. Excess sugar in our body cannot be disposed of in an unlimited number of ways. With our increasing sedentary lifestyles refusing to burn off much of this sudden and quick release of carbohydrate as we consume, sugar is rapidly converted to the same saturated fats we are constantly warned about (as you can see, limiting saturated fat in the diet does not prevent us from accumulating fat in our bodies).

Sugar has other unpleasant side effects. The constantly elevated insulin levels can eventually lead to decreased insulin sensitivity (Syndrome X) and another case of type II diabetes. Sugar also has an effect on cortisol and our adrenal glands. It causes an excess of these hormones leading to symptoms of stress and fatigue. Sugar also competes with the glucose carriers in our blood, which work with vitamins like vitamin C, causing disruption to our preciously balanced immune system and causing premature ageing of the skin.

Sugar can be thought of as nitro-fuel for the body. It releases a very quick but harsh burst of artificial energy. In active individuals requiring peak performance from athletic pursuits, simple carbohydrates can be a useful tool, especially in the area of pre and post workout drinks. Much like a drag-racer using nitro fuel, this substance can be used to replace muscle glycogen and spare muscle wastage due to overtraining effects. Unfortunately, few of us use sugar in this careful and controlled manner and are attempting to drive the finely balanced engines of our bodies on a fuel, which causes too much stress and strain on a system that was never designed to handle the excess we provide.

So, since low-carb diets almost completely eliminate sugar from our diets, we have already found one significant health benefit.

HOW THE KETO DIET WORKS?

Consuming fat > Glucose level decreases

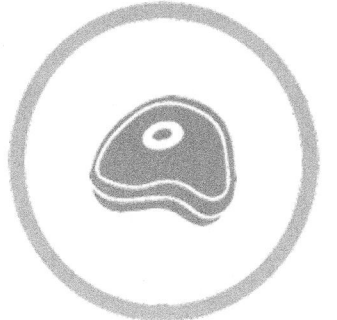 

Lipase releases triglyceride reserves

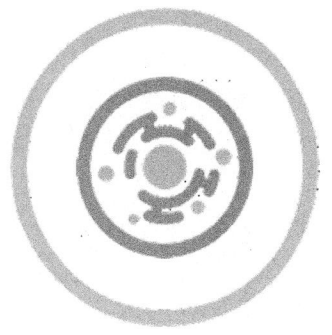 

Fat acids get in the liver

 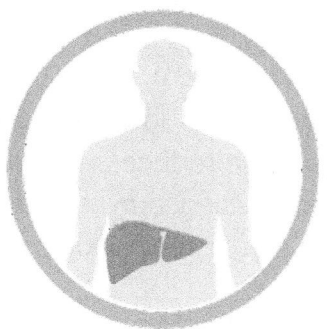 

Liver makes ketone cells > Energy appears

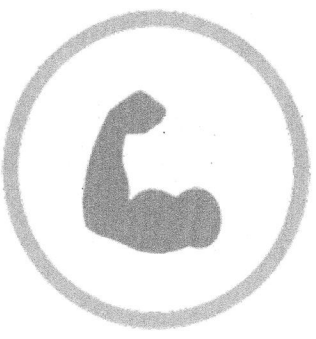

The Truth About Carbs And Fat Loss!

Before discussing the effects of the ketogenic diet, it is helpful to briefly talk about the characteristics of what we eat - carbohydrates and fats. It will help you to better understand some of the issues related to the keto diet later on.

So, what really is the truth about carbs and fat loss? If you go to fitness forums or read blogs in the market, you are likely to get a lot of conflicting information. Some of it is just flat out wrong, some of it is hype to support a new weight loss product, and some of it is right on target. The question is, how to choose?

There are generally two widely held beliefs when it comes to eating carbs and their effect on weight loss. The first belief is that carbs are inherently bad for losing weight and that carbs are easily turned into fat. Therefore, the anti-carb opinion is that to lose weight one should take in as few carbs as possible, which will promote the utilization of fat as fuel.

Then there is the "pro-carb" camp. They feel that limiting carbs is both unhealthy and will do little to promote fat loss. In addition, they would say a lack of carbs effects your ability to focus, upsets your mood, and can lead to over training in those who exercise.

So, which of these proponents are we to believe? The low-carb people? The pro-carb people? Let's peel back the onion on this and find out what the best approach to eating carbs is if you want to lose weight.

How Many Carbs Should You Eat In Order To Lose Weight?

Even the pro-carb enthusiasts would not say you should eat as many carbs as you like. And obviously, the low-carb enthusiasts would agree. But what is the optimal level?

First, it helps to understand that the number of calories you need to consume in order to lose weight should affect the amount of carbs you eat. There is plenty of proof to demonstrate that if you consume more calories than you expend, your weight will go up. Consume less than you expend and your bodyweight will go down.

This also explains why many people are successful on low-carb diets. The average American gets 50-60% of their calories from carbs. If we reduce carbs, we also reduce out total caloric intake and lose weight. For example, cutting our carb intake in half could reduce our daily calories by close to 30%, which is a sure recipe for losing weight.

Therefore, before you figure out how many carbs you should or should not have, it is best to figure out how many total calories you should eat. Once you have that number, we can come up with a really good rule of thumb for determining your calories from carbs. A good starting point is to portion your calories so that you get 40% from carbs and 30% from both proteins and fats.

This a moderate carb diet and will work well for most people. This approach will keep you from gaining excess weight due to carb and calorie intake, and it will help you maintain your exercise schedule without passing out from lack of fuel. In fact, you are likely to find that your performance in the gym or on the field is actually better following this approach.

Are There Such Things As Good And Bad Carbs?

Generally speaking, there is agreement that certain carbs are worse for your diet than others. Sugary foods, such as candy, cake, and soda pop are simple carbohydrates that get broken down by the body quickly. If they are not utilized quickly for fuel, they then get shuttled to storage for use later on. This storage area is the accumulated fat around our body and that's why a diet high in sugars leads to weight gain.

Most of us know by now that eating stuff like cake and candy is bad for us and will lead to putting on pounds if we are not careful. However, there is a grey area when it comes to carbs where people often make bad choices. For example, white bread and crackers might seem relatively healthy. But, most actually are high in carbs (it also means high in calories) due to the corn syrup and sugar that are used in making these products. The real nasty secret behind these kinds of ingredients are that they are the kinds of carbs that get broken down quickly and have greater potential to be stored as fats.

So, yes, some carb choices are better than others for fat loss. High sugar carbs should be replaced by better choices. Among the better choices are: fruits, vegetables, whole wheat, oats, barley, quinoa, rrown rice, lentils.

The other thing to note about the foods listed above is that they are more nutritionally dense and have fewer calories per serving than less optimal choices. It means that eating these foods will provide more value to your body in the form of vitamins, minerals, fiber, and all sorts of other good things that keep us healthy. In contrast, many processed foods tare calorie dense, but lack nutritional value.

A good recommendation to anyone who wants to burn off fat is to make these types of foods your primary source of carbohydrates and minimize other carbs.

The Truth About Fat And Fat Facts

Fat is probably the most contentious issue in nutrition. Are they as bad for us as we are led to believe? Are they really responsible for the often poor standard of health seen in the majority of the western world? Should we embrace the "low fat lifestyle"? The problem is that there is a huge amount of freely available information around, especially compared to pre-internet times. Unfortunately, much of it is a) out of date, b) incorrect, c) written by people with no formal training or qualifications or d) written using such technical language that for most of us it makes no sense!

Fats are classified according to their level of hydrogen content. All this actually means is that fats, which are said to be saturated, are packed to the gunnels with hydrogen molecules, and fats that are deemed unsaturated are missing some hydrogen molecules. The amount of hydrogen molecules present in a fat will dictate how a fat looks, tastes, and when we eat it. Fat should make up around 60-80% (in the keto diet) of our daily food intake. Very low-fat diets are actually quite unhealthy as we need a daily dose of fat for our bodies to perform at their best. Very low-fat diets are strongly linked to skin and hair problems, low birth weight babies, lowered testosterone levels in men, reduced brain function, impaired learning ability, lowered intelligence, and eye problems.

Let's take a look at the four main classifications of dietary fats.

1.   Saturated Fats

As mentioned before, these facts are saturated with hydrogen molecules, which make them very solid structures - they are often solid at room temperature e.g. butter and lard. They are chemically inert, which means they don't react much when exposed to heat, light, oxygen, or chemicals. Saturated fats are found mostly in animal products i.e. beef and dairy (milk, cheese, butter) as well as palm oil and coconut oil. Our bodies tend to use saturated fats for energy or energy storage (look down at your tummy - THAT'S saturated fat!!!)

Saturated fats are considered as the "bad boys" of the fat family but really this isn't the case. The worst thing we can say about saturated fats is they can make you fat if consumed in excess as they are very calorie dense. Being obese is associated with a host of negative health concerns but it's not the consumption of saturated fats that is the problem. Being overweight can be caused by over-consumption of carbohydrates or even protein. Eating fat can make you obese and being fat can be a health problem but let's not shoot the messenger! Some saturated fat in the diet is not just fine but is actually essential.

The body mostly uses saturated fat for energy and if it doesn't need the energy, it will store the fat around your body for later - often in places we'd prefer to be fat-free like our stomachs, legs, and bums. As mentioned previously, saturated fats are inert so they don't undergo any chemical changes when we eat them. Saturated fats don't clog your arteries, won't cause heart attacks, and are actually vital for mineral and vitamin absorption e.g. putting butter on your Sunday roast vegetables means the veggies become even better for you! Saturated fats are ideal for cooking as they don't turn rancid when heated (more on this later) and should make up around 30% of our daily fat consumption.

Speaking of saturated fats, how many of us have been told by "experts" to switch from butter to margarine to improve our health? This is a huge myth that I'd like to lay to rest right now. As we know, butter us made from cows' milk. Very little is added so it's safe to say that butter is a natural food. It consists mostly of saturated fat so is deemed by some as unhealthy but look closer at the alternative - margarine. Prior to the invention of refrigerators, margarine didn't exist. It was invented solely because butter doesn't spread when cold.

Margarine is a man-made food, more chemical than natural, contains all sorts of additives like E numbers, emulsifiers, acidity regulators, colors, artificial flavors, stabilizers etc. It's basically a chemistry set in a plastic pot. Butter, on the other hand, has no artificial ingredients, contains vitamins and minerals, is rich in CLA, which is an "anti cancer" super-fat, and also contains something called Wulzen Factor X. It is a substance, which prevents calcification of deposits in our arteries! So, in short, butter = good, margarine = bad. Even the so-called wonder-margarines that promise improvements for your health are no better for you than good old natural butter. Do like your grandparents did and eat butter in moderation - your heart and your taste buds will thank you for it! Incidentally, some cultures revere butter and actually prescribe it as a medicinal health food. It is given to soon-to-be mothers, growing children, the elderly and the sick as a cure all. Food for thought!

Here's a little experiment to try, which will hopefully show you that butter is best. Buy some margarine and some butter. Leave them both side by side on your kitchen worktop for a few days. After a while, you'll see the butter discolors very slightly (the outer surface oxidizes) but will pretty much stay unchanged. No fungus will grow on it (butter has anti-microbial properties, which can enhance gut health), it won't go off and, except for maybe a few fly foot prints (!), it will be completely unchanged. The margarine, however, will most likely have begun to separate, discolor noticeably, have fungus and bacteria growing on it, begin to smell bad, and actually go off. Don't eat it! The butter will be quite safe for consumption but the margarine won't do you any good at all.

2. Monounsaturated Fats

This type of fat is missing some of its hydrogen molecules and has a single bend in its chemical chain. This means that, unlike saturated fat, which is solid, straight and inert, monounsaturated fats are more reactive and liquid at room temperature. The body can use monounsaturated fats for energy but also for important chemical reactions in the body. They are good for our hearts, our hair and skin, and our overall health.

This reactivity is good because we can use monounsaturated fats for a host of healthy processes in our bodies but this reactivity also means monounsaturated fats can "go bad" and cause us more harm than good if they are over-heated, exposed to too much light or oxygen, or processed too aggressively. For example, the extraction method used when producing olive oil (the most common monounsaturated oil) can greatly affect its healthful properties. Extra virgin cold pressed olive oil is the Rolls-Royce of oils. It comes from the first pressing of the olives (hence "extra virgin") without the application of heat (hence "cold pressed") or solvents. This makes it very healthy. Anything other than extra virgin cold pressed olive oil will have been heated to high temperatures, had solvents used to increase oil yield, and come from a second or third pressing of the olives. All these factors mean our once healthy olive oil is now no longer good for us and may, in fact, be very bad for the body.

To preserve the healthy characteristics of monounsaturated oils (e.g. olive oil) it is important not to overheat them (stir frying is okay, long cooking times/high temperatures however will damage the oil), stick to extra virgin cold pressed oils where possible, and make sure oils are stored in an airtight dark glass container away from direct sunlight.

Olive oil is really best kept as a condiment and consumed raw but because it is only mildly reactive, it's okay to cook with it but only for short periods/lower temperatures. Saturated fats are better suited for longer cooking times and higher temperatures as heat doesn't affect them negatively. About 30% of our daily fat intake should be made up from monounsaturated fats.

3. **Polyunsaturated Fats**

This type of oil (e.g. sunflower oil) has lots of missing hydrogen molecules and, therefore, lots of bends in its chemical chain making it very reactive. These oils are so reactive that when we eat them, they are used almost exclusively for reactions in our bodies and very rarely for energy. Polyunsaturated fats are usually described as "Essential Fatty Acids" or EFA in short. They are often sold as supplements and are vital for the health of our hearts, nervous systems, joints, and brains. In fact, pretty much the entire body will benefit from regular consumption of EFA.

The reason polyunsaturated oils are considered so healthy is because of all the fats, they are the most reactive. No sooner have we eaten them they are whizzing around our bodies doing a myriad of useful functions. However, this reactivity is a double-edged sword. Polyunsaturated fats are very easily damaged by heat, light, and oxygen and should NEVER be heated. Heating polyunsaturated fats creates trans fats, which are the true "bad boy" of the fat gang (more about trans fats in a moment). They should be consumed raw, in their cold pressed extra virgin form only, and stored in a dark glass airtight bottle. They have a life span of around 4-8 weeks so should not be stored (even correctly) for longer than this to preserve their healthful properties.

As a side note — EFA are excellent anti-inflammatories. They can reduce the pain of some arthritic conditions very effectively. Cod liver oil has long been associated with healthy joints and is a great example of polyunsaturated oils doing an essential job. Around 30-40 % of our daily fat intake should be made up of polyunsaturated fats.

4. Trans Fats

Trans fats are "bent" unsaturated fats which have been straightened out artificially, which causes great confusion in our body's cells. In chemistry shape matters. Square pegs fit into square holes, round pegs into round holes. Trans fats are treated by the body as one thing when, in fact, they are something completely different. They end up going places they shouldn't and block the healthy fats from doing their job. It's as though a square peg has been jammed into a round hole, and this means other fats consumed a) can't do their healthy job and b) are now surplus to requirements and more likely to be stored around our middles.

Trans fats should be avoided at all costs. They're not hard to dodge if you follow these simple guidelines.

- Don't cook with polyunsaturated fats - use saturated fat or monounsaturated oils instead
- Avoid overheating monounsaturated fats - they do rancid easily
- Cut down on processed and takeaway foods - they often contain "hidden" trans fats
- Switch back to butter from margarine - there are no trans fats in butter!
- Avoid any food which has the word "hydrogenated" or "partially hydrogenated" listed on it's ingredients
- Cut back on shop-bought pies and pastries - homemade is best
- Keep your oils in dark glass airtight bottles
- Only buy extra virgin cold pressed oils.

Myths about the Ketogenic Diet

Carbohydrates Are The Most Important Macronutrient

It's simply not true. It is an ancient myth that has no fundament, no real study to prove it. Actual, as a medical term, means that the human body can't synthesize the nutrient itself, which means you have to get it through your diet. We all learn as kids in school that everything could be broken down in carbs if needed.

One prevalent saying is that we need carbohydrates to produce the fuel for a healthy and well functioning brain. What these people don't know is that this is only the case if you are going on a high-carb diet, which causes your brain to rely on more then usual amounts of carbohydrates. Our skeletal muscles burn fatty acids preferentially to spare glucose for the brain. However, once a person is keto-adapted, your brain switches to keto burn-mode and uses ketone bodies for over half its energy. If you look at people from African tribes, you won't see any health problems due to their diet. So, as you can see, carbohydrates are not an essential nutrient for a healthy lifestyle.

Keto Is Dangerous Due To Ketosis

It's a myth that will show you that your opponent has no idea about the term ketogenic diet. It is most likely because they confuse the terms ketosis and ketoacidosis.

Ketosis is what happens to your body when you use a controlled ketogenic diet. Insulin levels are regulated. It leads to the production of fatty acids and ketones triggered by either a rapid or decreased carbohydrates.

Ketoacidosis is caused by too low a concentration of insulin in the body. Without this, blood sugar levels immediately rise, leading to the release of stored fat from the fat cells. It causes your body to produce large amounts of ketones, which, combined with high blood sugar, interferes with the average acid-base balance of the system to the point that it can be too dangerous.

But with ketosis, the situation is different. So this is just another myth caused by a lack of knowledge.

High Protein Intake Will Damage Your Kidneys

Like the myths mentioned above, this one is based on a lack of knowledge. Nobody ever said that a ketogenic diet is low in carbohydrates and high in protein instead. The ketogenic diet is based on moderate protein intake and high fat intake. So no - your kidney will not be damaged by your high protein intake, it just isn't.

The Ketogenic Diet Is Just A Trendy Diet

The ketogenic diet is not a new diet. Anyone who says this is a trendy diet is ignoring the facts. In fact, the ketogenic nourishment has been considered a cure for epilepsy for almost 100 years. But going back even further, we see that low-carb diets are even older. The first low-carb diet was published in 1863. Then it also had great success.

In addition to being an "ancient concept" of diet, low-carb nutritional therapies have been proven effective in over 20 different scientific studies since 2000 alone. So we're talking about a hobby around for more than 150 years and has proven successful results for people. It doesn't look like a fancy diet at all.

Trendy diets may come and go every year, but the ketogenic diet isn't one of them. It has been around for a long time and will be a successful way to lose weight for a long time.

The Ketogenic Diet Is Hard To Follow

Some people say that following a ketogenic diet is more complicated than others because you have to remove entire food groups from your diet. It makes the person crave the missing food groups; therefore, he ends up breaking his diet. However, all diets exclude something, be it a food group or calories. However, the idea is that it is more challenging to stick to a ketogenic diet that you can eat until you are full.

On the other hand, people with calorie restriction cannot afford ever to enjoy food. It is a sure way to break your diet.

The Ketogenic Diet Will Ruin Your Physical Performance

Many people believe that carbohydrates are essential for maximum physical performance. Most top athletes eat a high carbohydrate diet, so it follows that this is a better diet for the best results.

Your physical performance will indeed decrease. But only at the beginning of the ketogenic diet. It is because your body is adjusting to using fat for energy. However, after you give yourself a few weeks to get used to the new changes, you will find that the ketogenic diet no longer slows you down. Several studies have confirmed that low-carb meal plans like the ketogenic diet improve physical performance in the long term, especially during endurance exercise.

One study, published in 2014 in the British Journal of Sports Medicine, found that when people are given a few weeks to adjust, they perform better on a low-carb diet. Other studies, including one published in 2014 in the Journal of the International Society of Sports Medicine, have shown that a low-carb diet is beneficial for muscle strength and mass.

Ketosis Will Disrupt The Body's Metabolism

This idea is also a confusion of two different metabolic terms. Ketosis is often confused with ketoacidosis. It is a process when your body synthesizes ketones from fat for fuel.

Ketoacidosis is a dangerous disease. It is caused by uncontrolled type I diabetes. When the bloodstream is filled with ketones to the point that it becomes acidic, if left untreated, it can be fatal. On a ketogenic diet, you will never go into a state of ketoacidosis. For ketoacidosis to occur, something must be wrong with your body.

Low Carbohydrate Intake Leads To Muscle Shrinkage

It is quite evident that the opposite is true. Several studies show that people who were in a calorie deficit while dieting high in carbohydrates and low in fat lost more lean muscle mass than people who followed the keto diet. The main factor in maintaining muscle mass is an adequate protein intake, which you will achieve with a ketogenic diet.

There will be many "nutritionists" who will say that you should be getting at least 100 grams of carbohydrates every day. Indeed, only in this case, our body will not inhibit muscle growth. It is valid only in one case - if your body is continuously high in carbohydrates, high in insulin and blood sugar, and no ketones that would give the brain the necessary energy.

Most Of The Weight Loss Comes From Water Weight

It is true that at the beginning of the ketogenic diet, you will lose a lot of excess weight. It will happen mainly due to the loss of water. It is because glycogen, which the body stores in the liver and muscles as a reserve (in case of blood sugar drops), binds to water.

Also, as blood sugar levels drop, so does insulin levels. This decrease in insulin allows the kidneys to excrete more sodium from the body, reducing water retention. As a result of these two factors working together, a significant amount of water is lost almost immediately. There is no reason to say that this is bad. If you don't need an extra five to ten pounds of water weight, why carry it around with you everywhere?

People On A Ketogenic Diet Suffer From Diseases Caused By Low Fiber Intake

First of all, the standard Western diet contains too little fiber to maintain healthy intestinal flora. Second, the ketogenic diet provides us with a wide variety of vegetables. These are spinach, broccoli, kale, parsley, and more. And these vegetables are the primary source of fiber for those on a ketogenic diet.

Don't let the myth of the lack of knowledge lead you astray!

Before Keto. Overview Of Various Diets

Before moving on to a detailed description of the keto diet, I suggest looking at the many other existing diets. We have a vast selection. So, let's choose!

Beverly Hills Diet - a diet consisting of grapefruit, eggs, rice, and kelp; it is deficient in minerals and vitamins.

Cambridge Diet - a very low calorie (300-600 kcal/day); protein/carb mixture with mineral imbalances; the dieter is close to fasting.

Complete Scarsdale Diet - this diet is unbalanced nutritionally; some days are calorically restricted; the dieter alters portions of carbohydrate, protein, and fat; the diet consists of low carbs (20-50 g/day) and high fat and protein; the diet has a high meat (saturated fat and cholesterol) content.

Dr. Atkin's Diet Revolution - this diet is unbalanced nutritionally; some days are calorically restricted; the dieter alters portions of carbohydrate, protein, and fat; carbs are very low (20-50 g/day), whereas fat and protein are high; there is high meat (saturated fat and cholesterol) consumption.

Dr. Linn's Last Chance Diet - this diet has a very low-calorie intake (300-600 kcal/day); it consists of a protein/carb mixture with a mineral imbalance; the dieter is close to fasting.

Dr. Reuben's The Save Your Life Diet - this is a calorically dilute diet consisting of high fiber (30-35g/day); the diet is low in fat and animal products; there is poor absorption of minerals because of too much high fiber.

F-Plan Diet - this is a calorically dilute diet consisting of high fiber (30-35 g/day); it is low in fat and animal products; there is low absorption of minerals because of too much fiber.

LA Costa Spa Diet - this diet promotes weight loss of 1-1_ lbs./day; there are various plans of 800, 1000, and 1200 kcal/day composed of 25% protein, 30% fat (mostly polyunsaturated), and 45% carbohydrate; the diets includes the four food groups.

Medifast Diet - this diet is balanced nutritionally, but provides only 900 kcal/day; use of liquid formulas makes this diet monotonous and expensive.

Nutrimed Diet/Medifast Diet - this is a nutritionally balanced diet, but it supplies only 900 kcal/day; the use of liquid formulas makes this diet monotonous and expensive.

Optifast Diet - this diet is nutritionally balanced, but supplies only 900 kcal/day; use of liquid formulas makes this diet monotonous and expensive.

Pritikin Permanent Weight-Loss Diet - this is a nutritionally unbalanced diet; some days are calorically restricted; the dieter alters portions of carbohydrate, protein, and fat; the diet consists of high protein (100 g/day); unless the foods properly chosen, it may be low in vitamin B12.

Prudent Diet - this is a balanced, low calorie (2400 kcal/day) diet for men; it is low in cholesterol and saturated fats; a maximum of 20-35% calories are derived from fat with an emphasis on protein, carbohydrates, and salt; there is ample consumption of fish and shellfish, and saturated fats are substituted with polyunsaturated fats.

Quick Weight Loss Diet - this diet is unbalanced nutritionally; some days are calorically restricted; the dieter alters portions of carbohydrate, protein, and fat, although there are low carbs (20-50 g/day), and high fat and protein; there is high meat consumption (saturated fat and cholesterol) with this diet.

San Francisco Diet - this diet begins at 500 kcal/day, consisting of two meals per day of one fruit, one vegetable, one slice of bread, and two meat exchanges; the second week limits carbohydrates, with most food coming from the meat group and with some eggs and cheese, and a few vegetables; week three includes fruit; in week four there is an increase in vegetables; week five the dieter add fat containing foods (e.g., nuts, avocados); week six includes milk; week seven includes pastas and bread, where the diet is maintained at about 1300 kcal/day; this diet avoids the issue of saturated fats and cholesterol.

Slendernow Diet - this diet is unbalanced nutritionally; some days are calorically restricted; the dieter alters portions of carbohydrate, protein, and fat; the protein is generally high (100 g/day); unless foods are properly chosen, there may be a deficiency in vitamin B12.

Weight-Watchers Diet - this diet is balanced nutritionally, at about 1000-1200 kcal; use of high nutrient-dense foods are consumed; economic and palatable food makes it one of the most successful diets with no real health risks.

Wine Diet - this diet is about 1200 kcal/day, containing 28 menus together with a glass of dry table wine at dinner; besides the medicinal components of wine, it is believed that individuals reduce portion sizes when wine is consumed with a meal; the diet is low in cholesterol and saturated fats; there is a focus on fish, poultry, and veal with moderate amounts of red meat.

Yogurt Diet - this diet consists of two versions, being 900-1000 kcal/day and 1200-1500 kcal/day; plain low-fat yogurt is the main dairy dish, consumed at breakfast, lunch, and as a bedtime snack; the diet is high in protein and it is low in cholesterol, saturated fat, and refined carbohydrates.

The Standard Ketogenic Diet (SKD)

The standard ketogenic diet focuses primarily on protein and fat; carbohydrate intake is minimal. As stated earlier, if you keep your daily carbs low enough, your body relies on fatty acids and molecules called ketones for energy, not glucose (sugar).

This shift in substrate metabolism has many benefits. These include improved cognitive function, more energy throughout the day, lower blood sugar, and a possible reduction in certain types of cancer. You will learn more about these benefits in the following chapters of the book.

The standard ketogenic diet is one of three different types of ketogenic diets. Like others, it is right for your health and well-being. But the kind of ketogenic diet you choose should depend on your goals.

The standard ketogenic diet is more suitable for health and longevity. Next, you will find out everything you need to start your SKD journey.

Your Ketogenic Diet Option. The type of ketogenic diet you go for depends on your goals. When choosing a type, your genetic and metabolic characteristics of the body will play an important role in this. Either way, you should start with a standard ketogenic diet for at least 2 weeks.

This will give your body a chance to adapt to ketosis. It will help you switch to new fuel sources. Naturally, provided that you give up a diet rich in carbohydrates.

After those first few weeks on a standard ketogenic diet, you will be able to answer many questions: how are you feeling, and which ketogenic diet to follow in the long run. Other possible options are the cyclic ketogenic diet (CKD) and the targeted ketogenic diet (TKD), which we'll talk about later.

How To Start Your Own Standard Ketogenic Diet?

Below are the necessary steps to calculate your energy requirements for your body, as well as the required level of macronutrient intake with a standard ketogenic diet. The first calculation steps will help you figure out your macronutrient needs when you are meeting SKD.

The typical starting point for most people looking to lose weight is a 500 calorie deficit per day. But it's important to understand that there is no one set of calories, regardless of whether you want to lose weight or build muscle.

In any case, you will have to increase or decrease your nutrient intake. This will depend on the rate of fat loss or muscle gain. Also, note that your calorie intake will fluctuate every day if you choose to use CKD or TKD.

The following example shows how to calculate macronutrient needs for someone with 180 lbs of lean body mass following a 2'200 calorie SKD.

1. Determine your calorie requirements with a basic metabolic rate [BMR] calculator [2200 calories in this case].

2. Consume roughly up to 1,5 grams of protein per pound of lean body mass [g/lb LBM]: 270 g protein daily for this person.

3. Carbohydrate consumption should be 0.1-0.2 g/lb LBM: 25 g carbohydrates on a standard ketogenic diet per day.

4. Fat intake comprises the remaining calories to reach 2'200: 2'200 – 1'180 = 1'020 calories / 9 calories per gram of fat = 115 g of fat daily.

Therefore, this person nutrient amount is: 270 g protein, 25 g carbohydrate, and 115 g fat.

Tip: It is best to distribute all macronutrients proportionally across three to five meals each day.

Thus, the standard ketogenic diet is very low in carbohydrates, high in fat, and moderate in protein.

Therefore, you need to avoid direct sources of starch and carbohydrates on a standard ketogenic diet. Avoid foods such as wheat, rice, potatoes, cereals, etc. on SKD.

Your diet should consist primarily of animal proteins, eggs, nuts, coconut, MCT oil, nut butters, vegetables, and greens.

The standard ketogenic diet is best for people who have a goal of improving overall health and extending life expectancy (from ketosis). If you train intensely, consider following the CKD or TKD.

The Cyclical Ketogenic Diet (CKD)

All diets take discipline, some more than others. The cyclical ketogenic diet (CKD) is no exception. In addition to a healthy dose of discipline, the CKD also requires some calculations and calorie watching.

We are all equal, yet no two bodies are the same. That is exactly why there is no "one size fits all" for this and many other diets.

Simply put, the CKD is a cycle between periods of eating varying levels of fat, protein, and carbohydrates. It includes 5-6 days of eating a diet consisting of high-fat, high-protein, and low-carbs. This is followed by 1-2 days of low-fat, high-protein and high-carbs.

Most of us have fueled up a car at some point in life (and watched as the price kept rising). So, we all should know that some cars run on gasoline, while others run on diesel.

Now, imagine having a car that let *you* decide what type of fuel it would run on! If gasoline hit rock bottom prices, fill up with gas. Otherwise use diesel - whichever is cheaper. This would be a dream come true for most drivers.

How excited would you get if I told you that our bodies already have that ability?

Conventionally, most of us have been getting our fuel from carbohydrates (aside from dieting). The common symptom from people suffering from "carb withdrawal" is a lack of energy. This is what happens when you decide to cut down on carbohydrates. Here is the exciting part... there is a way to tell your body to use fat for energy instead of carbs! If your eyes light up as you read that last sentence then keep reading...

Cyclical ketogenic diet sounds nice, but how does it lead to six-pack abs?

When you stop eating carbs (or substantially minimize your carb intake) your body says, "oh no! Now where am I going to get my energy from?"

If those carbs are replaced with healthy fat, it's like telling your body, "hey, carbs got to expensive... I'm switching you to fats instead."

The fancy name for having that "conversation" with your body is The Metabolic Switch - burning fat for energy, instead of carbohydrates. However, you can't just switch back and forth whenever you feel like it and expect to lose fat while discovering your six-pack abs in the mirror. There is a method to the madness. Keep reading...

Cyclic ketogenic diet - eat more fat to lose more fat!?

By now, you might be considering doing the metabolic switch and telling your body to use fat for energy. Congratulations, you now have to start eating more fat and protein while nearly eliminating any carbs (the less carbs you eat, the better).

The purpose of the cyclic ketogenic diet is to lose extra fat. Yes, it's true that you will be eating a lot of fat and protein; however, your body will also burn that extra fat you want to lose... if you eat the right amount of total calories (from fat and protein) per day. Confused? Then read the example below.

For example only (please do not use these numbers on yourself, it's only an example):

You need to eat a total of 1800 calories per day to maintain your current weight (60% from fats, 35% from protein, 5% from carbs). If you only eat 1300-1400 calories per day, your body says, "I STILL NEED MORE FUEL!"

Since you cut down on carbs and the majority of your diet is fat, your body starts looking for more fat for energy... and guess where it finds that extra fat? Yup, that's right, that stubborn body fat that you have been trying so hard to lose becomes an energy source! Your body says, "Hey, I found all this extra fat so I'm going to burn it for energy." Day by day, your body fat is reduced, and the mirror becomes your best friend.

Exercising also helps... but you already knew that.

The result of all of this is that your body is now trained to burn that extra fat and you can finally plan the return (or arrival) of your six pack abs. Go jump for joy, then come back to read the rest.

Cyclic ketogenic diet - carbohydrates are our friends sometimes...

This diet is "cyclic." In other words, there is a cycle that you should repeat. It involves eating carbs, so pizza and bread lovers rejoice!

Without going into too much detail, the purpose of 1-2 days of high carb intake is to refill the glycogen stores in your muscles. Glycogen is the main source of food for your muscles. As you use your muscles throughout the week (hopefully you use your muscles), glycogen reserves slowly begins to empty. Therefore, increasing carb intake for a couple days a week fills up your muscle energy tanks again. Now you're ready to hit the gym with full force!

Cyclic ketogenic diet - I could do all that, if I knew how much to eat...

The most time-consuming part of the CKD is planning your meals out. Ideally, you want to aim for 60% fat, 35% protein and 5% carbs. These percentages are based on the recommended total caloric intake for your body. So don't go eating 4000 total calories a day and expect the results you're after. There are calculations of lean body mass and body fat percentage that need to be done. Like I said before, the hardest part (aside from the actual diet) is doing the research. Learning to do everything yourself AND counting calories for every meal can be challenging... make your diet easier and more efficient by getting a computer to do all the hard work for you.

The Targeted Ketogenic Diet (TKD)

is not much different from the standard ketogenic diet (SKD). There is one crucial difference: how and when you eat carbs.

On standard keto, you don't worry about carbohydrate choices. You know your carbohydrate level is always low. On TKD, you consume your daily carbohydrate intake at a specific time - before, during, or after your workout. Is there any benefit at all from a targeted ketogenic diet? Can TKD get you out of ketosis? And is TKD right for you? Let's find out.

Benefits of a targeted ketogenic diet

Do the TKD correctly. As a result, you will be in ketosis most of the time. It means that TKD has virtually the same benefits as a standard or cyclical keto diet.

General benefits

Here's a short overview of the main advantages of the keto diet, which we'll learn in more detail. All of them are to a lesser extent applicable to a targeted ketogenic diet: weight loss, improved appetite control, increased energy efficiency during the day, lower blood sugar, lower insulin levels, improved fat burning, increased cognitive performance, decreased systemic inflammation, the therapeutic potential for certain cancers, and other benefits

TKD for sports and endurance

The targeted ketogenic diet has one significant advantage over the standard ketogenic diet. This is your improved physical performance. Eating adequate amounts of fast-digesting carbohydrates before, during, or after intense exercise can help you achieve better results. This will replenish glycogen stores and make your workout more efficient.

To get this benefit from TKD, you need to:

1. Adapt to fats. This usually happens a few weeks after starting the keto diet. This will make it easier for you to get in and out of ketosis.

2. Deplete glycogen. If you eat carbohydrates and do not deplete muscle glycogen during exercise, then the glucose from the carbohydrates will remain in your bloodstream (instead of being stored in the muscles). And an increase in blood sugar will bring you out of the ketogenic state.

In other words, you will only benefit from TKD if you burn your glycogen stores (during exercise). You are more likely to run out of glycogen stores if you engage in heavy glycolytic training on a regular basis.

This could be CrossFit, high-intensity interval training, or sprint. Long-term cardio training also depletes muscle glycogen. However, when you are fat-adapted, it takes a long time for muscle glycogen to deplete.

Therefore, TKD can only benefit those who have been on the keto diet for a long time.

Who is TKD suitable for?

Among keto diets, the target ketogenic diet is between the standard ketogenic diet and the cyclical ketogenic diet (CKD). The choice of SKD, CKD, or TKD depends on your activity level. It also depends on the goals you set.

Choosing the right type of keto diet

Let's start with the Standard Keto Diet. If you have a light daily exercise plan, such as yoga, walking, or light cycling, then SKD is your best bet. These activities are not intense, and your fat can fuel them.

Many people may have a complicated daily exercise plan on SKD. It depends on the person and their level of physical stamina.

Basically, the standard ketogenic diet is the best option for weight loss, therapeutic ketosis, and other keto benefits.

The main exception is athletic performance.

The cyclic keto diet is for serious athletes. If you choose this type, then this means eating a large amount of carbohydrates (from 400 to 500 grams). Only once or twice a week, and the rest of the time, ultra-low carb intake.

Overactive people like professional athletes (marathon runners, bodybuilders, athletes) constantly burn glucose and deplete glycogen.

Therefore, they can choose CKD. They will be able to return to ketosis relatively quickly after a carbohydrate load.

CKD is not for weight loss or therapeutic ketone production. CKD is designed for high octane performance.

TKD is also designed for athletes, but unlike other types of the keto diet, it is suitable for anyone - male or female. For those doing heavy, glycogen-depleting exercise, this could be CrossFit, sprints, high-intensity workouts, or long-distance running.

Additional carbohydrates during exercise can help replenish glycogen stores. They raise blood sugar levels and reduce exercise fatigue.

You can lose weight with TKD. But only if you eat the right carbohydrates at the right time. In doing so, you do the right workouts with a sufficient level of intensity.

But remember that the performance-enhancing effect of TKD is very individual. Humans have natural differences in the storage and use of glycogen. There are also major differences in fat adaptation and ketone production.

Because of this, some will work better on TKD than SKD. And vice versa. Even during hard training.

This is especially important for strength training.

So TKD is for strength training?

For strength training or muscle building, you'd better be on a standard ketogenic diet.

Some people still say "you need carbs to build muscle." It's based on the theory that you need insulin to grow muscle. Because insulin is a building hormone and blood sugar regulator.

But recent research suggests otherwise. In one recent study, bodybuilders gained more muscle mass on a ketogenic diet than on a high-carb diet.

It's time to question the theory of carbs for muscle gain.

To build muscle, you only need to do two things:

1. do strength training.

2. eat enough protein

A ketogenic diet can help you achieve your strength goals because your main ketone, Beta-Hydroxybutyrate, actively maintains muscle mass. It also works with leucine, an amino acid in muscle-building protein, to accelerate muscle synthesis.

The bottom line is that adding carbohydrates for TKD or CKD does little to improve strength training.

In fact, some data on strength training athletes have shown little benefit from refeeding carbohydrates.

This is because lifting weights does not deplete muscle glycogen. But running for two hours is another matter entirely. Again, extra carbohydrates can help.

And remember, the type of carbohydrates matters.

What you can eat and avoid on a targeted keto diet

When comparing macronutrients, TKD is similar to SKD.

Calories: This is about 60% healthy fats, 30% protein and 10% carbohydrates. High in fat, low in carbohydrates and moderate in protein.

Healthy fats include:

• Monounsaturated fats (olive oil, avocado, nuts),

• Saturated fats (butter, ghee, animal fat, coconut oils and MCT oils),

• Polyunsaturated fat (nuts and fish in moderation).

Pro-inflammatory vegetable oils should be avoided. They have a high content of omega-6 linoleic acid, especially when cooking.

Protein is simple.

A complete protein source such as whey protein or high quality pasture meat and wild-caught fish should be included. Complete proteins contain all nine essential amino acids. They promote muscle growth and usually come in the form of animal proteins.

You need few carbohydrates.

For TKDs, the standard recommendation is 15-50 grams of fast-digesting carbohydrates before, during, or after exercise. These simple carbohydrates come in two flavors - powdered (dextrose) and real food (glucose).

Why dextrose and glucose?

If you exercise hard enough, these simple sugars are burned during exercise and stored as muscle glycogen.

Important! Avoid eating fructose for TKD or any other form of ketogenic diet. Fructose goes directly to the liver and is stored as glycogen.

It doesn't improve performance. In addition, a high fructose diet has been shown to induce insulin resistance. It can also cause obesity and liver disease.

Add high quality MCT oil to your TKD routine. It is rapidly absorbed, passed to the liver and converted into ketone bodies - regardless of carbohydrate intake.

MCT will help you stay in ketosis with TKD.

How TKD Affects Ketosis

Ketosis is the primary goal of the keto diet and a unique metabolic state. When you are in ketosis, your cells burn fat to produce ketones for energy.

Compared to glucose, we can say that ketones burn cleaner. They are less inflammatory and more efficient energy producers.

Basic rules of ketosis: ketogenic diet, fasting, exercise. The main rule is limiting carbohydrates. It's the #1 way to get into ketosis. Restricting carbohydrates will lower your insulin levels. This tells your body to burn fat and produce ketones.

Will TKD get you out of ketosis?

Eating carbohydrates (in any amount) raises blood sugar levels. This reduces the production of ketones.

So the answer is yes. Swallowing a packet of dextrose - even before or after a hard workout will get you out of ketosis.

So, it's new target. Return to ketosis as soon as possible.

The time you need to return to ketosis depends on several factors:

1) Fat adaptation. Before starting TKD, you need to adapt to fat.

Once your mitochondria learn to burn fat, it will be easier for them to return to this mode after coming out of ketosis.

2) Type of exercise. Intense exercise - sprint, crossfit, others - are called glycolytic. This is because they require glucose for fuel. And if you eat carbs before sprinting, those sprints will use up your blood glucose. Therefore, you can return to burning fat and making ketones.

But even on TKD, do low-intensity aerobic exercise. These exercises do not require glucose for fuel. Therefore, they are ideal for adapting to fats and producing ketones. Keep your heart rate at 180 minus your age (this is a working method).

3) Insulin sensitivity. The faster your blood sugar drops, the faster you will return to ketosis. This depends in part on your insulin sensitivity.

Keto-friendly carbs

The truth is, simple starches and simple sugars mean a quick end to your ketosis (ketogenic state).

For a standard ketogenic diet, low glycemic carbohydrates are best. These are berries, zucchini, artichokes and asparagus.

A low glycemic index refers to the effect of food on blood sugar levels. The lower the better.

These foods are low on the glycemic index because they are rich in fiber. The more fiber carbohydrates contain, the less they will raise blood glucose levels.

Also eating fiber: helps gut bacteria work (this keeps the gut and flushes out toxins), reduces the risk of stroke and cardiovascular disease, keeps the immune system in good working order, and helps prevent diabetes

High-fiber carbohydrates limit spikes in blood sugar and insulin levels. They help you stay in ketosis.

But on TKD, your goals are different.

You need these carbohydrates right during your workout. Therefore, they must be high on the glycemic index.

One option is dextrose powder. If you don't like dextrose, try simple starches like white rice or white potatoes. Avoid fructose.

Should I try TKD?

If you are new to the standard ketogenic diet, then you need to give your body about 4-6 weeks. This time is necessary in order to adapt to fat as fuel.

During this adaptation period, you may develop the keto flu. Low energy levels, poor sleep, or decreased physical activity are also often reported.

It's normal. And the most important thing now is not to increase the amount of carbohydrates. Also, don't try TKD or CKD. Take electrolytes instead. Add some low-intensity exercise. Eat non-starchy vegetables.

These symptoms will disappear soon. Also consider reducing intense glycolytic exercise during the initial phase. Once you get used to the fat, you can return to hard training. SKD best reflects the benefits of a low-carb lifestyle.

But if your performance is diminishing, try experimenting with a targeted ketogenic diet. Additional carbohydrates will help: Replenish muscle glycogen and provide glucose for intense workouts.

How to start TKD: step by step

Below you will find basic guidelines.

Go to standard keto first. Be aware that if you are not fat adapted, you cannot easily return to ketosis. To perform a TKD correctly, you will need at least 4-6 weeks of SKD experience.

Determine your own (unique) amount of carbohydrates. Different people switch to keto in different ways. Some can eat more than 50 grams of carbs and still produce ketones. Others cannot.

You will need to measure your ketone levels throughout the day to determine your unique carbohydrate intake. Ketone test strips are the best way to do this. Start small. Less than 25 grams of net carbs per day. Net carbs = grams of carbs - grams of fiber.

If your ketones consistently exceed 0.5 mmol/L, then you should cut out more carbohydrates. Try and experiment. When you try TKD, eat all carbs just before, during, or after your workout.

Minimize your carbohydrates. The goal of TKD is to eat as little carbs as possible. This is necessary to improve your productivity.

Play it. Again, start small. Consume 15-30 grams of carbohydrates before training. If you need more carbs, divide by 2. Eat them before and after training. This will reduce the spike in blood sugar.

To minimize the time without ketosis, do not exceed 50 grams of carbs per day.

Eat Carbohydrates Before or During Workout. This kind of carbohydrate intake (before or during your workout, not after) may work best for TKD.

That's why: Supplemental glucose assists in glycolytic exercise. It potentially improves your productivity; Intense exercise burns excess glucose. Therefore, you will quickly return to the ketogenic state.

Stick to protein and fat after exercise to stimulate muscle protein synthesis.

Eat fast-digesting carbohydrates. On SKD, you should prioritize low glycemic carbohydrates. These are berries, carrots and zucchini, greens, they have a high fiber content.

On TKD, your goals are different. You need these carbohydrates right during your workout. Therefore, they must be high on the glycemic index.

The best option is dextrose powder. If you don't like dextrose, eat simple starches. This is white rice or white potatoes. The main thing to remember is to avoid fructose.

Maintain your calorie intake. If your goal is to lose weight, you should maintain a constant TKD energy intake. If you add carbs before exercise, then you must subtract fatty calories from somewhere else. It's simple - a gram of carbohydrates contains 4 calories, and a gram of fat contains 9 calories.

If you eat 9 grams of extra carbs, subtract 4 grams of fat from your meal. Both contain 36 calories.

Smart supplements. Ketosis can deplete your electrolytes. These are minerals that support hydration, regulate PH levels, and activate muscle and nerve tissue.

If you experience muscle cramps or fatigue when exercising on TKD, then the cause may be a lack of electrolytes - magnesium, potassium, sodium, chloride, and calcium. Therefore, taking full spectrum electrolyte supplements can help.

Other supplements will also be helpful: creatine helps preserve muscle glycogen, L-citrulline increases nitrous oxide production by allowing more oxygen to enter the muscles, and MCT oil enhances ketone production and fat burning even in the presence of carbohydrates.

You can try these supplements one at a time. You can try them all together; only you decide.

Your commitment to TKD

A targeted ketogenic diet doesn't have to be lifelong. Try it for a week, two or three.

See how you feel. Track the changes.

Has TKD improved your exercise and quality of life? Has it helped improve your health?

Remember. TKD is not for everyone. Perhaps not for you.

But if you feel like your workout is suffering (even after adapting to keto), consider trying this type of keto diet.

Keto VS Other Diets

Ketogenic Diet

General Nutrition: Depending on the variation of the keto diet you choose, you will consume most of your calories from fat (75 percent to 90 percent), limited calories from protein (5 percent to 20 percent) and about five percent of calories from carbohydrate. This makes it hard to reach your daily intake of certain nutrients, such as fiber and other vitamins and minerals that you would get from consuming fruits and vegetables, which are limited to the plan.

Cost/Accessibility: This is not a commercial diet so there is no subscription fee or required foods to purchase. However, many of the keto diets recommend eating foods that are more expensive, such as grass-fed beef and specialty oils like avocado oil or MCT oil.

Weight Loss: While some studies have shown significant weight loss on a ketogenic diet, other studies have found that this eating style is no better than low-fat or other low-carb diets for long-term weight loss results. In addition, no-calorie targets are provided on a keto diet. Therefore, it is possible to consume more calories on this eating plan and gain weight as a result.

Sustainability: The ketogenic diet is often criticized as being hard to maintain for the long-term. Because the eating program is substantially different from a typical American diet, some consumers have a hard time maintaining the program when eating out or socializing.

Other Low-Carb Diets

There are many diets that fall into the low-carb category. Some consumers simply cut carbs for weight loss or improved health.

General Nutrition: There is no specific guideline for carbohydrate intake on a low-carb diet, but in general, you might consume 30 percent of your calories or less on a low-carb eating plan. This provides substantially more carbohydrate than a ketogenic diet. In addition, many low-carb diets are high in protein. As a result, you consume fewer calories from fat. On these eating plans, quality carbohydrates are often emphasized, meaning that you choose whole grains, fruits, and vegetables rather than processed foods that are high in sugar. As a result, you are more likely to meet nutritional goals on a low-carb diet than you are on a keto diet.

Cost/Accessibility: There is no single low-carb diet, but many commercial diets follow a low-carb eating style (such as the South Beach Diet and others). While you might choose to join one of those subscription programs for a fee, there is no cost involved in simply cutting carbs from your meals. Additionally, since low-carb eating has become more popular, many traditionally high-carb foods are now manufactured and sold in low-carb versions. This eating style is more accessible and is likely to be less expensive than a keto diet.

Weight Loss: Many different low-carb eating plans have been studied with mixed results in terms of weight loss. In some studies, low-carb diets have been compared to low-fat diets or to low-glycemic diets. While there have been various study results, researchers often conclude that the diets most likely to produce weight loss are the diets that consumers can stick to for the long-term.

Sustainability: A low-carb diet is likely to be more sustainable than a very low-carb, high-fat diet, such as the ketogenic diet. A low-carb diet provides a more balanced approach to eating and allows for a wider variety of foods overall.

What We Can And Can't Eat On The Ketogenic Diet

When you are switching to a ketogenic diet for weight loss, you must be careful. The most important one is that you must not end your regular meals abruptly. Instead, you should take a gradual approach. Most of us consume meals that comprise more than 50% carbs, and when you switch to ketogenic diets abruptly, you may have to cope with some side effects, such as dizziness, headache, fatigue, and irritability. For this reason, you should aim at cutting down your carb intake by 10-20% daily until you comfortably switch to ketogenic diets.

Increasing your water intake can help you switch effectively into the ketogenic diet phase, and the reason being that high-carb diets usually increase water-retention capacity. When you switch to ketogenic diets, you may lose more water than usual. While some side effects of abrupt switching to these nutrition plans can be mild, most of them will disappear within a few hours or days.

What To Eat?

The ketogenic diet approach is simple and straight-forward: eat real food and avoid high carbs. You should consider eating natural and nutritious foods, such as eggs, meat, nuts, dairy, vegetables, and fish. From your shopping list to eating habits, ketogenic diets must pass through everything. Here is a guide to what you should consume:

Meat. Many types of meats are recommended. These include beef, game meat, turkey, and chicken. Make sure you mix the fatty part of the meat with the lean and skin portion. If possible, try to consume organically raised animals and make sure the meat is properly cleaned before cooking.

Fish. These include all kinds of fishes and shellfish. Excellent choices include salmon, herring, and mackerel, but try as much as possible to avoid breading.

Eggs. All kinds of eggs can be consumed but more importantly, organically raised poultry eggs are recommended. Consumed on a ketogenic diet, they can be boiled, fried, or made as omelets.

Natural fats and high-fat sauces. You may consider cooking your meals with butter and cream because they make your foods taste good and can make you feel satiated the more. Hollandaise sauce is also recommended. However, you must check all the ingredients used in making the sauce or simply make one by yourself. You can also make use of coconut or olive oil in place of butter and other forms of cooking oils.

Vegetables cultivated above the ground. The ones that grow above the ground are excellent sources of essential minerals and vitamins. You should consider cauliflower, cabbage, brussels sprouts, broccoli, eggplant, asparagus, olives, zucchini, mushrooms, spinach, lettuce, avocado, cucumber, peppers, onions, and tomatoes.

Dairy Foods. These products must be selected if you are not allergic to some foods, such as milk. If you have lactose intolerance, then you should consider talking to your doctor about the choices you can make. For dairy products, you must select full-fat or medium-fat options such as cream (about 40% fat), butter, Greek yoghurt, Turkish yogurt, high-fat cheese, sour cream, and Greek cheese. You need to be careful with the use of skimmed and regular milk because they contain milk sugar. Similarly, try as much as possible to avoid flavored, low-fat products and sugary foods.

Nuts and seeds. These are highly nutritious foods with lots of protein. They can be your best companions when watching the TV. Thus they are suitable replacements for candies and other unhealthy sugary snacks. Some of the best nuts and seeds you should consider include peanuts and groundnuts.

Berries. They must be consumed in moderation, especially if you are sensitive to them. Berries are generous and delicious when finished with whipped cream. There are no limits to the choices of berries you can consider; strawberries, cranberries, blueberries, and blackberries are some of the best.

Liquids. Water is highly recommended; it keeps you hydrated even though your body's water retention capacity may be lowered while consuming the ketogenic diet. Water will sustain your system by transporting nutrients to all parts of your body. Try as much as possible to avoid caffeinated drinks because they are diuretic in nature, and you may have to urinate all the time — this means you will remain dehydrated.

Also, read the labels of all food items before buying them at the grocery stores. The basic rule is this: your diet should be no more than 5% carbohydrates.

What To Avoid In The Ketogenic Dieting?

The ketogenic diet works best to help you lose weight if you stick with recommended food categories, as highlighted above. You must try as much as possible to avoid or to limit the following:

Sugar. It is the worst of them all. Sugars come in different forms. Therefore, you must avoid foods and beverages, such as carbonated soft drinks, buns, cakes, pastries, sugary breakfast cereals, and ice cream. If possible, try as much as possible to avoid artificial (not keto-friendly) sweeteners.

Starch. Just like processed sugars, starches also contain high-carbs and must be avoided if possible. Starchy foods to avoid include pasta, potatoes, bread, rice, porridge, french fries, potato chips, and muesli. Be careful with legumes and lentils because they contain a significant amount of starch. Likewise, whole-grain foods may contain hidden sugar. If you must consume root vegetables, then you should exercise moderation.

Margarine. Margarine is processed with some synthetic materials, including hydrogen. Thus they contain a high amount of Omega-6 fatty acids — these have no health benefits in addition to the fact that they taste so bad. Margarine has been clinically linked to several diseases, including worsening of asthma symptoms, inflammatory diseases, and the worsening of several other food allergies.

Fruits. If you must consume fruits, they must be half unripened ones, and the reason being that ripe fruits are so sweet and contain lots of sugar. You should treat ripe fruits as natural forms of candies; therefore, they must be consumed sparingly.

Once in a while, you may consider eating dark chocolate because it is made up of 70% cocoa. You must drink water or tea without sugar, and if you must take coffee, then try the one with full-fat cream.

If you have a sufficient amount of time to work out, especially early in the morning, then you should go for low-impact exercises. Some cardio workouts, weight-lifting, or stretching exercises can keep you going and speed up your metabolism for the rest of the day.

ALLOWED FOOD
SHORT LIST

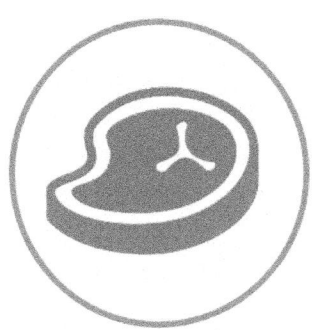 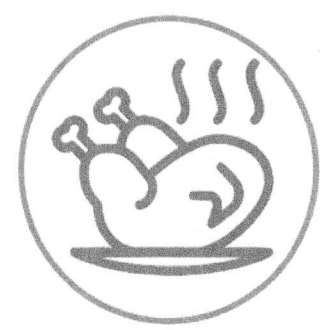 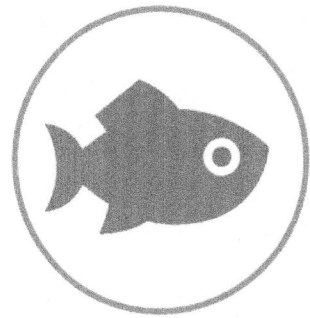

MEAT — **POULTRY** — **FISH**

 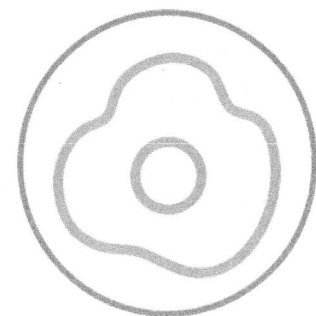 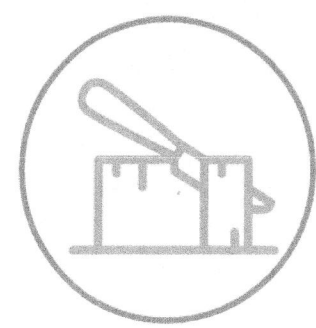

CHEESE — **EGGS** — **BUTTER**

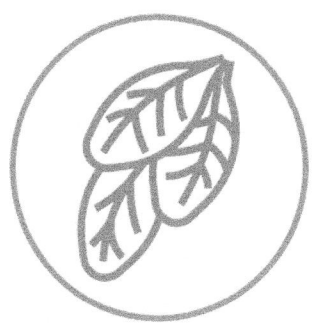 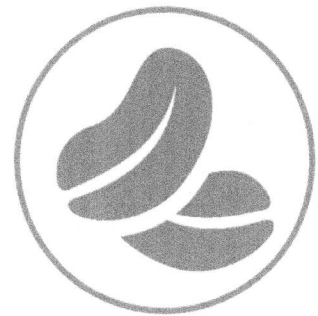 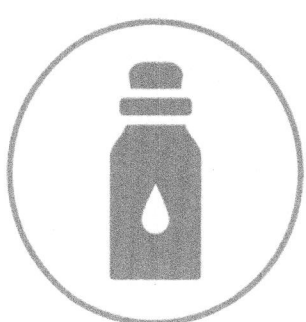

GREENS — **NUTS** — **OIL**

Food Lists

Repetition will help us avoid mistakes in the future. Therefore, I propose to take another look at the list of foods that you can eat on a ketogenic diet. That is somewhat similar to Atkins. However, there is greater emphasis on fats, usually "good" fats. On the keto diet, you can have: Olive oil, Coconut oil, Nut oils, Butter, Ghee, Grass fed beef, Chicken, Fish, Other meats, Full fat cheese, Eggs, Cream, Leafy greens, Non-starchy vegetables, Nuts, Seeds.You can also get a whole range of snacks that are meant for keto followers. As you can see from this list, fruits are restricted. You can have low sugar fruits in a limited quantity (mostly berries), but will have to forego your favorite fruits as these are all sweet and/or starchy.

This diet includes no grains of any kind, starchy vegetables like potatoes (and all tubers), no sugar or sweets, no breads and cakes, no beans and lentils, no pasta, no pizza and burgers, and very little alcohol. This also means no coffee with milk or tea with milk - in fact, no milk and ice-creams or milk based desserts.

Many of these have workarounds as you can get carbohydrate free pasta and pizza, you can have cauliflower rice and now there are even restaurants that cater to keto aficionados.

If you are wondering if this diet is safe, its proponents and those who have achieved their weight loss goals will certainly agree that it is. These are the benefits of the keto diet you can expect: loss of weight, reduced or no sugar spikes, appetite control, seizure controlling effect, blood pressure normalizes in high blood pressure patients, reduced attacks of migraine, type 2 diabetes patients on this diet may be able to reduce their medications, some benefits to those suffering from cancer.

Apart from the first four, there is not sufficient evidence to support its effectiveness or otherwise for other diseases as a lot more research is required over the long-term.

In the next chapters you will find the complete food list to enjoy and to avoid.

FOOD TO AVOID
SHORT LIST

BREAD

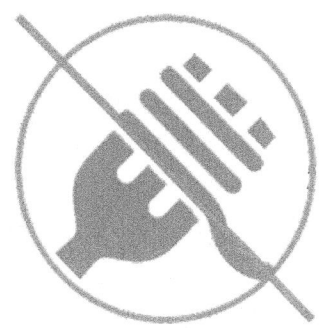
PASTA

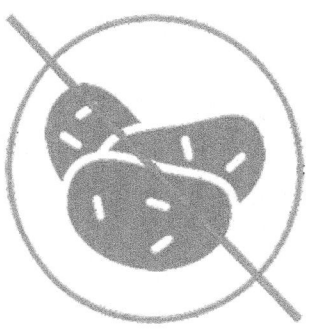
POTATO

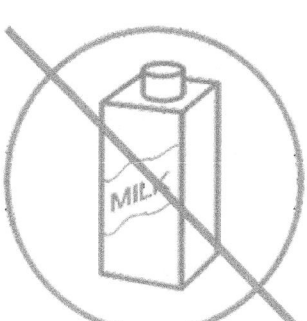
MILK

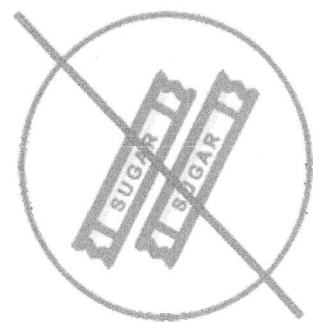
SUGAR

CORN

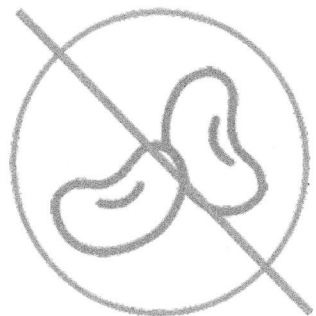
BEANS

PORRIDGE

ALCOHOL

Keto-Friendly Sweeteners

First of all, let's define what each of these top keto sweeteners have in common. We'll also find out how they follow the low-carb guidelines.

1. Low glycemic index (GI)

It indicates how much a food raises blood glucose levels. It ranges from zero to 100. Zero means no increase in blood sugar and insulin levels. 100 is the highest (like table sugar).

The goal and key principle of the ketogenic diet is to stay in a state of ketosis. Therefore, the best option is to get closer to zero GI for the sweeteners you use.

2. Sugar-free

The ideal keto diet is a lack of pure sugar. You are adjusting your body to burn fat for fuel instead of carbohydrates. Therefore, everything related to the addition of sugar should be prohibited. Even fruit should be severely restricted.

Therefore, zero or low-carb sweeteners are essential if you want to stay in ketosis.

The Best Low-Carb Keto Sweeteners

I believe there are 2 best sweeteners on the keto diet, but I mainly use 1 of them:

1 is Stevia

It is an extract from the stevia plant, which contains no calories or carbohydrates, and also has a zero glycemic index. One of its benefits is that it is almost 300 times sweeter than sugar. This means that you need very little of this sweetener to make your food sweet.

In addition, stevia has health benefits. It doesn't affect blood sugar and contains no carbohydrates or calories. On the other hand, it contains compounds that reduce oxidative stress in the body.

The liquid stevia and powdered form are most commonly used to sweeten drinks, salad dressings, and desserts. Stevia used to have a bitter taste, but today, most popular brands have fixed this problem. Therefore, it has become much more pleasant to use, and it is much easier to give up sugar.

When shopping for stevia, it is important to avoid additional filler ingredients. Because many commercial products add fillers like maltodextrin, dextrose, cane sugar, or artificial sweeteners. But along with a decrease in nutritional value, they raise blood sugar levels. They can also contain hidden carbohydrates or have other unwanted side effects.

Therefore, pure stevia (in liquid or powder form) is the best choice for a keto diet.

2 is Erythritol

Erythritol is also a good sugar substitute. But its downside is that it is classified as sugar alcohol. This may sound daunting, but remember that it is found naturally in many foods, mainly fruits and vegetables. It also does not cause negative side effects when used in moderation. The structure of erythritol gives it a sweet taste without the side effects of sugar.

You will see on the label of this product that it contains carbohydrates. This may be confusing, but it is not a cause for concern. Why? Because your body cannot digest the sugar alcohol in erythritol. Therefore, 100% of the carbs that are in erythritol are subtracted from the total carbs to get net carbs.

Erythritol use

The glycemic index of erythritol is zero like in stevia. But it has more calories - about 0.24 calories per gram. That's not a lot, as it only accounts for 6% of the calories in sugar. Erythritol is not as sweet as stevia. Therefore, you will need a little more to get the same sweetness.

You can find 100% pure erythritol in the store or in combination with other ingredients. Just make sure erythritol is free of additives that increase carbohydrates and affect blood sugar levels.

Other keto-friendly sweeteners

You can also use other keto-friendly sweeteners, but before that do take a closer look at each of them. You will also need to choose which one is right for you. Remember, it shouldn't cause side effects or interfere with your keto goals.

Sucralose. It is an artificial sweetener that is not metabolized. That is, it passes through your body undigested. Therefore, the body does not receive calories or carbohydrates from it.

Xylitol. Another type of sugar alcohol that is commonly found in many foods is sugarless gum or mints. It is as sweet as sugar, but it contains only 3 calories per gram. Similarly to other sugar alcohols, the carbs in xylitol are not considered net carbs because it does not raise blood insulin levels to the same extent as sugar.

Monk Fruit. It is a natural sweetener. It extracted from the monk fruit - a plant that grows in southern China. Depending on the concentration of mogrosides (the antioxidants that make it sweet), the monk fruit sweetener is almost 200 times sweeter than sugar.

Allulose. It is a natural sugar substitute. This natural sweetener tastes like sugar but has zero calories, zero net carbs, and zero glycemic index.

FOOD TO ENJOY

MEATS:
Beef
Goat
Lamb
Organ meats
Pork
Veal
Venison

POULTRY:
Chicken
Duck
Goose
Ostrich
Partridge
Pheasant
Quail
Squab
Turkey

GREENS & SALADS:
Arugula
Iceberg
Kale
Leafy greens
Lettuces
Parsley
Romaine
Spinach
Swiss chard

FISH:
Catfish
Cod
Flounder
Halibut
Herring
Mackerel
Mahi-mahi
Salmon
Trout
Tuna
Walleye

SHELLFISH:
Clams
Crab
Lobster
Mussels
Oysters
Prawns
Shrimp
Snails
Scallops

HEALTHY FAT AND OILS:
Avocado oil
Butter and ghee
Coconut butter
Coconut oil
Flaxseed oil
Lard
Mayonnaise
MCT oil
Olive oil
Sesame seed oil
Walnut oil

NUTS & SEEDS:
Almonds
Brazil nuts
Chia seeds
Flaxseeds
Hazelnuts
Macadamia
Peanuts[1]
Pecans
Pumpkin seeds
Sesame seeds
Sunflower seeds
Walnuts

DAIRY:
Almond milk (unsweetened)
Coconut milk (unsweetened)
Eggs
Ghee
Greek yogurt (full-fat)
Heavy (whipping) cream
Sour cream

SWEETENERS:
Stevia
Liquid Stevia
Erythritol
Allulose
Monk fruit
Sucralose
Xylitol

CHEESE:
Blue cheese
Brie
Cheddar
Cottage cheese
Cream cheese
Feta
Gouda
Mozzarella
Parmesan
Provolone

FRUITS & BERRIES:
Avocado
Blackberries
Blueberries
Cranberries
Lemons
Raspberries
Strawberries

VEGETABLES:
Asparagus
Bell peppers
Broccoli
Cabbage
Cauliflower
Celery
Cucumbers
Garlic[1]
Green beans
Onions[1]
Scallions
Tomatoes[1]
Zucchini

[1] - in moderation

FOOD TO AVOID

DAIRY:
Almond milk (sweetened)
Coconut milk (sweetened)
Soy milk
Milk
Yogurt

NUTS & SEEDS:
Cashews
Chestnuts
Pistachios

GRAINS:
Amaranth
Barley
Buckwheat
Flour & corn tortillas
Oats
Corn
Buckwheat
Oatmeal
Pumpernickel
Pasta
Rice
Rye
Sandwich wraps
Sorghum
Sourdough
Quinoa
Wheat
White
Whole grains
Wild rice

FRUITS:
Apples
Apricots
Bananas
Cherries
Grapes
Fruit Juices
Mangos
Melons
Nectarines
Oranges
Pineapples
Peaches
Pears
Pineapple
Plums
Tangerines
Dried fruits such as raisins dates and dried mango
Fruit smoothies (carb count will vary by fruits used)
All fruit juices (excluding lemon and lime juice)

VEGETABLES:
Potatoes
Sweet potatoes
Baked potatoes
Yams
Peas
Corn
Artichoke
Parsnips
Cassava (Yuca)
Squash

LEGUMES:
Baked beans
Chickpeas
Lima beans
Pinto beans
Black beans
Black-eyed peas
Lentils
Green peas
Kidney beans
Cannellini beans
Great Northern beans
Lima beans
Navy beans

BEVERAGES:
Colas
Cocktails (margaritas screwdrivers piña coladas)
Energy Drinks (not sugar-free)
Fruit juices
Frappuccino
Hot Chocolate
Ginger Ale
Grape Soda
Lemonade
Mocha
Non-light beers
Root Beer
Sports Drinks
Sweetened iced tea
Tonic Water (not sugar-free)
Vitamin Water

WHEAT OTHER NAMES:
Bulgar
Bran
Burghul
Couscous
Durum
Einkorn
Emmer
Farina
Farro Flour
Graham flour
Kamut
Orzo
Semolina
Spelt
Triticale
Wheat berries

FLOURS STARCHES & THICKENERS:
Arrowroot
Cornmeal
Cornstarch
Cassava
Chickpea flour
Gram
Cottonseed
Dal
Fava bean
Inulin
Lentil
Manioc
Modified starch
Powdered cellulose
Sago
Taro
Soy
Vegetable starch

Make Your Own Decision About Dieting

With so many different diets available, how are we to know what works and what is safe? The only way to be sure is to discover the author's background and the research behind the diet's methodology. Every good diet should give a background about the author and his/her credentials and experience in the fields of nutrition and biochemistry. However, even a vast resume does not mean a credible and safe diet. But it does suggest, at least, that the author has some knowledge of nutrition. Providing research behind the diet proves that it is not something the author invented, so long as the research is not self-serving and altered to fit a hypothesis.

Some diets may not need a great deal of tests and studies behind them, simply because they are based on fundamentals. For example, many women's magazines have articles on dieting and weight loss, but they are common sense suggestions that most people concerned about weight should know already: "eat smaller meals", "cut down on sugar and fat", etc., are typical philosophies. More structured diets should give some scientific reasons for its suggested success, preferably case studies and research performed on everyday test subjects, as well as athletes.

Since we have established the importance of eating a balanced diet in accordance to selecting healthy foods and obtaining RDA minimums, it is possible now to rate the nutritional therapy in accordance to those specific criteria. Begin with a score of 200 and subtract 10 points from the total for each statement below in which the diet concedes.

An ideal diet should maintain a score of 200, but a score of 160 or greater is acceptable.

1. The diet does not include the food groups in adequate amounts. Some fad diets eliminate one or more of the food groups. Do not deduct 10 points if a food group's nutrients (e.g., carbs, proteins, fats, fiber, vitamins, and minerals) are adequately substituted with that of another food group.

2. The diet does not provide at least 45% of its calories from carbohydrate sources. In order to prevent ketosis, at least 150g of glucose/day is required. That's 33-50% of total calorie intake on a 1200-calorie diet. Keep in mind that is the minimum. For highly active individuals, that amount should increase to 60% at times, i.e., immediately after exercise.

3. The carbohydrate content exceeds 20% concentrated sugars. At least 80% of carbohydrate sources should be complex and, preferably, in the form of vegetables, seeds, and legumes.

4. The protein content exceeds 30%. A very high intake is unnecessary; it places additional strain on the urinary system, and it is a poor source of energy. Thirty percent is more than

adequate, even for growing children and teenagers. The only group that requires higher protein intake are those who recently suffered a severe injury (e.g., leg amputation), infection, or surgery. However, these individuals will be under the care of a physician with a special high protein diet.

5. Protein content accounts for 15% or less of total calories. Although unnecessary in large amounts, protein still has many vital functions, including tissue repair and the formation of enzymes.

6. Fats exceed 30% of total intake. Besides increasing the risk of cardiovascular disease, high fat diets have not been demonstrated to decrease weight better than other methods of 'proper' eating.

7. Total fat consumption is less than 15% of total calories. Fat in moderate amounts is essential for a healthy diet, and such nutrition plan provides taste to many foods. Fat intake below 15% for long periods, for most individuals, is unrealistic.

Fat intake that is too low can also be detrimental to children and teenagers who require ample calories for continued growth.

8. Total fat consumption is less than 25% essential fatty acids, and saturated fat is more than 30% of total fat consumption. Deduct 10 for each.

9. The diet does not suggest common foods, meaning foods you should be able to obtain at any grocery store or market.

10. The foods for the diet are expensive or monotonous. Some diets require the purchase of 'their' foods or expensive 'organic' foods only obtained through health food stores. Some products taste so bad they are difficult to tolerate repeatedly (e.g., seaweed). Deduct 10 for each.

11. The diet consists of an inflexible meal plan. It does not allow for substitutions or deviations, requiring a person to live under 'house arrest' with the same food selections every day.

12. The diet provides less than 1200 calories per day. Less than that and the body's basic functions may not be getting the energy, vitamins and minerals needed to work properly, and the dieter almost is certain to feel hungry all the time. Diets below 1200 calories should be reserved for those under the supervision of a dietitian or licensed physician.

13. The diet requires the use of supplements. If it provides adequate energy and it is well balanced, supplements are unnecessary. 'Fat accelerators,' such as ephedrine, may increase the rate of weight loss, but the diet should be able to stand on its own merit. Some

clinics promote a vast array of herbal preparations and fat accelerators, and this is where these clinics make their money — not in their knowledge and ability as nutritionists.

14. The diet does not recommend a realistic weight goal. Diets should not be promoting the body of a Greek god or a supermodel. They should not be suggesting that a person lose 100 pounds (even if 100 pounds overweight) nor should diets recommend weight loss below an ideal weight.

15. The diet recommends or promotes more than 1-2 lbs/week weight loss. Do not expect to lose more than 1-2 pounds of fat a week — it is physically impossible unless chronically obese, at which point 3 pounds may be possible. If more than two pounds is lost per week, the body change is due to a loss of water and/or muscle tissue. Gimmicks that promise 10 pounds in 2 weeks are either simply not true or else something other than fat is being lost. Also keep in mind that the more fat a person wishes to lose and the less a person has, the more difficult and slower it will be to lose additional fat.

16. The diet does not include an evaluation of food habits. Dieting should be a slow process by which a person changes normal eating habits. It should not include looking for quick fixes and quick plans promising short cuts and extreme changes — a person would never stay with these programs and such diets do not work long-term. The number of calories eaten, the food selections, and their amounts should be reevaluated on a regular basis... perhaps once every 1-2 months to determine the program's effectiveness.

17. Regular exercise is not recommended as part of the plan for proper weight loss. Weight loss occurs twice as fast with exercise, and without exercise there is a greater tendency to lose lean muscle tissue as well as fat. This is not ideal.

Conclusion

You now have a basic understanding of what the ketogenic diet is and how it differs from others. And I hope you have already taken the first step towards deciding whether to choose keto as your lifestyle or not.

In this part of the book, we've covered the basic concepts:

- What is the keto diet and its short history
- How does it differ from other diets
- The truth about carbs and fats
- How it works
- What types of this diet exist
- What to eat and what to avoid.

We've also covered the most common myths regarding the keto diet. And now you know exactly what you can believe and which beliefs are false.

Next, we'll take a look at the keto diet from its good side. We will move on to its main advantages, the main benefits that the keto diet provides.

CHAPTER 2.
KETO GENERAL BENEFITS

How The Body Adapts To The Ketogenic Diet — The Main Reason for Many of the Benefits

From The Cell's Point of View. Carbohydrates are the body's preferred fuel source. When its consumption is restricted, the body reacts as if it is fasting. This stimulates new energy pathways to provide energy for the cells. One of these energy pathways is called ketogenesis, and its result is an alternative fuel source called a ketone body.

These ketones bodies can be used by almost every cell in your body for fuel (except for the liver and red blood cells). However, sugar and ketone bodies affect the body in many different ways.

For example, burning sugar for fuel creates more reactive oxygen species. These reactive oxygen species cause damage, inflammation, and cell death when they accumulate. This is why consuming too much sugar is known to impair brain function and cause plaque build up in the brain.

On the other hand, ketones provide a more efficient energy source and help protect neuron cells in the brain. This is partly because burning ketones for fuel decreases the production of reactive oxygen species and enhances mitochondrial function and production.

The healthy cells that are struggling to survive are helped by the carbohydrate restriction as well. Without access to carbohydrates, a cellular process called autophagy is activated. This process up-regulates many factors that improve cell health and resilience, clean up the cell from damage, and elicit anti-inflammatory processes.

The combination of autophagy and ketone burning are essential in helping people with cancer and brain disorders like epilepsy, migraines, and Alzheimer's.

From The Body's Perspective. Now, let's zoom out and look at how the ketogenic diet changes the body. It all begins with a change in insulin levels.

By restricting carbohydrates, we take the biggest stimulator of insulin out of the diet. This decreases insulin levels, increases fat burning, and reduces inflammation. The combination of these three changes addresses the primary drivers of many chronic diseases — insulin resistance, inflammation, and fat accumulation.

The Mechanisms Behind The Ketogenic Diet. From a mechanistic level, here is why the ketogenic diets can lead to benefits that reach beyond caloric restriction:

On a cellular level:

- Ketones burn more efficiently than sugar.
- Carbohydrate restriction triggers autophagy and anti-inflammatory processes.
- Burning ketones for fuel creates less reactive oxygen species.
- Ketone usage enhances mitochondrial function and production.

In the body:

- Insulin levels decrease because dietary carbohydrate isn't stimulating its release.
- Fat burning increases because the body needs to use alternative fuel sources.
- Inflammation is reduced because inflammatory fat levels decrease and less reactive oxygen species are formed.

The combination of the cellular and bodily effects of the ketogenic diet provides us with a basis for why they may be useful in the treatment of the conditions we mentioned earlier. However, this is only biochemistry. Is the ketogenic diet scientifically proven to help people with those conditions?

How The Ketogenic Diet Benefits Us All

We spent the majority of this article going over how the ketogenic diet helps people with specific conditions, but there are some benefits that everyone can experience. (The ketogenic diet is fun for the whole family.) Below, you'll find four primary benefits of the ketogenic diet.

Boosts Brain Function

Following the consumption of a ketogenic diet, brain cells become more efficient, brain inflammation is reduced, and health-promoting neurotrophic factors are activated. This is caused by the combination of carbohydrate restriction and ketone use.

Ketones, in particular, give the brain the opportunity to balance the neurotransmitters called glutamate and GABA (gamma-Aminobutyric acid). Glutamate is the primary excitation neurotransmitter (promotes stimulation) in the body and GABA is the main inhibitory neurotransmitter (reduces stimulation) in the body.

Brain fog and a lack of focus can be caused by having too much glutamate and very little GABA. This will happen if your brain has to use glutamate and glutamic acid for fuel, which leaves little left over to be processed into GABA. By giving the brain another form of energy when you break down ketones, you're able to balance out the neurotransmitter production.

This balance (increase in GABA production) helps to reduce the excess firing of neurons in the brain, leading to better mental focus. An added benefit of more GABA production is a reduction of stress and anxiety and an increased sense of calmness.

Increases Energy

As we mentioned before, research has shown that those who follow a ketogenic diet will develop better mitochondrial function and produce less reactive oxygen species.

Better mitochondrial function equates to more energy for your cells while having less reactive oxygen species increases energy efficiency. In others words, the ketogenic diet allows you to get the most out of your cells so that you can get the most out of life.

Help To Weight Loss

Weight loss is the biggest reason that people begin any sort of diet in the first place, and high-fat and low-carb nutrition plans have been used for centuries for those who tend to carry a little extra weight. One of the most incredible benefits of the ketogenic diet is that it suppresses your appetite. When you have a decreased appetite and lower insulin levels, your body's fat levels will also reduce. When you enter ketosis, you will also burn fat and use your fat storages as energy. It is a win-win for most people. On a regular diet, your body uses carbohydrates to create "life energy." In return, your body stores the fat in unwanted places. On the ketogenic diet, this will not be an issue at all, and you will begin to lose weight.

Decreases Inflammation and Pain

Without excess damage being caused by reactive oxygen species, the inflammatory processes of the body don't have to be used to repair damage as frequently. This reduces inflammation levels in the body. A pleasant side effect of theses anti-inflammatory benefits is that people with chronic pain may notice a reduction in pain as well.

Increase Your Performance

Different studies have found that the ketogenic diet is beneficial in helping athletes increase their overall performance. It can be due to the lower lactate load in the body, as well as lowered oxidative stress when the body is fueled by fat. Other studies have found that higher levels of ketones in the blood lead to increased energy over thirty minutes.

Helps Build More Lean Muscles While Losing Fat

The main reason for this is that people placed on Ketogenic diets have been found to force their bodies to use up more water. Secondly, the lowered Insulin hormones will cause the kidneys to remove excess sodium. The combined effect of these is that there is a speedy loss of weight within the shortest possible period.

Improves Body Composition

Many studies conclude that caloric restriction is inferior to the ketogenic diet when it comes to weight loss. For example, one study split 132 people into two groups: a low-carbohydrate diet (30 grams or less of carbohydrates a day) group and a calorie-restricted, low-fat diet group.

After six months of this dietary intervention, the researchers concluded that "severely obese subjects with a high prevalence of diabetes and the metabolic syndrome lost more weight in a six-month period on a carbohydrate-restricted diet than on a fat and calorie-restricted diet."

If you restrict carbohydrates, then you will drop the extra pounds. This is wonderful for people who want to lose fat, but what about people who want to gain muscle?

The ketogenic diet is perfect for increasing muscles mass. This is because you will be consuming much more protein than many other diets. To find out the right amount of protein for you, use our keto-calculator.

Treating Epilepsy — The Origins Of The Ketogenic Diet

Our journey through the research on the ketogenic diet starts in 1924 with Dr. Russell Wilder. At the prestigious Mayo Clinic, Dr. Wilder designed a carbohydrate-restricted diet to treat epilepsy in children, and the research at the time indicated that it was highly effective.

The first high-quality study on epilepsy and the ketogenic diet wasn't published until much later, in 1998. In this study, researchers recruited 150 children, and nearly all of them had more than two seizures per week despite taking at least two seizure-reducing medications. The children were provided with a ketogenic diet for a one-year trial. After three months, about 34% of the children, or slightly over one-third, had over a 90% decrease in seizures.

After six months, 71% of the children remained on the ketogenic diet, and about 32% had over a 90% reduction in seizures. After a full year, 55% stayed on the diet and 27% experienced at least a 90% decrease in seizures.

Thus, the researchers stated that the ketogenic diet is "more effective than many of the new anticonvulsant medications and is well tolerated by children and families when it is effective." Not only was the ketogenic diet helpful, but it was more helpful than some commonly used drugs.

More recently, a meta-analysis was published in the Journal of Neurology that assessed the impact of the ketogenic diet in treating epilepsy. It included a total of 19 studies with a total of 1084 patients. After analyzing the data, the researchers noted that the patients who stayed on the diet had a 2.25 times greater probability of treatment success (at least a 50% reduction in seizures).

The Ketogenic Diet In Reversing Type 2 Diabetes

Insulin resistance is a widespread problem that, if not properly managed, can lead to prediabetes and eventually type 2 diabetes. Thankfully, abundant research suggests that modifying your diet to a low-carbohydrate or ketogenic diet can help people lower their insulin to healthy levels and reverse insulin resistance.

In fact, after analyzing the data from 10 randomized trials on using diet to treat diabetes, researchers found that a low-carbohydrate diet has a greater effect on blood sugar control in type 2 diabetics than high-carbohydrate diets.

They even found a distinct relationship between carbohydrate restriction and blood sugar lowering. Less carbohydrate consumption meant better blood sugar levels.

It's that simple — put people with prediabetes or type 2 diabetes on a low-carbohydrate ketogenic diet, and their health improves, blood sugar levels drop, and insulin sensitivity increases. Even studies that put healthy individuals on a ketogenic diet found similar improvements.

Controlling Type 1 Diabetes with the Ketogenic Diet

Type 1 diabetes causes the same blood sugar control issues as type 2 diabetes, but in an entirely different way. Type 1 diabetics cannot produce enough insulin or any insulin at all, which requires them to have insulin administered exogenously. On top of that, the perfect diet will not be able to reverse this disease as the ketogenic diet can for type 2 diabetes.

However, there may be a perfect diet to help manage type 1 diabetes. One case report of a 19-year-old male with this diagnose found that a paleolithic ketogenic diet may have the ability "to halt or reverse autoimmune processes destructing pancreatic beta cell function [in type 1 diabetes]." In other words, a ketogenic diet consisting of low-carbohydrate whole-foods may be able to reverse type 1 diabetes!

Although it is a stretch to say that a paleolithic ketogenic diet can make a reverse, a recent critical evaluation of the literature confirms that the ketogenic diet is the best-documented diet for controlling type 1 diabetes.

The group of 26 leading researchers stated that there is "…evidence supporting the use of low-carbohydrate diets as the first approach to treating type 2 diabetes and as the most effective adjunct to pharmacology in type 1. They represent the best-documented, least controversial results."

Improving Blood Pressure With the Ketogenic Diet

According to the World Health Organization, high blood pressure is estimated to cause about 12.8% of the total of all deaths. Luckily, the ketogenic diet may be the solution, according to a 2007 study.

In this study, researchers compared the impact of a low-carbohydrate diet and three other diets on blood pressure and other measures of cardiovascular fitness in women. After the 12 month trial, all subjects who successfully completed their respective diet experienced notable reductions in body mass, triglycerides, and LDL cholesterol. Those in the low-carbohydrate diet group, however, had the best results.

These participants decreased their systolic blood pressure by an average of 7.6 mm Hg — twice more than any other group. Their diastolic pressure also decreased by 2.93% from 75 mm Hg to 72.8 mm Hg.

These findings were confirmed in another interesting study. Researchers compared the effects of the low-carbohydrate diet to the effects of a combination of a low-fat diet and orlistat (a weight-loss and blood pressure lowering medication) on blood pressure. The researchers stated that the low-carbohydrate dietary intervention "was more effective for lowering blood pressure."

Does this mean that you should throw away your blood pressure medication and dive into the ketogenic diet? Not just yet — you should first consult with your dietitian or doctor to see if cutting some carbs is a suitable strategy for you

Booster Of The Digestive Health

While on the ketogenic diet, you will increase the level of fiber in your diet via (mostly) non-starchy vegetables and healthy fruits. By increasing the amount of fiber in your diet, you can improve your digestive health. Also, you will be able to lower your risk of gastric ulcers, colorectal cancer, cramping, bloating, diarrhea, and constipation.

The Power To Improve The Alzheimer's Disease

Many studies on Alzheimer's disease patients agree with the biochemistry as well. In fact, a group of scientists reviewed the literature and concluded that "high carbohydrate intake worsens cognitive performance and behavior in patients with Alzheimer's disease." This means that eating more carbohydrates cause more problems in the brain. Will the opposite (eating fewer carbs) improve brain function?

Recent studies on the ketogenic diet provide evidence that it may be able to reverse Alzheimer's disease. Experiments on ketone supplementation specifically found that the ketone body, β-hydroxybutyrate, improved memory function of Alzheimer's patients.

Scientists validated this finding by giving MCT oil (a fat found in coconut oil that is usually converted into ketones in the liver) to Alzheimer's patients and tested their memory. They found that the Alzheimer's patients experienced greater memory recall that directly correlated with their blood levels of ketone bodies.

Other benefits that ketone bodies have on brain health are:

- They prevent neuronal loss.
- They preserve neuron function.
- They protect brain cells, against multiple types of injury.

Parkinson's Disease Symptoms Reduced By Ketogenic Diet

One recently published clinical study tested the effects of the ketogenic diet on symptoms of Parkinson's disease. In this study, patients experienced a mean of 43% reduction in Unified Parkinson's Disease Rating Scale scores after a 28-day ketogenic diet.

All participating patients reported moderate to very good improvement in symptoms. The researchers hypothesize that these results are partly due to the increase in essential fatty acid consumption that is common with ketogenic diets.

Improve Cholesterol Levels And Reverse Heart Disease With The Ketogenic Diet

Although the ketogenic diet tends to be high in saturated fat (commonly thought to increase cholesterol), it has been found to improve cholesterol levels and reduce the risk of heart disease.

In a recent meta-analysis published in the British Journal of Nutrition, researchers investigated the impacts of very-low-carbohydrate ketogenic diets (VLCKD) on key metrics of cardiovascular health including HDL cholesterol. The authors defined a VLCKD as a diet of less than 50 g of carbohydrates.

After examining 12 studies including 1257 patients, they found that the VLCKD increases HDL by double the average increase in HDL of the low-fat dieters. As a result, the authors concluded that carbohydrate-restricted diets confer cardiovascular benefits because they improve levels on HDL in the body.

However, one of the most important risk factors for heart disease is the "bad" LDL cholesterol. How does the ketogenic impact LDL cholesterol levels?

In a 2006 study, researchers assessed the effects of carbohydrate restriction on LDL cholesterol in a group of 29 men for a 12-week weight-loss intervention. Their LDL cholesterol levels improved, leading to the conclusion that weight loss induced by carb restriction favorably alters the secretion and processing of plasma lipoproteins, rendering VLDL, LDL, and HDL particles associated with decreased risk for atherosclerosis and coronary heart disease.

In another study on women, researchers confirmed that the ketogenic diet resulted in favorable changes in LDL particles consistent with lower cardiovascular disease risk. However, the total LDL cholesterol did not change. This is why it is important to test the levels of different LDL particles. Looking at the LDL number itself may be misleading, especially on the ketogenic diet.

A Potential Treatment For Polycystic Ovary Syndrome And Infertility

Polycystic ovary syndrome (PCOS) is responsible for as much as 70 percent of infertility issues in women.

The primary cause of this condition is elevated insulin levels. When insulin levels are high, they cause the ovaries to produce more androgens (like testosterone) and decrease the production of sex-hormone binding globulin — a glycoprotein that prevents testosterone from freely entering cells.

With more androgen production and less sex-hormone binding globulin, free testosterone can freely float through the blood and interact with cells. Depending on what cells it influences, this can result in hair growth on the chest and face, mood swings, fatigue, low sex drive, acne, infertility, and other PCOS symptoms.

As androgen levels continue to increase, they stimulate 5-alpha reductase activity — an enzyme that converts testosterone to a more potent metabolite called dihydrotestosterone. This makes PCOS symptoms even worse.

The research on how diet affects PCOS is minimal, but there is one compelling study on the ketogenic diet and women with PCOS. In this study, five overweight women ate a ketogenic diet (20 grams of carbohydrates or less per day) for 24 weeks. The results were astounding — average weight loss was 12%, free testosterone decreased by 22%, and fasting insulin levels dropped by 54%. What's even more impressive is that two of the women became pregnant despite previous infertility problems.

Although this is a small study, the results are clearly backed by the fact that the ketogenic diet has been found in many other studies to help reverse insulin resistance and reduce insulin levels, the two main causes of PCOS.

Reverse Non-Alcoholic Fatty Liver Disease With The Ketogenic Diet

Non-alcoholic fatty liver disease is associated with type 2 diabetes, obesity, heart disease, and hyperlipidemia, and it probably will not develop unless one or more of these issues are present as well.

We've already explored how the ketogenic diet helps with diabetes, heart disease, and hyperlipidemia. Does this mean it helps with non-alcoholic fatty liver disease as well?

A recent pilot study put five patients on the ketogenic diet (less than 20 grams per day of carbohydrate). At the end of six months, the average weight loss was 28 pounds (but this wasn't the most surprising finding). Each patient underwent a liver biopsy, and four of the five patients had a reduction in liver fat, inflammation, and fibrosis. However, this is a small pilot study that also used supplements, so the results are not conclusive. What does the rest of the research say?

In a 2016 meta-analysis and systematic review, the researchers found that the low carbohydrate diet decreased fat in the liver significantly, but liver function tests did not improve significantly. When we look closely at the studies in the meta-analysis, they either found no effect on liver enzyme levels or a significant effect. In other words, the liver function of some people stayed the same on the low-carbohydrate diet while others improved significantly. Why the difference?

My guess is that if subjects were required to eat more fibrous foods (like low-carbohydrate vegetables), then they probably would have had results similar to the small pilot study.

The Ketogenic Diet Helps Cancer Patients

Recently, there has been more talk about the potential of ketogenic diet being a cancer treatment, but what does the available literature have to say about that?

A recent meta-analysis looked at the literature on 32 glioma patients (people that had a tumor in their brain or spinal cord) treated using the ketogenic diet as an alternative or complementary therapy. The researchers noted that some patients were more responsive to the ketogenic diet than other patients.

The best response was in a 3-year-old girl who had complete remission after five years of treatment with a ketogenic diet. Two other patients also experienced complete remission after the diet, while another experienced cancer progression after stopping the diet.

These are incredible results, but we must remember that these results are due to a combination of a ketogenic diet and conventional treatment, not the ketogenic diet alone.

It is evident, however, that the ketogenic diet is one of the best diets for cancer patients. According to dietitian Heidi H. Pfeifer at the MGH Center for Dietary Therapy, the ketogenic diet may be effective because of the following two reasons.

First, the ketogenic diet deprives cancer cells of their primary source of energy — glucose. While many of the cancer cells are starving, the body is running on ketones, which the cancer cells cannot use for fuel.

Second, the ketogenic diet suppresses insulin like growth factor (IGF-1). This molecule is associated with the formation and progression of cancerous cells. IGF-1 levels are increased when we eat more carbohydrates. Because the ketogenic diet is much lower in carbohydrates, scientists suspect that this suppresses IGF-1 production, slowing the formation of cancerous cells.

Prevent And Reduce The Severity Of Migraines

The first study on the Ketogenic diet and how it affects migraines came a few years after its first use for epilepsy in 1928. The study was done on 28 patients, and only 9 of them showed "some improvement" although most of them admitted poor compliance.

In a review of the research on the ketogenic diet and migraines (over seventy years later), the scientists concluded that the ketogenic diet "ameliorates headaches and reduces drug consumption in migraineurs, while the SD [standard low-calorie diet] is fully ineffective on migraine in a short term observation."

The researchers hypothesized that the positive effects that the ketogenic diet has on migraines are due to how ketone bodies inhibit neural inflammation and enhance brain mitochondrial metabolism. The ketone bodies do this by blocking high concentrations of glutamate (commonly found in both migraine and epilepsy sufferers) and reducing oxidative stress.

Conclusion

Well, now you clearly understand how powerful the ketogenic diet is. It has unique effects on the body and inside of the cells and provide benefits that reach beyond what any other diet can provide.

The combination of carbohydrate restriction and ketone production reduces insulin levels, triggers autophagy (cellular clean-up), increases mitochondrial production and efficiency, reduces inflammation, and burns fat.

And I am sure that you have found something that bothered you for a long time and could not get rid of. Let's agree that this list of benefits is really long, and this type of diet inspires confidence.

Well, in this chapter, we found out what wonderful prospects the keto diet offers for our body, our brain, and our well-being.

Among them:

- Boosts brain function
- Increases energy
- help to weight loss
- Decreases inflammation and pain
- Increase your performance
- Helps build more lean muscles while losing fat
- Improves body composition
- Helps to cure many different diseases
- And much more.

Next, we'll take a look at the keto diet from the other side. We will look at how safe this diet is, its side effects, and what you need to be careful with. Hopefully, in the next chapter, I can answer your other questions about this diet.

CHAPTER 3. COMMON CONCERNS WITH A KETO DIET

Dawn Effect Of The Ketogenic Diet

Normal fasting blood sugars are less than 100 mg/dl and most people in ketosis will achieve this level if they are not diabetic. However, in some people fasting blood sugars tend to increase, especially in the morning while on a keto diet. This is called the "dawn effect" and is due to the normal circadian rise in morning cortisol (stress hormone) that stimulates the liver to make more glucose. If this happens, make sure you are not consuming excessive protein at dinner and not too close to bedtime. Stress and poor sleep can also lead to higher cortisol levels. If you are insulin resistant, you may also need more time to achieve ketosis.

Low athletic performance. Keto-adaptation usually takes about 4 weeks. During this persiod of time, switch to something that is less vigorous instead of doing intense workouts or training. After the adaptation period, athletic performance usually returns to normal or even better, especially for endurance sports.

Keto-rash is not a common side effect of the diet. Probable causes include production of acetone (a form of ketone) in the sweat that irritates the skin or nutrient deficiencies including protein or minerals. Shower immediately after exercise and make sure you eat nutrient dense whole foods.

Ketoacidosis. This is a very rare condition that occurs when blood ketone levels go above 15 mM. A well-formulated keto diet does not cause ketoacidosis. Certain conditions such as type 1 diabetes, being on medications with SGLT-2 inhibitors for type 2 diabetes, or breastfeeding require extra caution. Symptoms include lethargy, nausea, vomiting, and rapid shallow breathing. Mild cases can be resolved using sodium bicarbonate mixed with diluted orange or apple juice. Severe symptoms require prompt medical attention.

Who Should Be Cautious With A Keto Diet?

For most people, a keto diet is very safe. However, there are certain individuals who need to take special care and discuss with their doctors before going on such a diet.

- Those taking medications for diabetes. Dosage may need to be adjusted as blood sugar goes down with a low-carb diet.
- Those taking medications for high blood pressure. Dosage may need to be adjusted as blood pressure goes down with a low-carb diet.
- Those who are breastfeeding should not go on a very strict low-carb diet as the body can lose about 30 g of carbs per day via the milk. Therefore, have at least 50 g of carbs per day while breastfeeding.
- Those with kidney disease should consult with their doctors before doing a keto diet.
- Those with liver disease should consult with their doctors before doing a keto diet.

How Safe Is The Keto Diet?

Just like any other diet that restricts foods in specific categories, the keto diet is not without risks. As you are not supposed to eat many fruits and vegetables, beans, lentils and other foods, you can suffer from lack of many essential nutrients. Since the diet is high in saturated fats and, if you indulge in the 'bad' fats, you can have high cholesterol levels upping your risk of heart disease.

In the long-term the keto diet can also cause many nutritional deficiencies since you cannot eat grains, many fruits and vegetables. Moreover, you miss out on fiber as well as important vitamins, minerals, phytonutrients, and antioxidants among other things. You can suffer from gastrointestinal distress, lowered bone density (no dairy and other sources of calcium), kidney, and liver problems (the diet puts added stress on both the organs).

The major benefit of the keto diet is that it does work so you lose weight, but then again, it is a diet and like all diets, it is a short term solution. It is not really a sustainable nourishment plan in real life situations. More importantly, your goal is not just to lose weight — anyone can lose weight. The more necessary goal is to keep the lost weight off.

The keto diet can be an effective way to reduce excess body fat but there are several cons that should be noted by anyone wanting to follow any eating plan. In fact, the keto diet has serious risks. For one thing, it's high in saturated fat, which has been linked to heart disease. Additionally, a nutrient deficiency and constipation could occur since the keto diet is very low in fibrous foods such as fruits, vegetables, and whole grains.

Liver problems for those with existing liver conditions could possibly worsen since the keto diet puts stress on the liver, and kidney problems could also occur.

If you are considering going on the keto diet, work with a knowledgeable practitioner or seek out a registered dietitian with experience in prescribing it and following you to avoid any adverse effects.

Is Keto Safe For Long-Term?

If you are willing to forego your usual dietary staples and are really keen to lose weight, you may be tempted to try out the keto diet. The biggest issue with this diet is poor patient compliance thanks to the carbohydrate restriction, so you have to be sure that you can live with your food choices. If you simply find it too difficult to follow, you can go on a version of the modified keto diet that offers more carbs.

However, the keto diet is definitely effective in helping you lose weight. According to a recent study, many of the obese patients were successful in losing weight. Any problems that they faced were temporary. If you do not have any significant health problems except for obesity and have been unsuccessful in losing weight following any conventional diet, the keto diet may a viable option. You must be absolutely determined to lose the weight and be prepared to go on a restricted diet as specified. Even if you have any medical problems, you can take your doctor's advice and a nutritionist's guidance and go on this diet.

Another study that was carried out for a longer time showed that going on the keto diet is beneficial in weight loss and also results in reduced cholesterol levels with a decrease in the bad cholesterol and an increase in the good cholesterol.

Is The Keto Diet Safe For You?

Given all the buzz, adopting a ketogenic diet may be the perfect weight loss plan, especially if you have diabetes, or want to try this approach to lose those troublesome extra pounds. After all, it's a very low-carb meal plan that promises effective weight loss while also lowering your blood sugar to the point where you could possibly stop taking medication. By all accounts, the "keto" diet, as it's widely known, may even reverse type 2 diabetes, at least for some lucky individuals.

Another advantage to the keto diet: It can help reduce systemic inflammation, which can have a variety of negative effects on your entire body.

Unlike some of the other popular low-carb nutrition plans, which typically are high in animal protein, the keto diet focuses on getting to the body to burn stored body fat instead of sugar as the main fuel. When body fat is broken down in the liver instead of glucose, an energy byproducts, known as ketones, are produced.

Most doctors and nutritionists have agreed that the keto diet is good for weight loss over the short-term. As for the long-term, more studies are needed. Do keep in mind that obesity is not an apt choice as it comes with its own risk of health problems.

In any case, if you decide to start the keto diet, it will be better to consult your doctor before starting. Especially if you taking medications for diabetes, taking medications for high blood pressure, have some kidney or liver disease.

Are There Any Side-Effects Of This Diet?

When you initially start the keto diet, you can suffer from what is known as keto flu. These symptoms may not occur in all people and usually begin a few days after being on a diet, when your body is in a state of ketosis. Some of the side-effects are:

- Nausea
- Cramps and tummy pain
- Headache
- Vomiting
- Diarrhea and/or constipation
- Muscle cramps
- Dizziness and poor concentrations
- Insomnia
- Carbohydrate and sugar cravings.

These may take up to a week to subside as your body get used to the new diet regime. You can also suffer from other problems when you start the keto diet. You may find that you have increased urination, so it is important to keep yourself well hydrated. You may also suffer from keto breath when your body reaches optimal ketosis and you can use a mouthwash or brush your teeth more frequently.

Usually the side effects are temporary and once your body acclimatizes to the new diet, these should disappear.

Short-Term Side Effects

There are several short-term side effects that are most evident at the beginning of therapy, particularly when patients commence the diet with an initial fast.

Hypoglycemia is a common side effect in this instance, and noticeable signs may include:

- Excessive thirst
- Frequent urination
- Fatigue
- Hunger
- Confusion, anxiety and [or] irritability
- Tachycardia
- Lightheadedness and shakiness
- Sweating and chills.

Additionally, patients may also experience some constipation and low-grade acidosis. These effects tend to improve when the diet is continued, as the body adapts to the new diet and adjust the ways in which it sources energy.

Alteration in Blood Composition. As a result of the changes in dietary consumption and the body's adaptive mechanisms to cope with the reduced carbohydrate intake, there are several changes in the blood composition of individuals following the ketogenic diet.

In particular, the levels of lipids and cholesterol in the blood are commonly higher than what is considered to be normal. More than 60% of patients have raised lipid levels and more than 30% have high levels of cholesterol.

If these changes are profound and there is some concern about the health of the child, slight changes to the diet can be made for the individual patient. For example, saturated fat sources can be substituted for polyunsaturated fats. In some cases, it may be necessary to lower the ketogenic ratio and reduce the proportion of fat to carbohydrate and protein in the diet.

Long-Term Effects

When the ketogenic diet is continued for extended periods of time, there are other adverse effects that become more evident and have a greater impact on individuals.

Kidney stones, also known as nephrolithiasis, are a common complication for children following the diet, with approximately 5% of patients suffering from the condition. It is, however, treatable and the current recommendations suggest that the diet should be continued. The formation of kidney stones is believed to be linked to hypocitraturia and hypercalciuria when acidosis causes the bone to demineralize. Additionally, low pH in the urine can encourage the formation of crystals and, eventually, kidney stones.

There is some evidence that supplementation with potassium citrate reduces the incidence of kidney stones, as it binds to and reduces the level of calcium in the bloodstream. More research on this is required, however.

Additionally, patients have an increased risk of bone fractures. This arises from the altered levels of insulin-like growth factor 1 and the effects of acidosis. Acidosis leads to the erosion of bone, weakening the bones and leaving them prone to fractures.

In order to manage these side effects, supplementation of vitamins and minerals are routinely administered to patients following the ketogenic diet. This commonly comprises of a multivitamin, calcium, and vitamin D supplements.

Side Effects in Adults. For adults following the ketogenic diet, the most common complications include weight loss, constipation, and increased levels of cholesterol and triglycerides. Women may also experience amenorrhea or other disruptions to the menstrual cycle.

What To Do About Keto Diet Side Effect

Take it easy with physical activity

Although many people find that their energy and stamina improve on a keto lifestyle, trying to do too much in the early stages can worsen keto flu symptoms.

Well-known ketogenic researcher Dr. Steve Phinney has conducted studies in endurance athletes and obese adults demonstrating that physical performance decreases during the first week of very-low-carb eating.

Fortunately, his research also shows that performance typically recovers — and often improves — within 4 to 6 weeks.

Walking, stretching, or doing gentle yoga or other mind-body exercise should be fine and may even help you feel better. But when your body is already under stress from trying to adapt to a new fuel system, don't place an additional burden on it by attempting any type of strenuous workout. Take it easy for the first few weeks and then slowly increase your exercise intensity.

Don't consciously restrict food intake

Some people find that they aren't very hungry the first week of keto because they are nauseated or have a headache that reduces their appetite. Yet others may get pretty hungry and worry that they're eating too many calories to achieve the kind of fast weight loss they've heard about.

The keto diet begins with induction, its strictest phase that allows for maximum fat burning and getting into ketosis quickly. On this diet, as long as carbs are restricted to 20 or fewer grams per day, you can eat as much of the allowed foods you need to feel full.

Once you're steadily in ketosis, your appetite will likely go down, and you'll naturally end up eating less.

Eat as much of the allowed foods as needed until you're no longer hungry and have keto snacks like hard-boiled eggs available in case hunger strikes between meals. On the other hand, make sure to avoid getting overly full by eating slowly and paying attention to hunger and fullness signals.

Other Cautions And How To Avoid Them

The keto flu. Symptoms of the keto flu:

- Fatigue
- Headache
- Irritability
- Difficulty focusing ("brain fog")
- Lack of motivation
- Dizziness
- Sugar cravings
- Nausea
- Muscle cramps.

The cause. The keto flu occurs as your body transitions from burning sugar to burning fat for most of its energy needs.

Switching from a high-carb diet to a very-low-carb diet lowers insulin levels in your body, one of the primary goals of a ketogenic diet. When insulin levels are very low, your liver begins converting fat into ketones, which most of your cells can use in place of glucose.

When your body is mainly using ketones and fat for energy, you're in a state of ketosis. However, it takes your brain and other organs some time to adapt to using this new fuel. When your insulin levels drop, your body responds by excreting more sodium in the urine, along with water. Because of this, you'll likely find yourself urinating a lot more often in the first week or so of keto eating.

This change is responsible for some of the rapid – and usually very welcome(!) – weight loss that happens in the early stages of a keto diet. However, losing a lot of water and sodium is responsible for many of the unpleasant symptoms of keto flu.

It's well known that response to the keto transition is very individual. Some people may feel fine or slightly tired for a day or two after starting keto. At the other extreme, there are those who develop symptoms that strongly impact their ability to function for several days.

However, the keto flu doesn't have to be unbearable for anyone if the proper steps are taken to remedy it.

More About Keto Flu

It happens when you're not being able to reach ketosis. Although the ketogenic diet is safe for healthy people, there may be some initial side effects while your body adapts.

Make sure you are not eating too much protein and there are no hidden carbs in the packaged foods that you consume. Also, you may be eating the wrong kinds of fat, such as the highly refined polyunsaturated corn and soybean oils.

When in ketosis, the body tends to excrete more sodium. If one is not getting enough sodium from the diet, symptoms of a keto-flu may appear, such as feeling light-headed, dizziness, headaches, fatigue, brain fog, and constipation.

A ketogenic diet can also change the water and mineral balance of your body, so adding extra salt to your meals or taking mineral supplements can help. This is easily remedied by drinking 2 cups of broth (with added salt) per day. If you exercise vigorously or the sweat rate is high, you may need to add back even more sodium.

The first week is usually when people attempting a keto diet fail and quit. Just remember that this happens to everyone early in the process, and if you can get past the first week, the hardest part is over. There are a few remedies you can use to help you get through this rough spell: taking electrolyte supplements, staying hydrated, drinking bone broth, eating more meat, and getting plenty of sleep. Also, you can try a regular low-carb diet for the first few weeks. This may teach your body to burn more fat before you completely eliminate carbs. For minerals, try taking 3,000–4,000 mg of sodium, 1,000 mg of potassium and 300 mg of magnesium per day to minimize side effects.

Keto flu is an unfortunate event that occurs to everyone as the body expels the typical day-to-day diet. You just have to power through. At least in the beginning, it is important to eat until you're full and avoid restricting calories too much. Usually, a ketogenic diet causes weight loss without intentional calorie restriction.

The Simplest Cure For The Keto Flu

Symptoms of the keto flu usually disappear by themselves within a few days to weeks, as the body adapts. But rather than suffering needlessly during this time, why not address the cause and start feeling better right now? The first step is by far the most important, and it's often all that's needed.

Top tip: increase your salt and water intake.

Since loss of salt and water is responsible for most keto flu issues, increasing your intake of both can help reduce your symptoms significantly and often eliminate them altogether.

During the first few weeks of your keto lifestyle, whenever you develop a headache, lethargy, nausea, dizziness or other symptoms, drink a glass of water with half a teaspoon of salt stirred into it. This simple action may alleviate your keto flu symptoms within 15 to 30 minutes. Feel free to do this twice a day or more, if needed.

Or for a tasty alternative, drink consommé, bouillon, bone broth, chicken stock. or beef stock — and stir in a spoonful of salted butter, if you like. Or, if you're using low-sodium bone broth or stock, add a pinch or two of salt.

In addition, make sure you're drinking enough water. The larger you are, the more water you'll probably lose in the early stages of keto and the more you'll need to replace. A good rule of thumb is to drink a minimum of 2.5 liters of fluid every day during your first week of keto. This doesn't mean you must drink at least 2.5 liters of plain water in addition to your other beverages. Although drinking plenty of water is important, coffee and tea will contribute toward your fluid intake as well.

Still, try to keep your caffeine intake modest (about 3 cups of coffee per day), as high amounts may potentially increase loss of water and sodium.

Getting enough water, sodium, and other electrolytes like magnesium and potassium can also help with another issue people often experience in the early stages of a keto diet: constipation.

More fat = fewer symptoms

Increasing salt and fluid intake usually resolves most of the keto flu side effects. However, if you continue feeling poorly after following those recommendations, try eating more fat.

Due to decades of misinformation about fat being unhealthy, fat phobia is common among people who are new to low-carb eating. But if you sharply cut back on carbs without upping your fat intake, your body will think it is starving. You'll feel tired, hungry, and miserable.

A well-balanced keto diet includes enough fat to ensure you're not hungry after a meal, therefore, you can go for several hours without eating, and have ample energy.

Be sure to increase your intake of fat at the start of your keto journey until your body adapts to using fat and ketones for most of its energy needs. Once you're fat adapted, let your appetite guide you in cutting back on fat a bit and seeing how much you need to feel satisfied.

In short: When in doubt, add butter or other fat to your food. And check out our top 10 tips for boosting fat intake. You can also follow our keto recipes, which have enough fat in relation to carbs and protein.

Slower transition. Has adding more water, salt, and fat not helped very much? Are you still feeling achy, tired and off?

We recommend you try to endure keto eating for a few more days until the symptoms pass. Research suggests that a very-low-carb diet is best for weight loss and metabolic issues like type 2 diabetes.

Keto flu symptoms are only temporary – they'll be long gone once you're a fat burner. You can, however, slow down the transition to ketogenic eating by consuming a few more carbs, such as following a more moderate low-carb diet that provides 20 to 50 grams of carbs a day. Eating slightly more carbs may potentially slow down weight loss and result in less rapid and dramatic health improvements.

However, it can still lead to better health, especially if you are cutting out sugar and processed foods. And keto flu will no longer be an issue. Once you've adapted to low-carb eating, feel free to try eating less than 20 grams of carbs again to see whether your body prefers this or slightly higher carb intake.

Conclusion

There are medical guidelines that should make you think about starting keto - or at least inform your doctor before trying it.

There are also a number of side effects that can throw you off the keto lifestyle path. Knowing your enemy by sight, you can prepare for this. As a result, the effects like keto flu will not come as a surprise to you. If they occur, you'll know what to do about it.

Hopefully, in this part of the book, I have answered questions about the precautions to take before deciding on a keto diet:

- To be cautious with a keto diet
- How safe is the keto diet
- Safety for short and long-term
- Side-effects of this diet and other difficulties you will have to face and will have to overcome.

I am sure that they will not be able to lead you astray. Therefore, in the next part of the book, I will talk about the state of ketosis - the basic state and meaning of the keto diet. So let's get started!

CHAPTER 4.
ALL ABOUT KETOSIS

Short Introduction To Ketosis

I have good news for all of us: many people can lose weight this way. On the other hand, some people find it difficult to enter this state and maintain a lifestyle with ketosis.

The word "keto" comes from the word "ketones," which are small molecules that the body can use as fuel. These are produced when your blood sugar becomes lower in supply. You can lower your blood sugar by eating fewer carbohydrates, higher fat concentrations, and a moderate amount of protein. These ketones (fuel) are produced in the liver from the fats you will be eating on this diet. However, the brain is not able to function off fat alone. It is why your body converts these fats into ketones.

Today, there is a belief that your brain needs carbohydrates to function correctly. However, scientific studies have shown that this isn't necessarily true. Studies have shown that your brain can work just as well on ketones as it does with your current diet, if not better. As exampled by many people on the ketogenic diet, more focus and energy running off ketones was reported as compared to other diets.

What Is The Ketosis?

When the body is fueled completely by fat it enters a state called "ketosis," which is a natural state for the body. After all of the sugars and unhealthy fats have been removed from the body during the first couple of weeks, the body is now free run on healthy fats. That has many potential benefits-related to rapid weight loss, health, or performance. In certain situations like type 1 diabetes, excessive ketosis can become extremely dangerous, where as in certain cases paired with intermittent fasting can be extremely beneficial for people suffering from type 2 diabetes. Substantial work is being conducted on this topic by Dr. Jason Fung M.D. (Nephrologist) of the Intensive Dietary Management Program.

Ketosis is a metabolic state in which fat provides most of the fuel for the body. It occurs when there is limited access to glucose (blood sugar), which is the preferred fuel source for many cells in the body. It is most often associated with ketogenic and very low-carb diets. Also, happens during pregnancy, infancy, fasting, and starvation.

To go into ketosis, people generally need to eat fewer than 50 grams of carbs per day and sometimes as little as 20 grams per day. This requires removing certain food items from your diet, such as grains, candy, and sugary soft drinks. You also have to cut back on legumes, potatoes, and fruit.

When eating a very low-carb diet, levels of the hormone insulin go down and fatty acids are released from body fat stores in large amounts. Many of these fatty acids are transferred to the liver, where they are oxidized and turned into ketones (or ketone bodies). These molecules can provide energy for the body.

Unlike fatty acids, ketones can cross the blood-brain barrier and provide energy for the brain in the absence of glucose.

Ketones Can Supply Energy for the Brain. It's a common misunderstanding that the brain doesn't function without dietary carbs. It's true that glucose is preferred and that there are some cells in the brain that can only use glucose for fuel.

However, a large portion of your brain can also use ketones for energy, such as during starvation or when your diet is low in carbs. In fact, after only three days of starvation, the brain gets 25% of its energy from ketones. During long-term starvation, this number rises to around 60%.

In addition, your body can use protein to produce the little glucose the brain still requires during ketosis. This process is called gluconeogenesis. Ketosis and gluconeogenesis are perfectly capable of fulfilling the brain's energy needs.

Ketosis Is NOT the Same as Ketoacidosis. People often confuse ketosis and ketoacidosis. While ketosis is part of normal metabolism, ketoacidosis is a dangerous metabolic condition that can be fatal if left untreated.

In ketoacidosis, the bloodstream is flooded with extremely high levels of glucose (blood sugar) and ketones. When this happens, the blood becomes acidic, which is seriously harmful. Ketoacidosis is most often associated with uncontrolled type 1 diabetes. It may also occur in people with type 2 diabetes, although this is less common. In addition, severe alcohol abuse may lead to ketoacidosis.

What Are Ketones?

Although a ketogenic diet has been used to greatly improve people's quality of life, there are some out there who do not share the majority's way of thinking. But why is that exactly? Ever since we can remember we have been taught that the only way to get rid of the extra weight was to quit eating the fat filled foods that we are so accustomed to eating every day. So instructing people to eat healthy fats (the key word is healthy) you can certainly understand why some people would be skeptical as to how and why you would eat more fat to achieve weight lost and achieve it fast. This concept goes against everything we have ever known about weight loss.

Ketones serve a number of functions in the body. The primary role and, arguably, the most important to ketogenic dieters, is to replace glucose as a fat-derived fuel for the brain. A commonly held misconception is that the brain can only use glucose for fuel. Quite to the contrary, in situations where glucose availability is limited, the brain can derive up to 75% of its total energy requirements from ketone bodies.

Ketones also decrease the production of glucose in the liver, and some researchers have suggested that ketones act as a 'signal' to bodily tissues to shift fuel use away from glucose and towards fat. These effects should be seen as a survival mechanism to spare what little glucose is available to the body.

A second function of ketones is as a fuel for most other tissues in the body. By shifting the entire body's metabolism from glucose to fat, what glucose is available is conserved for use by the brain. While many tissues of the body (especially muscle) use a large amount of ketones for fuel during the first few weeks of a ketogenic diet, most of these same tissues will decrease their use of ketones as the length of time in ketosis increases. At this time, these tissues rely primarily on the breakdown of free fatty acids (FFA).

In practical terms, after three weeks of a ketogenic diet, the use of ketones by tissues other than the brain is negligible and can be ignored. A potential effect of ketones is to inhibit protein breakdown during starvation through several possible mechanisms, discussed in detail in the next chapter. The only other known function of ketones is as a precursor for lipid synthesis in the brain of neonates.

Key Benefits Of Ketosis

Effects on Epilepsy. Epilepsy is a brain disorder characterized by recurring seizures. It's a very common neurological condition, affecting around 70 million people worldwide. For the majority of patients, anti-seizure medications can help control the seizures. However, around 30% of patients continue to have seizures despite using these medications.

In the early 1920s, the ketogenic diet was introduced as a treatment for epilepsy in people who don't respond to drug treatment. It has primarily been used in children, with some studies showing remarkable benefits. Many epileptic children have had massive reductions in seizures on a ketogenic diet, and some have even seen complete remission.

Effects on Weight Loss. The ketogenic diet is a popular weight loss diet that is well-supported by science. In fact, many studies have found that ketogenic diets lead to much greater weight loss than low-fat diets. One study reported 2.2 times more weight loss for people on a ketogenic diet, compared to those on a low-fat, calorie-restricted diet.

What's more, people tend to feel less hungry and more full on a ketogenic diet, which is attributed to ketosis. For this reason, it is generally not necessary to count calories on this diet.

Other Health Benefits of Ketosis. Ketosis and ketogenic diets may also have other therapeutic effects. They are now being studied as a treatment for a wide variety of conditions:

Heart disease. Reducing carbs to achieve ketosis may improve heart disease risk factors like blood triglycerides, total cholesterol and HDL cholesterol.

Type 2 diabetes. The diet may improve insulin sensitivity by up to 75%, and some diabetics are able to reduce or even stop diabetes medication.

Metabolic syndrome. Ketogenic diets can improve all major symptoms of metabolic syndrome, including high triglycerides, excess belly fat and elevated blood pressure.

Alzheimer's disease. A ketogenic diet may have benefits for patients with Alzheimer's disease.

Cancer. Some studies suggest that ketogenic diets may aid in cancer therapy, possibly by helping to "starve" cancer cells of glucose.

Parkinson's disease: A small study found that symptoms of Parkinson's disease improved after 28 days on a ketogenic diet.

Acne. There is some evidence that this diet may reduce the severity and progression of acne.

Ketosis Health Effects

There are a few potential side effects you may experience from ketosis and ketogenic diets.

Although extremely rare, there have been a few cases of breastfeeding women developing ketoacidosis likely triggered by a low-carb or ketogenic diet. Also, some epileptic children have developed kidney stones on the diet.

People who are taking blood sugar lowering drugs should consult with a doctor before trying a ketogenic diet, because the diet may reduce the need for medication. Sometimes ketogenic diets are low in fiber. For this reason, it is a good idea to make sure to eat plenty of high-fiber, low-carb vegetables.

All that being said, ketosis is generally safe for healthy people. Nevertheless, it will not suit everyone. Some people may feel great and full of energy in ketosis, while others feel miserable.

Ketosis Phases

It's going to take you at least one or two weeks to make the change to the keto diet. You're going to be adapting to a carb-less diet, and so is your body. Your whole life, you've been running your body mainly on carbs, so it's going to take some time to adapt.

However, once you have made the switch, you'll feel better. Also, because this diet stabilizes your blood sugar, it supports your energy.

The first phase lasts about 8 hours from the last intake of carbohydrates. The body still uses glucose, which came with the las intake of carbohydrates. Still, after 10 hours, about 50% of the energy begins to come from the splitting of fatty acids.

The second phase lasts from 1 to 2 days in the lack of carbohydrates. The body receives the energy of cleavage fatty acids and liver glycogen (usually, liver glycogen is consumed after 12-16 hours from the last intake of carbohydrates).

The third phase lasts for a week. The body receives energy from the cleavage of fatty acids and glucose formed by gluconeogenesis from protein, lactate, pyruvate, and glycerol. In this phase, there is a high probability of increased use of protein for gluconeogenesis.

The fourth phase comes in 5-7 days approximately. The fourth phase is almost a full adaptation of the body and entrance to ketosis. In this phase, the decay of intrinsic protein and protein that comes with food slows down, and the brain already receives about 75% of the fuel it needs from ketones.

Now we know that the fewer carbohydrates and the longer they are gone, the closer our organism to ketosis. It is crucial to understand. Even a minimal amount of glucose in the early days will withdraw your body from ketosis. Therefore, it is important not to deceive yourself and not eat sweet, do not matter how much you like it.

Main Types Of Ketosis

There are a few ways to enter ketosis besides the widespread practice of lowering your carb intake and consuming foods that are higher in fat. This specific type of ketosis is known as nutritional ketosis. Below, we will outline several other ways of entering ketosis if you feel the more popular way doesn't fit your lifestyle.

Type 1 of Ketosis [Carbohydrate-Restricted]. It is one of three variations of nutritional ketosis and one of the most popular. Diet is critically important in this version of ketosis; however, the macronutrient distribution can change drastically in individuals. When on high-fat and low-carb diet, there is an increase in fat oxidation, so this diet is best for those who are looking for a sustainable, long-term approach to the ketogenic diet.

Type 2 of Ketosis [Supplemental]. The main benefits of a ketogenic diet are that it takes little more than limiting carbohydrate intake to be effective. It is especially true at the levels of ketones that can be a bit difficult to maintain while on the ketogenic diet. For those who have trouble keeping their levels steady, there are supplements for this. As mentioned earlier, there are supplements known as MCTs, which help you to maintain and increase ketone levels for a more extended period. If you have chronic health issues and are attempting to cure them with a change in your diet, you will want to consider this version of the ketogenic diet.

Type 3 of Ketosis [Fasting]. Ketosis occurs when blood glucose and insulin levels drop in your body. At this point, the fat oxidation begins to increase, allowing your body to produce the ketones. At first, this will only be about .1 mmol/L to .3 mmol/L. As you continue to fast, the number of ketones will increase. If you are looking for a jumpstart way to enter ketosis, this is the best option for you.

Signs Of Ketosis

There are several symptoms that you may experience. So, we suggest going to the doctor's office to test if you are in a state of ketosis officially. However, if you choose to skip going to the doctor, there are several signs of ketosis you can detect by yourself. Watch for the following symptoms to make sure you are in ketosis:

Dry Mouth. As your body enters ketosis, you may find your mouth becoming drier than usual or that you feel thirstier. Ultimately, you will want to be sure that you are well-hydrated while on the ketogenic diet.

Increased Urination. As you drink more liquids, you will also notice an increased need to urinate. Additionally, acetoacetate, one of the ketone bodies, can build up in your urine. You can take an at-home urine test to determine the number of acetoacetates in your urine.

Ketone Scent. One of the more prevalent symptoms of the ketogenic diet is the ketogenic smell. For many people, this is what is known as "ketone breath," but it can also be produced via sweat. For some, this scent is fruity, but for others, it can smell like nail polish remover.

Loss of Hunger. For those looking to lose weight, this may be an exciting symptom for you to experience. Many people on the ketogenic diet experience a reduced appetite, which is mostly due to the way that the body burns energy by using fat storage while in ketosis. Some people have even reported eating one or two meals a day while on the ketogenic diet and still feeling satisfied.

Ketones Measuring

Measuring your ketone level is going to be vital during this diet. You must keep your body in a state of ketosis so that you don't have to keep fasting to get back into it.

Judging from Symptoms of Ketosis. It doesn't cost money, but it isn't as reliable as the other methods, nor does it give you the same levels of ketones. The typical symptoms that your body is entering ketosis can vary from person-to-person, but here are the most common:

1. Increased urination.

2. Dry mouth and increased thirst. It's okay to counter this by drinking more water. You can also add salt to your diet unless salt causes you issues or you have problems with high blood pressure.

3. Acetone breathe. Acetone is a ketone that can be excreted through the breath; it has a fruity smell. This symptom usually is temporary.

4. Increased energy. You might experience a temporary decline in power when you first go onto the diet as your body adjusts to the change. But often, once your body makes the adjustment to the diet and enters ketosis, you'll experience higher levels of energy.

5. Reduced hunger. Because fat is a steadier and more reliable source of energy than glucose, once you start entering ketosis, you're apt to experience fewer and milder hunger pangs.

Urine Strips. Urine strip is the easiest and cheapest way to determine whether you've entered ketosis. However, you won't know the ketone levels. You can buy these strips online or from any drug store. The instructions can vary from brand to brand, but you just pee in a cup and dip the strip into it for about fifteen seconds. If you're in ketosis, the strip will turn a different color, as per the instructions. This is the cheapest and easiest way to measure your ketones. If you are just beginning the ketogenic diet, this may be the best option for you, as you simply have to stick the strip into a cup of your fresh urine. The strip's color will then change depending on the level of ketones that are in your system at that moment. If the strip turns a dark purple color, you will know that you are indeed in a state of ketosis.

One problem with urine strips is that they only are entirely reliable for at most a few weeks because your body then becomes more efficient at reabsorbing ketones from urine, so that you won't be losing as many ketones to your urine. You should make sure that you use the urine strips daily from the beginning of your diet and continue using them after you start getting positive results. And then, if you start getting adverse effects, you can switch to a different method for monitoring your ketone level.

Breath Analyzer. These instruments determine ketosis levels from your breath. Like urine strips, they give you a color code for a general ketone level rather than an exact measurement, and they aren't always completely reliable. You can get them for about $150 online or in drug stores.

The breath analyzer is a device that can measure the number of ketones on your breath, so this may be a suitable device for you to check your body's ketosis level if you are short on time. This device is both reusable and straightforward, unlike urine strips; however, it may not always be reliable. It is because the number of ketones on your breath can change depending on the time of day and may even vary from breath to breathe. If you do not need an exact number, this still may be a good option for you!

Blood Ketone Meter. These babies measure ketone levels and are much more reliable than the other three choices. They're similar to the test diabetics use for testing their blood sugar. You prick the side of your finger to get a drop of blood and then put the fall on a strip for a machine to measure. It's usually an easy and straightforward process. Just follow the instructions and dispose of the needles correctly.

These meters cost about $100 and include several strips. If you are not queasy at the sight of blood, the ketone meter blood test may be a good option for you. It is the most reliable method currently available, but the device itself tends to be relatively expensive. Additionally, if you have low pain tolerance, this will not be a feasible option as you will need to prick your finger for each test.

How To Enter Ketosis?

Let most of your fat calories come from the healthy kinds of alternatives, mainly monounsaturated fats, saturated fats, and omega-3.

If your net carb limit is low, you should avoid fruits and other low-carb treats, but don't starve yourself. Ensure that you eat whenever you are hungry.

While it helps to keep an eye on your calorie intake, you should never ignore your body's needs. Drink at least 2-3 liters of water daily.

Stock up on healthy foods like non-starchy vegetables, meat, eggs, coconut oil, avocado, macadamia nuts, bone broth and other fermented foods, saturated fats, and unsaturated fats.

Avoid processed fats like vegetable oils, fully and partially hydrogenated oils, margarine, trans fats, soybean oil, corn oil, and canola oil.

Raw and organic dairy products are also right as long as you don't have any allergies. However, you should try to avoid milk due to its high carb content or opt for unpasteurized full-fat dairy if you have to.

Increase your electrolyte intake. The ketogenic diet may cause sodium, calcium, and potassium deficiencies. So, you should increase your intake of mushrooms, salmon, and avocados for potassium; nuts or magnesium supplements for magnesium; and salt or bone broth for sodium.

Avoid processed foods because of containing hidden carbs such as sorbitol, maltitol, preservatives, additives, and artificial sweeteners. Always read the labels when shopping.

If you are using any medications that contain sugars or sweeteners, ask for the sugar-free variety. Make sure you always plan your diet to avoid temptation and intuitive eating.

Shop weekly and get rid of anything that is not allowed on a diet from your home. Have salads and hard-boiled eggs available in case you feel like snacking.

Let us now get to the specifics; what should you eat and what should you avoid while on a ketogenic diet to get into a state of ketosis effortlessly? Let's start with what to eat.

Conclusion

Adopting the keto diet can deliver a shock to your system for obvious reasons. Some people might even get what's known as the keto flu during the first few days. Symptoms can include decreased energy, mental sluggishness, hunger pangs, insomnia, and nausea.

Should you want to avoid the early pitfalls of a ketogenic diet, you can start by supplementing your virtual no-carb diet with a low-carb diet. In other words, slowly reduce your carb intake during the first few weeks so that your body can adjust accordingly.

Also, keto can affect your water and mineral balance, so consider adding more salt to your diet and/or taking mineral supplements. Recommended dosages of mineral supplements are 3,000–4,000 mg of sodium along with 1,000 mg of potassium and 300 mg of magnesium per day.

So, now you know that the word "keto" comes from the word "ketones", which are small molecules that the body can use for fuel.

Also, you know:

- What is the ketosis and what are ketones
- Key benefits of ketosis and its health effects
- Ketosis phases and types
- Signs of ketosis and ketones measuring.

To sum up, now you know how to enter ketosis. Next, we'll take a look at key principles to be on the keto diet: fundamental rules, frequent mistakes, and possible difficulties with keto diet.

CHAPTER 5.
KEY PRINCIPLES OF THE KETO DIET

Fundamental Rules To Be On A Keto

Know What Foods You'll Eat And Avoid On The Ketogenic Diet

In following a keto meal plan, you'll be severely limiting carbs. Start off with between 20 and 30 grams of carbohydrates per day, says the New York City–based dietitian Kristen Mancinelli, RD, author of The Ketogenic Diet: A Scientifically Proven Approach to Fast, Healthy Weight Loss.

Also make sure that you know what foods have mostly carbs, fat, and protein, so you can make the right choices. For instance, it's not just bread, pasta, chips, cookies, candy, and ice cream that contain carbs. Beans may contain protein, but they're also very high in carbohydrates. Fruit and veggies also mostly contain carbs. The only foods that don't contain carbs are meat (protein) and pure fats like butter and oils (including olive oil and coconut oil).

Examine Your Relationship With Fat — Keto Involves Lots of It!

"People are afraid of fat because they've been told that it'll kill them," says Mancinelli. What is confusing is that research today remains mixed. Some studies suggest that replacing saturated fat with polyunsaturated fat (and avoiding unhealthy trans fat) is important for mitigating heart disease risk, while others (for example, an article published in June 2018 in BMJ) suggest that total fat and types of fat weren't associated with cardiovascular problems.

Deciding exactly how to eat then becomes confusing. What is helpful, the authors note, is to remember that food is more than a single nutrient, and it's the overall quality of the diet that counts. They do say that high-fat, low-carb diets still need more research to assess their long-term health benefits and risks.

To prepare for a high-fat diet, which can be uncomfortable at first, start making small adjustments to what you eat every day, she suggests, like ordering a burger on lettuce leaves and subbing green veggies for fries.

Instead of potatoes or rice with your meal, opt for a nonstarchy veggie. Start cooking with more oil, such as olive or avocado oil. Realize that old dieting habits — like making a plain skinless grilled chicken breast — just don't make sense on a keto diet because you won't get enough fat.

"Slowly start pushing out carbs and getting in fat. If you're afraid of fat, a ketogenic diet won't work for you," she says.

Switch Up Your View of Protein — This Is A Moderate-Protein Diet

One of the most common misconceptions about the keto diet is that you can eat as much protein as you'd like. But this is not a diet where you watch carbs only — you also have to keep your protein intake moderate, says Ginger Hultin, a Seattle-based registered dietitian, a spokesperson for the Academy of Nutrition, and the owner of ChampagneNutrition. Protein can be converted into glucose, and, therefore, overeating protein can take your body out of ketosis. Think of your ratios as a small portion of meat topped with a generous amount of fat rather than the other way around.

Hone Your Cooking Skills to Make Fresh Fare, as High-Carb Processed Foods Aren't Okay on Keto

Look at a variety of keto websites and cookbooks for keto-approved recipes you'll love. Mancinelli recommends finding four to five recipes with foods you know you'll like. "That way you're not standing around wondering what to eat, and turn to carbs," she says.

Try Bulletproof Coffee — It's One of the Best Keto-Friendly Drinks

"Made by mixing coconut oil and butter into your coffee, this drink will help keep your hunger at bay, giving you time to plan your next meal," advises Mancinelli.

Just note that coconut oil has the potential to send LDL, or "bad," cholesterol levels soaring, so if you have heart disease or at an increased risk for it because of family or personal health history, you'll likely want to avoid this drink. To be on the safe side, check with your doctor.

Talk to Your Family About Your Weight Loss Goals on the Diet

Tell them your plan. You may not be able to eat what they're eating during family mealtimes, so you'll want to prepare them (and yourself) for what your new habits will look like. Because this diet is often done only short term (three to six months), you can assure them that it's temporary.

If you get pushback, announce: "I've done my research, I've figured out it's safe, and I really want to try this," recommends Mancinelli. They don't have to like what you're doing, but it does help if they have your back. In a study published in September about obesity, having the support of friends and coworkers helped dieters more successfully lose weight and maintain that loss over a two-year period. It also can't hurt if everyone knows your goals on a keto diet, so they're less likely to push office treats or suggest splitting a side of fries when you're out to dinner.

Know What Side Effects to Expect [for Example, the 'Keto Flu']

For all the attributes of a ketogenic diet (like weight loss), there's one big side effect you have to be prepared for: the keto flu. It is a term that refers to the period after you start the diet when your body is adjusting to burning fat for energy. "Some people have no problem with it and others are miserable," says Mancinelli.

In the first week or 10 days, you may feel extremely lethargic in your limbs. Walking upstairs may feel impossible. You may deal with mental fog. Often, keto causes constipation or potentially diarrhea because of a change in fiber intake.

For that reason, you should pick a start date when your week isn't crazy with deadlines and obligations; choose a slower time when you can rest as needed. Along the same lines, you'll want to be sure to take it easy with exercise for the first week or two as your body adjusts to burning more fat rather than carbs for fuel.

Up Your Electrolytes to Prevent or Mitigate Unpleasant Keto Side Effects

In ketosis, Mancinelli explains, your kidneys excrete more water and electrolytes. Make sure you're getting the sodium and potassium your body needs to function well. Salt your foods, drink salted bone broth, and eat nonstarchy veggies, such as asparagus, kale, bell peppers, and arugula.

Acknowledge When Keto Might Not Be Right for You

Now that ketogenic diets have become popular, many keto hybrid diets have sprung up, including plant-based versions (one is "ketotarian," which is predominantly plant-based but includes the option of eggs, ghee, fish, and shellfish). While this approach can be healthy, Hultin cautions against trying keto as a vegan.

In addition, there are medical conditions that should make you think twice about starting keto — or at least talk to your doctor before trying it out. Those include people on insulin, as well as those on oral and noninsulin injectable medications for high blood sugar or high blood pressure, says Hultin. Even struggling with GI issues may be a barrier to starting. "One of the side effects of a ketogenic diet is constipation, so if that's a struggle, there's serious reason not to go on this relatively low-fiber diet," says Hultin.

Last consideration: If existing personal dietary restrictions require you to avoid foods like soy, eggs, nuts, dairy, or seafood, a ketogenic diet may be too limiting for you. Coming from a place of elimination in an already restrictive diet can make it incredibly tough to follow, she says.

Have an After Plan Because Keto Isn't Meant to Be a Long-Term Weight Loss Solution

A keto diet is not a forever diet. It's designed to be short-term. While Mancinelli says that some people go on a keto diet a few times per year, others will use it to lose weight and change their eating habits.

A whopping 46 percent of American adults still eat what's considered a "poor" diet in American Heart Association standards, notes a study published in June 2016 in JAMA, which was based on a survey of nearly 34,000 people. For some people, going on a keto diet is an effort to change those poor habits, but there's the risk of falling back into your old ways once the diet is over. Don't go straight back to a standard American diet because you'll likely lose any health benefits and regain the weight.

Your ultimate goal should be "to shift your diet to a healthier pattern that involves eating less bread, less pasta, less flour, and less sugar, as well as more nonstarchy veggies," she says.

Think about what that will look like for you once the keto diet is over. How will you use this temporary diet as a springboard to bettering your long-term health?

Use The Macro Calculator

If you ask, how does this calculator help you? I'll answer - this "device" will help you identify your unique needs so you can: reach your weight loss goals, achieve indicators of weight gain, easily go into ketosis and stay there, accurately track your macros on a keto diet, stop guessing what and how much you need to eat, enjoy optimal health.

There are many calculators and applications that will calculate your macro. You just need to open the search bar or app store and enter 'the macro calculator'.

I will not advise which application or website to use because everyone has their own preference, which will be the most convenient. I only recommend taking turns using 2-4 calculators and then settling on a specific one, which is right for you.

Almost all of them work according to the same principle. Here I will briefly talk about it so that you have an understanding of this. It's simple - you only need to enter a few key details.

How The Macro Calculator Works?

Step # 1: enter your basic information: gender, age, height, and weight.

The calculator uses this data to find the so-called base metabolic rate (BMR). That is, the basic amount of energy that you expend while resting. In fact, it shows how much energy your body burns without doing absolutely anything.

Basically, calculators use the Mifflin-St Jora formula because this is one of the most accurate formulas.

Why does your data affect your BMR:

Gender: Body composition is different for men and women.

Age: Your BMR decreases with age, especially after 30-35 years.

Height and weight: To calculate, you need to know your unique body composition.

The device then calculates your resting energy consumption.

Step # 2: enter your activity level

Physical activity level (PAL) shows how much energy you expend on average daily. It depends on what kind of lifestyle you are going - passive or active.

The calculator combines your BMR and your PAL to determine your total daily energy expenditure (TDEE). It shows the number of calories your body burns in 24 hours.

Your TDEE tells the calculator how many calories you need to eat daily to cover your expenses.

Step # 3: set your goal

Here you can tell the calculator what you want to keep, lose, or gain weight. Depending on the goal, you have to choose a calorie deficit or an excess.

For example, if you choose a 10% calorie deficit, your total daily calories will be 10% less than you actually need. This will help you lose weight in moderation.

If you add 10% excess calories, then your daily calories will be 10% higher. This will help you gain weight.

Here's how the calorie scale works:

To maintain weight: Keep the bar at 0%.

To moderately lose weight: Move the scale between 10 and 20% (calorie deficit).

To lose a lot of weight: Move the scale between 20 and 50% (calorie deficit). But from my own experience, I do not recommend doing this because it is a great burden for the body. After a while, a "breakdown" may occur. Therefore, it is better to keep the level up to 20%.

To gain weight in moderation: Stay between + 10% and + 20% of your BMR level. If you are using a specialized calculator, there are a few more details to fill in - body fat percentage, protein ratio, or total carbohydrate intake.

At the initial stage, this is not very important because these characteristics are needed for "advanced users". And when you follow a keto diet for a long time, you can go back and study these indicators in more detail.

It must be remembered that for the classic ketogenic diet, the following proportion should be observed:

70-80% fat / 20-25% protein / 5-10% net carbs *
* net carbs are grams of carbs in food minus grams of fiber in food.

Below you can see a table in which the rate of consumption of fats, proteins, and carbohydrates for a ketogenic diet is calculated. You will be able to use its data when calculating how many calories you need to consume per day.

Day calorie Target	2'500 calories	2'250 calories	2'000 calories	1'750 calories	1'500 Calories	1'250 calories
Fat 75% of calories	208 g	188 g	167 g	146 g	125 g	104 g
Protein 20% of calories	125 g	113 g	100 g	88 g	75 g	63 g
Carbs 5% of calories	31 g	28 g	25 g	22 g	19 g	16 g

Be aware that your personal calorie intake may be below or above these values. Therefore, the specific grams of each of the macronutrients will look different to you.

Frequent Mistakes Of Beginners And How To Avoid Them

Cutting Your Carbs and Increasing Your Fat Too Much Too Quickly

One day you're eating cereal, sandwiches, and pasta. Then on the next you decide to hop on keto and eat only 20 grams (g) of carbohydrates a day, which is often the recommended amount to start with (a medium apple has 25 g of carbs, for reference). That may be a drastic change for your body.

Consider easing in. "Prior to starting a keto diet, individuals may benefit from tapering down their carbohydrate intake instead of reducing carbs cold turkey," says Lara Clevenger, a ketogenic dietitian-nutritionist with a private practice in New Smyrna Beach, Florida.

Not Drinking Enough Water on Keto

For all the focus on what you're eating, don't forget about what you're sipping. Dehydration is an increased possibility on keto. "The drastic decrease in carbohydrate intake on the ketogenic diet can cause shifts in your fluid and electrolyte balance. Carbs are stored along with water in the body, so as these stores are depleted, that water is lost along with them," says Alyssa Tucci, RDN, nutrition manager at Virtual Health Partners in New York City.

She also says that the body flushes out the buildup of ketones in urine, which also depletes water and sodium from the body. Tucci recommends waking up to a large glass of water and sipping regularly throughout the day to reach a goal of consuming half of your body weight in ounces of water daily.

Not Preparing Yourself for the Keto Flu

As your body transitions from a carbohydrate burner to a fat burner, you may experience what's known as the "keto flu," or flu-like symptoms (including muscle cramps, nausea, aches, and fatigue) during the first two weeks of the keto diet (it doesn't happen to everyone). If you're not prepared for this feeling, you may think something is drastically wrong and give up the diet completely.

More than that, you can help yourself through the transition period of low energy by planning out your meals or meal prepping, says Clevenger. She also recommends eating foods rich in potassium, magnesium, and sodium, as well as hydrating to help ease keto flu symptoms.

Forgetting to Eat Foods Rich in Omega-3 Fatty Acids

While fat reigns supreme on the diet, don't just turn to bacon, cheese, and cream. When choosing your fats, aim to include more anti-inflammatory omega-3s, particularly EPA and DHA, the types that are found in salmon, sardines, oysters, herring, and mussels, says Clevenger.

If seafood isn't your thing, you can also take cod liver oil or krill oil. Other healthy fats are a good choice, too. If you haven't stocked up on avocado, olive oil, and seeds, such as chia seeds and flaxseed, definitely do. They're not only keto friendly — they also offer healthy polyunsaturated and monounsaturated fat that your body needs to perform at its best.

Not Salting Your Food Enough

With people consuming more sodium than ever in a diet rich in processed food, you're probably not used to hearing the call to eat more salt. But on keto, it's necessary. Not only does the clearance of ketones cause the body to lose sodium, but you may be getting much less table salt (which is comprised of 40 percent sodium and 60 percent chloride) now that you've kicked out the top source of salt in the standard American diet: packaged, processed foods, including bread, chips, crackers, and cookies.

"Chances are, if you're following a ketogenic diet, you will need to prepare most, if not all, of your own meals and snacks from scratch, so simply season with salt," says Tucci.

Going It Alone and Not Clearing the Diet With Your Doc

Many followers of the keto diet try it because they're hoping to use it therapeutically for a medical condition. If that's you, talk to your doctor first and make sure they're on board with your plan — especially if you're also taking medication, says Clevenger.

"Some medications may need to be adjusted by your healthcare practitioner as your signs and symptoms improve," she says. Just one example is insulin, as a lower dose may be needed now that you're severely limiting carbohydrates.

Not Paying Attention to Your Veggie Intake

Vegetables have carbohydrates. And that means that you have to watch how much you eat — even lettuce. If you're not careful or are eating them as a free-for-all, you could overconsume carbs, and thus get kicked out of ketosis. On the other hand, you may be skipping veggies altogether if counting every baby carrot is getting too complicated. But it's important to get in vegetables (these contain fiber that prevent constipation, a potential side effect of keto) while minding portions and properly counting carbs.

Go for non-starchy options in a rainbow of colors for a variety of nutrients, says Tucci, like leafy greens, cucumber, tomato, broccoli, cauliflower, bell peppers, and asparagus.

Getting Caught Up in Carb-Counting and Forgetting That Food Quality Matters

When it seems as if the sole goal of keto is to drastically cut carbs, the rest can feel like an afterthought. "Reducing your carbohydrate intake is great, but focusing on higher-quality products when budget allows will help improve your health, too," says Clevenger.

That means choosing omega-3 rich foods like wild salmon, grass-fed, local or organic meats, and snacking on whole foods rather than processed keto-approved treats. It also means trying to follow a balanced diet as best you can by incorporating as many nutrient-rich fruits and veggies as you can. Many registered dietitians aren't a fan of keto because it may lead to nutrient deficiencies.

Possible Difficulties with Keto for beginners

May lead to the keto flu

Carb intake on the keto diet is typically limited to fewer than 50 grams per day, which can come as a shock to your body. As your body depletes its carb stores and switches to using ketones and fat for fuel at the start of this eating pattern, you may experience flu-like symptoms.

May stress your kidneys

High fat animal foods, such as eggs, meat, and cheese, are staples of the keto diet because they don't contain carbs. If you eat a lot of these foods, you may have a higher risk of kidney stones.

That's because a high intake of animal foods can cause your blood and urine to become more acidic, leading to increased excretion of calcium in your urine.

Some studies also suggest that the keto diet reduces the amount of citrate that's released in your urine. Given that citrate can bind to calcium and prevent the formation of kidney stones, reduced levels of it may also raise your risk of developing them.

Additionally, people with chronic kidney disease (CKD) should avoid keto, as weakened kidneys may be unable to remove the acid buildup in your blood that results from these animal foods. This can lead to a state of acidosis, which can worsen the progression of CKD.

What's more, lower protein diets are often recommended for individuals with CKD, while the keto diet is moderate to high in protein

May cause digestive issues and changes in gut bacteria

Since the keto diet restricts carbs, it can be difficult to meet your daily fiber needs. Some of the richest sources of fiber, such as high carb fruits, starchy vegetables, whole grains, and beans, are eliminated on the diet because they provide too many carbs.

As a result, the keto diet can lead to digestive discomfort and constipation. A 10-year study in children with epilepsy on the ketogenic diet found that 65% of participants reported constipation as a common side effect.

What's more, fiber feeds the beneficial bacteria in your gut. Having a healthy gut may help boost immunity, improve mental health, and decrease inflammation.

A low carb diet that's lacking in fiber, such as keto, may negatively affect your gut bacteria — although current research on this topic is mixed.

Some keto-friendly foods that are high in fiber include flax seeds, chia seeds, coconut, broccoli, cauliflower, and leafy greens.

May lead to nutrient deficiencies

Since the keto diet restricts several foods, especially nutrient-dense fruits, whole grains, and legumes, it may fail to provide recommended amounts of vitamins and minerals.

In particular, some studies suggest that the keto diet doesn't provide enough calcium, vitamin D, magnesium, and phosphorus.

A study that evaluated the nutrient composition of common diets revealed that very low carb eating patterns like Atkins, which is similar to keto, provided sufficient amounts for only 12 of the 27 vitamins and minerals your body needs to obtain from food. Over time, this may lead to nutrient deficiencies.

Notably, guidelines for clinicians who manage people on a very low calorie keto diet for weight loss recommend supplementing with potassium, sodium, magnesium, calcium, omega-3 fatty acids, psyllium fiber, and vitamins B, C, and E.

Keep in mind that the nutritional adequacy of this diet depends on the specific foods that you eat. A diet rich in healthy low carb foods, such as avocados, nuts, and non-starchy vegetables, provides more nutrients than processed meats and keto treats.

May cause dangerously low blood sugar

Low carb diets like keto have been shown to help manage blood sugar levels in people with diabetes. In particular, some studies suggest that keto may help decrease levels of hemoglobin A1c, a measure of average blood sugar levels.

However, individuals with type 1 diabetes may be at a high risk of more episodes of low blood sugar (hypoglycemia), which is marked by confusion, shakiness, fatigue, and sweating. Hypoglycemia can lead to coma and death if not treated.

A study in 11 adults with type 1 diabetes who followed a ketogenic diet for over 2 years found that the median number of low blood sugar events was close to 1 per day.

Individuals with type 1 diabetes typically experience low blood sugar if they are taking too much insulin and not consuming enough carbs. Thus, a low carb keto diet may increase the risk.

Theoretically, this could also happen to individuals with type 2 diabetes who are taking insulin medications.

May damage bone health

The keto diet is also associated with impaired bone health. Several studies in animals link the keto diet to decreased bone strength, likely due to losses in bone mineral density, which may occur as your body adapts to ketosis.

In fact, a 6-month study in 29 children with epilepsy on the keto diet discovered that 68% had a lower bone mineral density score after going on the diet.

Another study in 30 elite walkers determined that those who followed keto for 3.5 weeks had significantly higher levels of blood markers for bone breakdown, compared with those who ate a diet higher in carbs.

May increase your risk of chronic diseases and early death

The ketogenic diet's effect on your risk of chronic illness, such as heart disease or cancer, is hotly debated and not entirely understood.

Some evidence suggests that high-fat, low-carb diets that focus on animal foods may lead to poor health outcomes, while diets that emphasize vegetable sources of fats and proteins provide benefits.

A long-term observational study in over 130,000 adults linked animal-based low-carb diets to higher rates of death from heart disease, cancer, and other causes. On the other hand, vegetable-based low-carb diets were associated with a lower rate of death from heart disease and other causes.

Another study in over 15,000 adults found similar results but tied both low and high-carb diets to a greater all-cause death rate, compared with moderate carb diets in which carbs comprised 50–55% of total daily calories.

Yet, more substantial studies are needed.

Make a concrete nutrition plan

Implementing a Keto Diet Plan

You can excel on the keto diet plan by writing how much of each nutrient group you need and then recording the numbers throughout the day. Here are how the numbers will work on your keto diet plan:

Caloric Intake – daily caloric intake will dictate how many grams of fat, protein, and carbs you will ingest per day. Caloric intake is dictated by what your fitness goals are: weight loss, maintenance, or healthy weight gain.

After you've established what fitness goals you'd like to hit (weight loss, maintain, or weight gain), you can use this calories calculator to get concrete caloric numbers. If you're working from the daily caloric intake perspective, this number (caloric intake) will be your compass for finding the right intakes of fats, proteins, and carbs. Here's how:

Keto Diet Plan Nutrition

Example Daily Caloric Intake: 2000 Calories

Fats	Protein	Carbs
9 Calories Per One Gram Of Fat	4 Calories Per Gram Of Protein	4 Calories Per Gram Of Carbohydrates
70–75% Of Caloric Intake Should Be Fat	20–30% Of Caloric Intake Should Be Protein	5–10% Of Caloric Intake Should Be Carbs
70% Of 2000 = 1400 Calories	20% Of 2000 = 400 Calories	10% Of 2000 = 200 Calories
1400/9 = 155 Grams Of Fat Per Day	400/4 = 100 Grams Of Protein Per Day	200/4 = 50 Grams Of Carbs Per Day

Now that you know your numbers, you can focus on which foods will help you achieve them. Anyone who wants to accomplish a goal knows the tools they need for the job. For example, the mechanic knows what tools he needs to fix the car in his shop.

The painter knows the exact utensils she'll need to complete the masterpiece.

Similarly, you need to know what types of foods will help meet the caloric requirements that you have set up for yourself up for success.

Fats:

Avocados: 29 g Total fat [Per one avocado]

Saturated fat 4.3 g, Polyunsaturated fat 3.7 g, Monounsaturated fat 20 g

Salmon: 27 g Total fat [Half a fillet]

Saturated fat 6 g, Polyunsaturated fat 8 g, Monounsaturated fat 7 g

Chicken Thigh: [One thigh without skin] 10 g Total fat

Saturated fat 2.6 g, Polyunsaturated fat 1.9 g, Monounsaturated fat 3.9 g

Ribeye Steak: [One steak] 63 g Total fat

Saturated fat 28 g, Polyunsaturated fat 3 g, Monounsaturated fat 31 g

Coconut Oil: [One tablespoon] 14 g Total fat

Saturated fat 12 g, Polyunsaturated fat 0.2 g, Monounsaturated fat 0.8 g

Olive Oil: [One tablespoon] 14 g Total fat

Saturated fat 1.9 g, Polyunsaturated fat 1.4 g, Monounsaturated fat 10 g

Organic Grass Fed Butter: [One tablespoon] 11 g Total fat, Saturated fat 7 g

Proteins:

Chicken thigh [One thigh without skin]: 28 g Protein

Ribeye steak [One steak]: 69 g Protein

Salmon [Half a fillet]: 40 g Protein

Egg [One egg]: 6 g Protein

Peanut butter [Smooth, salted, one tablespoon]: 3 g Protein

Tuna [One can]: 42 g Protein

Carbs [What to avoid] no carbs while you're on the keto diet plan:

White bread [One slice]: 15 g Carbs

Pizza [Average of one slice]: 36 g Carbs

Banana [One medium banana]: 27 g Carbs

Grapes [One cup red or green]: 27 g Carbs

Big Mac [One sandwich]: 44 g Carbs (yikes!)

Potato chips [One oz.]: 15 g Carbs

Flour [One cup]: 95 g Carbs

The Fats, proteins, and carbs listed above are in no way exhaustive. These are just examples of items that could be easily added to (or subtracted from) an everyday routine. You have to take it upon yourself to be cognizant of the nutrition facts of each food and/or beverage you consume.

If you grab a box of random "protein bars" and just assume that they're good for you – that's on you. And because we want you to succeed, we're going to give you an example keto diet plan.

Example Keto Diet Plan

Example Target Caloric Numbers: 2000 Calories [155 g Fat / 100 g Protein / 50 g Carbs]

Breakfast:

2 Eggs [Scrambled]: 182 Calories [14 g Fat / 12 g Protein / 2 g Carbs]

2 Slices of Bacon: 86 Calories [6.6 g Fat / 6 g Protein / 0.2 g Carbs]

1 Half Avocado: 161 Calories [14.5 g Fat / 2 g Protein / 8.5 g Carbs]

1 Tablespoon Coconut Oil: 117 Calories [14 g Fat / 0 g Protein / 0 g Carbs]

Total Daily Nutrition Breakdown: 546 Calories [49.1 g Fat / 20 g Protein / 10.7 g Carbs]

Lunch:

Half Salmon Fillet: 412 Calories [27 g Fat / 40 g Protein / 0 g Carbs]

Cooked in 1 Tablespoon Butter: 102 Calories [12 g Fat / 0.1 g Protein / 0 g Carbs]

3 Cups Spring Mix: 19 Calories [0 g Fat / 1.9 g Protein / 2.9 g Carbs]

1 Tablespoon Ranch Dressing: 73 Calories [8 g Fat / 0.2 g Protein / 1 g Carbs]

1 Tablespoons Peanut Butter [Dessert]: 94 Calories [8 g Fat / 4 g Protein / 3 g Carbs]

Total Daily Nutrition Breakdown: 1246 Calories [104.1 g Fat / 66.2 g Protein /17.6 g Carbs]

Snack:

Macadamia Nuts [half cup]: 481 Calories [51 g Fat / 5.5 g Protein / 9.5 g Carbs]

Dinner:

1 Chicken Thighs [Without skin]: 206 Calories [10 g Fat / 28 g Protein / 0 g Carbs]

1 Side Caesar Salad: 151 Calories [12.61 g Fat / 4.5 g Protein / 5.8 Carbs]

Total Daily Nutrition Breakdown: 2084 Calories [178 g Fat / 104 g Protein / 33 g Carbs]

How Many Meals Should Eat On The Keto Diet

This is completely subjective to your schedule. In the 21st century, work shifts are ever-changing, and off days aren't slotted in the typical weekend as much as they once were.

Look at your daily schedule and see what type of eating schedule will be most advantageous to you. As long as you've met your caloric intake through the proper proportion of fats, proteins, and carbs by bedtime, viva you!

But we all know you're going to snack. At least at first. It's best to try to hard schedule snacks, giving yourself concrete times to indulge in a keto-friendly snack. Random snacking almost always goes too far. You wake up dazed and confused, covered in the remnants of what was a chocolate ice cream cake.

If you're desperately unorganized, fear not! You too can execute a successful keto lifestyle! If you've led a life of falling off the proverbial wagon, with your peers rolling their eyes at the notion of you starting a new diet – this your opportunity to prove them wrong.

The lynchpin to a successful ketogenic diet is discipline. As Jocko Willink says, "Discipline equals freedom." The moment you surrender to the discipline of the ketogenic diet is the moment you open up your life to the freedom of great health – not depending on meds, "comfort food," or crash diets.

Best Keto Products

Cheese Crisps for a High-Fat Snack

It can be difficult to find low-carb prepackaged keto snacks to take on the go. Most chips, cookies, and crackers traditionally are filled with carbs and processed sugars. Thankfully, keto-friendly products are becoming more common and accessible — like KetoLogic Keto Crisps.

Cheese is a keto diet staple. Because of its high-fat, low-carb macronutrient ratio, cheese (in its hundreds of varieties) has become the go-to snack for anyone on keto. But even though it's a go-to, it's not necessarily a to-go type of snack. You don't want cheese melting in your backpack.

KetoLogic Keto Crisps are an easy-to-carry, low-carb snack made entirely from locally sourced milk. As a gluten-free, sugar-free, keto-friendly product, the crisps can be consumed by virtually anyone (aside from lactose intolerant individuals). With only 1g of carb per serving, its safe to say it won't take you out of ketosis.

They come in three flavors, including cheddar, buffalo, and chili lime. Whether you are at school, work, the gym, or on the road, these snacks are portable enough to bring anywhere.

Instead of reaching for those greasy potato chips, reach for some cheese instead.

Beef Jerky for a Low-Carb Snack

Like cheese, another snack you'll see on the desks of keto dieters is beef jerky, mostly because of the high protein content and low amount of carbohydrates.

Beef jerky is an easily portable source of protein that's easy to carry anywhere. Problem is, it can be really difficult to find beef jerky that doesn't contain much sugar, and thus, excess carbs. We like Epic's beef, apple, bacon bar. We know... beef jerky in a bar seems weird. But it's even more convenient than a pouch, and also enables portion control.

This bar only has 4g of carbs per serving — far less than many other brands. It also has 9g of protein and 13g of fat, so it's pretty keto-friendly.

Epic uses 100% grass-fed, free-range beef for its bars; not only does it taste good (it's got bacon!), but you can feel good eating it.

Creatine To Support Muscle Growth

Creatine has been one of the most frequently researched supplements of all time. Thousands of studies have shown creatine to be effective for supporting muscle strength, power, and size.

As the supplement of choice for athletes, creatine can help improve athletic performance in several ways. Over 22 studies showed an average muscle mass increase of 8% compared to placebo groups. Increases in bench press (one repetition maximum) also increased from 3% to 45%. Substantial evidence has suggested that creatine supplementation can be far more effective at increasing muscle strength and weightlifting performance than resistance training alone.

Another benefit of creatine use is increased lean muscle tissue mass. A meta-analysis on 22 studies showed an average lean muscle mass increase of 1.37kg compared to placebo groups.

With so many brands of creatine in the marketplace, be sure to choose a high-quality product proven to work. Optimum Nutrition Creatine Monohydrate is made with a pure creatine monohydrate, and is easily mixed and blended. The beauty of the product is that it's unflavored, allowing it to work with many different types of supplements (like right into your protein shake post-workout).

Creatine works well as part of the keto diet, especially if you are looking to increase muscle growth or enhance strength performance. It's great for all you endurance athletes out there too. In one study, supplementing with creatine and carbohydrates showed benefits for power outputs in the closing sprints of time trials. That means better performance at the end of the race.

If you are a highly active individual, be sure to add creatine to your supplementation stack.

Salt For Electrolytes

As mentioned before, one temporary side effect of the keto diet is the keto flu.

The body often needs a bit of time to transition from using carbohydrates to using fat as its main energy source. During the period of adaptation, the body can experience flu-like symptoms known as the keto flu. The reported symptoms include mood swings, irritability, fatigue, and dizziness. Studies have compared the effects of carbohydrates on the brain to addictive drugs like cocaine, so it's no surprise these feelings stemming from carbohydrate withdrawal can last several days or weeks.

Once carbohydrate is drastically decreased, electrolytes are processed differently as glycogen is drastically reduced.

On keto, less insulin is released, causing the kidneys to excrete more sodium. As your body begins to lose sodium, this can also impact the balance of other key electrolytes in your body because those electrolytes are excreted in the urine. And water alone is generally not sufficient for replenishing electrolyte levels. Due to the excretion of electrolytes (such as sodium), it's important to use supplementation as a means of getting back to normal levels.

Using a sodium-based product such as Fyr Salt is one way to combat these imbalances. As an unrefined pink salt with trace materials, it can help replete what's lost from low-carb dieting.

Supplementing with sodium-based products such as Fyr Salt can help protect the function of a number of physiological processes, including: nerve function, regulation of blood volume and blood pressure, control of water retention.

With it's great taste, clean natural ingredients, and ketogenic diet support, Fyr Salt can help improve electrolyte balance and may help reduce symptoms of the dreaded keto flu. Try adding Fyr Salt to your diet — it's more than just your everyday table salt.

MCT Oil Powder for Sustained Keto Energy

Medium Chain Triglycerides or MCTs, have almost become synonymous with the keto diet.

In case you were unaware, triglycerides are a type of fat (lipid) found in your blood. These medium-chain triglycerides aren't actually exogenous ketones, but they are easily converted into ketones by the body. One product that can help your keto diet journey is MCT oil or MCT oil powder.

MCTs are rapidly digested and shuttered to the liver to be used for energy or to be converted into ketones that power the brain and body.

MCTs can help you stay in ketosis or get to ketosis quicker — as they're a healthy source of fat that is less likely to be stored as body fat.

Consuming MCT-based products as part of a ketogenic diet can produce several other health benefits including:

1. May improve weight loss: a study showed that people who consumed MCT oil with breakfast were less likely to overeat compared to a placebo group.

2. Can increase energy expenditure: one study showed MCT consumption helped to increase energy expenditure (burn more calories) compared to dieting alone.
3. May reduce the risk of heart disease: a study on healthy overweight men who consumed MCT oil had a 14% decrease in LDL (bad) cholesterol compared to a control group.
4. May positively benefit diabetic patients: a study on overweight type 2 diabetic patients using MCTs showed a reduction in body weight, waist circumference, and insulin resistance compared to a placebo group that used LCTs.

It seems MCT supplementation can have several benefits, from increased energy to weight loss. But you might be wondering — what's the best method of consuming MCTs?

Sure, MCT oil is one option, but it may also cause gastrointestinal distress in individuals with sensitive stomachs, especially with the increase of fat into the diet early on in keto. One alternative is a powder-based MCT source.

MCT oil powders are created through a process known as spray drying. Liquid MCT oil is spray dried and microencapsulated with a powder carrier shell to give it a powder-like appearance.

Blueberries For A Sweet Treat

Switching to a keto diet means you'll be consuming way less carbohydrates. Berries tend to have fewer carbs than other fruits making them the most keto-friendly option. If you want to enjoy fruit, be sure to pick a low-carb choice, such as blueberries.

Berries have the highest antioxidant levels of all fruits and veggies. A study done on common fruits found berries to have the highest cellular antioxidant activity out of more than 25 fruits researched. Increased antioxidant intake can decrease oxidative stress and may also reduce the risk of cancer.

Although berries can provide valuable antioxidants, they can also rot quickly. Buying frozen fruit or freezing the fruit yourself is one way to keep your favorite snacks handy and not in the trash can. We like Wyman's frozen blueberries. They're a snack you can keep in the freezer anytime you need to scratch that dessert itch.

Peanut Butter for Healthy Fat

All-natural peanut butter can be considered keto-friendly due to its healthy fats and relatively low carb content. The naturally sweet and salty treat can be a high-fat, high-protein food source that fits into a ketogenic diet.

One natural choice is Skippy Natural Creamy Peanut Butter spread. Free of preservatives and artificial flavoring, Skippy Natural provides a smooth taste without any unwanted additives.

Peanut butter is also extremely versatile. You can use it for topping veggies, creating fat bombs, or even eat it straight out of the jar in a moment of desperation.

One thing to be mindful of is portion sizes. Peanut butter is easy to overeat because it's so tasty; be sure to accurately measure serving sizes and enjoy in moderation.

Whey Protein To Hit Your Macros

Whey protein is a proven supplement capable of helping you meet dietary protein goals. If you are trying to build and maintain muscle, keep protein levels high enough to activate protein synthesis.

Some benefits of whey protein supplementation includ enhanced whole body anabolism, improved recovery after strenuous resistance exercise, increased lean muscle mass.

The problem is, many proteins on the market contain excess fillers such as maltodextrin (added sugar) resulting in higher carb content. Finding a great tasting low-carb, keto protein can be difficult, but there are viable options currently on the market.

Muscle Feast has created a keto-friendly whey protein without any added chemicals or fillers. It contains 21.5 grams of protein and only 89 calories per serving. Made with grass-fed dairy, it has everything you want and nothing you don't. With only contains 2 g of carbs per serving, it's the perfect keto-friendly protein option.

Whether you are searching for a high protein meal replacement or a convenient protein powder on the go, Muscle Feast Whey Protein has you covered.

Keto Testing Device To Measure Ketosis

Testing and understanding blood ketone levels is a fundamental element of biohacking and optimizing your keto diet to the best degree.

One of the latest innovations for keto dieters is the creation of a new ketosis measurement device. There are a few options (including blood and urine testing devices). Still, none are as easy-to-use as a breath-analyzing device: simply breathe into the device and measure ketone levels instantly.

With the help of a smartphone app, you are able to track ketosis in real time without any painful finger pricking or unsightly urine tests. The Keyto Breath Sensor is a pocket sized ketone measurement system providing instant readings. One of the downsides — those instant readings are a range of ketosis (similar to urine tests). Blood tests give an exact measurement of ketosis, but it's understandable people don't want to prick their fingers every time they want to check for ketone levels.

Still, the Keyto Breath Sensor is convenient. It allows you to stay accountable and keep your keto goals on track. Stick to your keto diet using the most simple and portable ketone measurement device to date.

Ketone Ester For Deep, Rapid Ketosis

The main goal of the keto diet is ketone production. Ketosis is generally defined as blood ketone levels above 0.5mM.

As you may already know, ketones can be produced either endogenously (meaning, the body produces its own ketones, usually via diet or fasting) or through an exogenous ketone supplement. Exogenous ketones are consumed through external means as a way of raising blood ketones and sustaining ketosis even without the help of a high-fat diet.18 studies have shown exogenous ketone drinks to be a practical, efficacious way of achieving ketosis.

Exogenous ketones that can be used to get into a deeper state of ketosis within minutes, inducing levels of ketosis usually seen in fasting for days or dieting for weeks.

Exogenous ketone supplements (specifically BHB monoesters) have several benefits, including improved cognitive performance, better regulated blood glucose, increased glycogen resynthesis, higher use of muscle fat stores.

Getting back into ketosis with ketone esters makes a big difference. It helps get me back on track and powers me through my day.

Because ketone esters can provide near-instant ketosis, they can be used to supplement your natural ketone production. Maybe you cycle off keto during the weekends (many people do). That's where exogenous ketones can be so useful — they helps you skip keto flu symptoms by providing the body with exogenous ketones as you ramp back into endogenous ketone production.

How To Determine If A Product Is Keto-Friendly

It can be difficult to decipher whether or not products are keto-friendly. When researching different food products, keep a few things in mind.

1. Look at nutritional labels for ingredients containing hidden carbs, such as sugars or high-fructose corn syrup.
2. Review serving sizes on all products. A relatively small serving size may make a product appear to be low in carbs, when actually it's not.
3. Practice moderation. No matter what foods you enjoy, it can be easy to overeat if you do not practice self-discipline.

By following these few steps, you can determine if a product is keto-friendly and fits into your dietary needs.

Which Keto Products Are Right for You?

No products are a one-size-fits-all when it comes to the ketogenic diet — and thus, your keto needs. The key is trying different products and determining which ones best fit your lifestyle.

A word of caution: don't sacrifice taste for quality. There are numerous keto-friendly products on the market that will make your taste buds happy without breaking ketosis. Find the best products to fit your diet, whether it's food or supplements, to achieve and maintain ketosis.

Limit Sugar

Few ingredients send our blood sugar and insulin on a rollercoaster like sugar. While some may be able to enjoy it in very small amounts, like in one or two squares of dark chocolate, we should otherwise try to eliminate added sugars from our diet.

Why are there so many names for sugar? This is one of the games that food companies play. If food manufacturers call sugar something else, you will be less likely to recognize it and more likely to buy.

Some food manufacturers will even use a couple of different kinds of sugar in a product so it will have less of each kind. That way, they can list the sugary ingredients farther down on the ingredient list, so buyers won't know how much sugar is in there. Tricky, right?

What might sugar be called in the ingredient list on packaged foods?

Sounds like sugar: Barbados sugar, Beet sugar, Brown sugar, Cane sugar, Castor sugar, Coconut sugar, Coconut palm sugar, Confectioner's sugar, Corn Sugar, Date sugar, Demerara sugar, Golden sugar, Granulated sugar, Grape sugar, Icing sugar, Invert sugar, Muscovado sugar, Palm Sugar, Powdered sugar, Raw sugar, Turbinado sugar, Yellow sugar.

Sounds like syrup: Brown rice syrup, Buttered syrup, Carob syrup, Corn syrup, Corn syrup solids, Golden syrup, High fructose corn syrup, High maltose corn syrup, Malt syrup, Refiner's syrup, Rice syrup, Sorghum syrup.

Sounds cryptic: Barley malt, Cane juice, Cane juice crystals, Caramel, Dehydrated cane juice, Evaporated cane juice, Diastatic malt, Florida crystals, HFCS, Malt, Muscovado, Panocha, Rapadura, Scant, Treacle.

Sometimes special sugars (other than sucrose) are listed by their scientific name. And sometimes sugar finds its way into your food as a natural ingredient, like maple syrup. So watch for these possibilities, too:

Sounds like a chemical: Dextran, Dextrose, Diatase, Disaccharides, Ethyl maltol, Fructooligosaccharides, Fructose, Galactose, Glucitol, Glucose, Glucose solids, Isoglucose, Lactose, Levulose, Maltodextrin, Maltose, Saccharose.

Sounds natural: Agave nectar, Blackstrap molasses, Coconut nectar, Dates, Dried Fruit, Fruit juice, Fruit juice concentrate, Honey, Maple syrup, Molasses.

Limit starch

When eating low-carb, limiting or completely avoiding refined starch is key. Wheat and corn are the biggest sources of starch in our food supply, so keep your eye out for those two primary offenders. Some people may be able to do just fine with an occasional starchy vegetable or a small amount of starch in their recipes (i.e. as a stabilizer or thickening agent). Just keep an eye on the carb count and how it makes you feel (even better if you can check your blood glucose).

But if your goal is to avoid starch completely, you need to stay away from all grains and almost all kinds of flour, with the exception of nut flours. And you need to avoid starchy vegetables like beans and tubers, too.

So watch for ingredients like these and keep products made with them out of your cart:

Grains & grain-like seeds: Amaranth, Barley, Buckwheat, Corn, Oats, Millet, Rice, Rye, Quinoa, Sorghum, Teff, Wheat, Wild Rice.

Other names for wheat: Bulgar, Bran, Burghul, Couscous, Durum, Einkorn, Emmer, Farina, Farro, Flour, Graham flour, Kamut, Orzo, Semolina, Spelt, Triticale, Wheat berries, White flour.

Flours, starches, & thickeners: Arrowroot, Cornmeal, Cornstarch, Cassava, Chickpea flour or Gram, Cottonseed, Dal, Fava bean, Inulin, Lentil, Manioc, Modified starch, Powdered cellulose, Potato, Sago, Taro, Soy, Tapioca, Plantain or Banana, Mesquite, Starchy vegetables, Sweet potatoes & yams, Vegetable starch.

Limit industrial fat

All fats are not created equal. Reviewing the ingredient list on products at the supermarket — before you buy — can help you eat more healthy, naturally-occurring fat and avoid or limit industrial oils.

We encourage you to completely avoid artificially produced trans fats, usually listed as "partially hydrogenated" oil or vegetable shortening. These fats are banned in Europe and are in the process of being eliminated from the US food supply due to concerns about their health effects.

In addition, we suggest you minimize margarine and the highly-processed vegetable oils listed below. Unlike olive oil, coconut oil, and nut oils that are pressed and minimally processed, most vegetable oils are produced with high heat, solvents, deodorizers, and bleach.

These oils are high in omega-6 polyunsaturated fatty acids (PUFAs), which are less stable when heated.

Finally, there are concerns that consuming foods very high in omega-6 fatty acids is at odds with our evolutionary diet, potentially leading to negative health effects (though this is controversial).

Although there isn't convincing data to show industrial seed oils are detrimental to our health, the evolutionary and mechanistic concerns are enough for us to recommend mostly sticking to the less processed, more natural oils and fats.

Trans Fats To Avoid:

- Diglycerides
- Hydrogenated anything
- Interesterified oils
- Margarine
- Monoglycerides
- Partially hydrogenated anything
- Shortening
- Vegetable shortening (like Crisco).

Highly Processed Vegetable Oils To Minimize:

- Canola
- Corn
- Cottonseed
- Grapeseed
- Rice bran
- Soybean.

Unfortunately, refined vegetable oils are contained in so many products that you may struggle to find certain items (like salad dressing) that do not contain them. For homemade versions of sauces of all sorts, check out our sauces and dressings recipes — they're really easy and delicious.

Note that for avoiding trans fat, the ingredient list is a better guide than the nutrition facts label. Artificial trans fats may be present in small amounts, up to 0.49 grams per serving, and the nutrition facts label will still show 0 grams trans fat. Small amounts can add up, especially when serving sizes are small, so check the ingredients before assuming a product is trans fat free.

Probably you don't need to worry about the small amounts of naturally occurring trans fats in whole foods like meat and butter. It is the artificial trans fats that we need to avoid.

Minimize sugar replacements

There are three types of very low calorie sugar replacements that you might find in packaged foods: sugar alcohols, artificial sweeteners, and some natural sweeteners. There are pros and cons to each of these additives. I recommend that you minimize or avoid them if possible.

Here are the names of sugar replacements you might see on an ingredient list:

Sugar alcohols: Glycerol, Isomalt, Lactitol, Maltitol, Mannitol, Sorbitol, Erythritol (keto-friendly), Xylitol (keto-friendly).

Artificial sweeteners: Acesulfame, Alitame, Aspartame, Cyclamate, Neotame, Saccharin, Sucralose (keto-friendly).

Conclusion

Before starting any diet, it's important to see a GP, particularly those with health conditions, who are elderly, pregnant, on medication, and who have a high intensity job and rely on mental alertness or physical exertion.

But, whichever diet you start, the main thing is to know the basic principles of staying on this diet. Indeed, without knowing this, it is practically impossible to achieve any significant results or achieve the goals that you have set for yourself and that you are going to achieve through diet.

Now you know:

- Fundamental rules to be on a keto
- Frequent mistakes of beginners and how to avoid them
- Possible difficulties with keto for beginners

Moreover, you know that you should make a concrete nutrition plan, simple examples of keto diet plan, and how many meals should you eat on the keto diet.

Also, you know the best keto products and how to determine if a product is keto-friendly, which keto products are right for you, and a lot more…

You can now move on to the next chapter, where I will tell about keto-specific suggestions – for men, women, children, and sportsmen. There will also be some information on keto for diabetics.

CHAPTER 6.
KETO SPECIFIC

Keto For Women

Is The Keto Diet Effective For Women?

The ketogenic diet shows promise when used therapeutically to improve certain factors of health. Studies have shown that it can be used as a way to reduce body fat and improve blood sugar and even as a complementary treatment for certain cancers.

Although much of the research focuses on how well the keto diet works in men, a decent number of studies have included women or focused exclusively on the effects of the keto diet on women.

Keto And Weight Loss For Women

One of the main reasons why women turn to the keto diet is to lose excess body fat. Some research suggests the keto diet may be an effective way to encourage fat loss in the female population.

Studies have shown that following a keto diet may aid weight loss by increasing fat burning and decreasing calorie intake and hunger-promoting hormones like insulin — all of which may help encourage fat loss.

For example, one study in 45 women with ovarian or endometrial cancer found that women who followed a ketogenic diet for 12 weeks had significantly less total body fat and lost 16% more belly fat than women assigned to a low fat, high fiber diet.

Another study in adults with obesity that included 12 women demonstrated that following a very low calorie ketogenic diet for 14 weeks significantly reduced body fat, decreased food cravings, and improved female sexual function.

Additionally, a review of 13 randomized controlled trials — the gold standard in research — that included a population comprised of 61% women found that participants who followed ketogenic diets lost 2 pounds (0.9 kg) more than those on low fat diets after 1 to 2 years.

Although research supports the use of this very low-carb way of eating to enhance fat loss in the short term, keep in mind that there's currently a lack of studies exploring the long-term effects of the keto diet on weight loss.

Plus, some evidence suggests that the weight-loss-promoting benefits of the keto diet drop off around the 5-month mark, which may be due to its restrictive nature.

What's more, some research shows that less restrictive low carb diets may result in comparable effects and are easier to sustain long-term.

For example, a study that included 52 women found that low and moderate-carb diets that contained 15% and 25% carbs, respectively, reduced body fat and waist circumference over 12 weeks similar to a ketogenic diet that contained 5% carbs. Plus, the higher carb diets were easier for the women to stick to.

Keto and blood sugar control for women

The ketogenic diet typically limits carb intake to less than 10% of total calories. For this reason, the diet is favored by women with high blood sugar, including those with type 2 diabetes.

A 4-month study that included 58 women with obesity and type 2 diabetes found that a very low calorie keto diet caused significantly greater weight loss and reductions in fasting blood sugar and hemoglobin A1c (HbA1c) than a standard low calorie diet. HbA1c is a marker of long-term blood sugar control.

A 2019 case study in a 65-year-old woman with a 26-year history of type 2 diabetes and depression demonstrated that after following a ketogenic diet for 12 weeks, along with psychotherapy and high intensity exercise, her HbA1c dropped out of diabetic range. Her fasting blood sugar and her markers for clinical depression normalized. Essentially, this case study showed that the ketogenic diet reversed this woman's type 2 diabetes.

A study in 25 people that included 15 women showed similar results. After 34 weeks of following a keto diet, approximately 55% of the study population had HbA1c levels below the diabetic level, compared with 0% who followed a low fat diet.

However, it's important to note that currently, studies on the long-term adherence, safety, and efficacy of the ketogenic diet on blood sugar control are lacking.

Plus, many other less restrictive diets, including the Mediterranean diet, have been researched for decades and are well known for their safety and beneficial effects on blood sugar control and overall health.

Keto and cancer treatment for women

The ketogenic diet has been shown to be beneficial when used as a complementary treatment method for certain types of cancer alongside traditional medications.

One study in 45 women with endometrial or ovarian cancer found that following a ketogenic diet increased blood levels of ketone bodies and lowered levels of insulin-like growth factor 1 (IGF-I), a hormone that may promote the spread of cancer cells.

The researchers acknowledged that this change, along with the decrease in blood sugar seen in those following ketogenic diets, creates an inhospitable environment for cancer cells that may suppress their growth and spread.

Plus, research also shows that the ketogenic diet may improve physical function, increase energy levels, and decrease food cravings in women with endometrial and ovarian cancer.

The ketogenic diet has also shown promise when used as a treatment alongside standard treatments like chemotherapy for other cancers that affect women including glioblastoma multiforme, an aggressive cancer that affects the brain.

However, it's important to note that because of the highly restrictive nature of the ketogenic diet and the current lack of high quality research, this diet isn't recommended as a treatment for most cancers.

Keto For Men

Men occupy an interesting place in the health sphere. While there's a disparity — albeit one that's approaching parity — between men and women in the conventional medical literature, in the alternative health world, it's flipped. Women are a "special interest" group, and their specific health issues and special considerations related to diet and exercise receive a lot of attention. Often, it is a way to counteract the conventional imbalance and because women tend to be higher consumers of health information.

Play At The Margins

Historically, anthropologically, and biologically speaking, men can tolerate great variations in environmental intensity. They're usually (not always of course) the ones going to war, performing great feats of physical endurance and strength, willingly subjecting themselves to misery and pain, as well as being more violent and getting into the most trouble. Also, (in general) carrying more muscle mass, secreting more testosterone, and being physically sizeable than the opposite sex. We see this kind of sexual dimorphism play out across most mammals, and there's no reason to think humans are any different.

Most men don't have these extreme situations foisted on anymore, but we still thrive doing them. Try a 2-day fast. Do one meal a day. Eat a 3-pound steak, then no meat at all the next day. Eat a dozen eggs for breakfast (whenever that happens). Try lots of seemingly extreme experiments to see what works. It may be that you thrive doing the occasional intense bout of keto bravado. There is only one way to find out.

Whereas women tend to have a lower tolerance for perturbations in caloric intake for their potential impact on fertility status, men have far more leeway. Take advantage of that.

Be As Strict As Possible Early On

Don't mess around with carb refeeds, pre-workout carbs, or "just one donut hole" until you have a good thing going. Get those fat-burning mitochondria built. Stay strong and stay strict.

Manage Your Stress Levels

This is good general advice for everyone on any diet, but especially for men eating keto.

A big part of traditional masculinity (for better and worse) is stoicism — the ability to soldier on through a difficult situation. This is, on balance, often a good yet misunderstood trait, which gets a bad rap that it doesn't always deserve. Stoicism isn't unfeeling. At its healthiest, it's the ability to address the feelings without being ruled by them. It's feeling grief without letting your life fall to pieces. These are positive ways to respond to life's slings and arrows. But this can lead to a denial of the physiological ramifications of stress and a failure to manage them with anti-stress behaviors.

Keto does not make you impervious to stress. Being a man does not make you impervious to stress. There are still limits to the amount of stress we can tolerate, physiological ones that no one should try to transcend. At those levels, "mind over matter" stops working. Stress will spike cortisol, blunt testosterone, and make all that decidedly non-keto junk food all the more attractive and alluring.

Monitor Your Testosterone Levels

For the most part, going keto tends to improve testosterone levels. Moreover, it reduces body fat. Researchers have known for decades that carrying extra body fat depresses testosterone levels, and that losing the extra fat restores them. In fact, a recent study found that a man's body weight is such a fantastic predictor of low testosterone and poor sexual function that the authors recommend it should be used as a standard biomarker for evaluating testosterone levels. If keto is helping you lose body fat, it's probably improving your T levels.

It increases saturated fat and cholesterol intake. Both nutrients (yes, nutrients) are important building blocks for the production of testosterone. Studies show that low-fat, high-fiber diets lower testosterone in men, while diets higher in saturated fat increase it.

Once the initial exodus of body fat is over, though, you have to be more vigilant. Calories can dip too low. Deficiencies of micronutrients you haven't been thinking about may start to surface. And this can all impact your testosterone levels.

Make sure you're not starving yourself. Men are built to handle and even prosper from acute boluses of extreme caloric restriction or expenditure (fasts, heavy training), but extended bouts can destroy our hormonal profile. Just look at what happens to a seasoned bodybuilder preparing for competition with caloric restriction and intense training — their testosterone tanks and their cortisol shoots up.

Make sure you're getting adequate amounts of the pro-testosterone micronutrients: zinc, vitamin D (either through sun exposure, vitamin D-rich foods like wild salmon, eggs, cod liver oil, or supplementation), saturated fat, cholesterol, magnesium. Using a tool like Cronometer can help you track them and get your diet in order.

Don't Let Keto Take Over

Men tend to obsess over things that interest them. We scour the literature, try to optimize everything, spend every waking moment thinking about how to do something better; in this case, keto. We can get a little iron-willed and myopic if we don't watch ourselves.

Focus is all well and good, but not if it starts impeding your ability to handle other aspects of health that are no less important.

Don't stay up 'til 2 A.M. arguing on keto forums and reading PubMed abstracts. Get your sleep.

Don't become a recluse because none of your friends understand your "weird keto thing." Maintain your social relationships, your community.

Don't stop sprinting because you measured your blood glucose once after a hill session and it spiked. Exercise is equally important.

Keto For People Over 40/50/60

The keto diet has gained in popularity in recent years and has become a nutritional plan favored by individuals of all ages. That said, this dietary roadmap might precipitate particularly important health benefits to persons over age 40,50,60.

Keto Diet Overview

Scientifically classified the ketogenic diet, this nutritional plan stresses the decreased consumption of foods containing carbohydrates and an increased intake of fats. The reduced intake of carbohydrates is said to eventually place the bodies of participating dieters into a biological and metabolic process known as ketosis.

Once ketosis is established, medical researchers opine the body becomes especially efficient in burning fat and turning said substances into energy. Moreover, during this process, the body is thought to metabolize fat into chemicals categorized as ketones, which are also said to provide significant energy sources.

An accelerator of this is an intermittent fasting method where the restricting of carbs causes your body to access the next available energy source or ketones that are derived from stored fat. In this absence of glucose, fat is now burned by the body for energy.

There are a number of other specific ketogenic diets including:

Targeted (TKD): Those participating in this version gradually add small amounts of carbohydrates into their diet.

Cyclical (CKD): Adherents to this dietary plan consume carbohydrates on a cyclical basis like every few days or weeks.

High-Protein: High-protein diet observers consume greater quantities of protein as part of their dietary plans.

Standard (SKD): Typically, this most commonly practiced version of the diet intake significantly diminished concentrations of carbohydrates (perhaps as little as five percent of all dietary consumption), along with protein-laden foods and a high quantity of fat products (in some cases, as much as 75 percent of all dietary needs).

In most cases, the average dieter or someone who is new to the keto diet partakes in the standard or high-protein versions. The cyclical and targeted variations are usually undertaken by professional athletes or persons with very specific dietary requirements.

Recommended Foods

Keto diet adherents are encouraged to consume foods like meat, fatty fishes, dairy products (cheeses, milk, butter and cream), eggs, products possessing low carbohydrate concentrations, condiments (salt, pepper and a host of other spices), various needs and seeds, and oils (olive and coconut).

On the other hand, certain foods should be avoided or strictly limited. Said items include beans and legumes, many fruits, edibles with high sugar contents, alcohol, and grain products.

Keto Diet Benefits To Individuals Over 50

Keto diet adherents, especially those aged 50 and older, are said to enjoy numerous potential health benefits including:

1. Increased Physical And Mental Energy

As people grow older, energy levels might drop for a variety of biological and environmental reasons. Keto diet adherents often witness a boost in strength and vitality. One reasons said occurrence happens is because the body is burning excess fat, which in turn gets synthesized into energy. Furthermore, systemic synthesis of ketones have a tendency to increase brain power and stimulate cognitive functions like focus and memory.

2. Improved Sleep

Individuals tend to sleep less as they age. Keto dieters often gain more from exercise programs and become tired easier. Said occurrence could precipitate longer and more fruitful periods of rest.

3. Metabolism

Aging individuals often experience a slower metabolism than they did during their younger days. Long-time keto dieters experience a greater regulation of blood sugar, which can increase their metabolic rates.

4. Weight Loss

Faster and more efficient metabolism of fat helps the body eliminate accumulated body fat, which could precipitate the shedding of excess pounds. Additionally, adherents are also believed to experience a reduced appetite, which could lead to a diminished caloric intake.

Keeping the weight off is important, especially as adults age. They may need less calories daily compared to when in their 20s or even 30s. Yet, it is still important to get nutrient rich food from this diet for older adults.

Since is common for aging adults to lose muscle and strength, a high protein specific ketogenic diet may be recommended by a nutritionist.

5. Protection Against Specific Illnesses

Keto dieters over age 50 could reduce their risk of developing ailments such as diabetes, mental disorders like Alzheimer's, various cardiovascular maladies, various kinds of cancer, Parkinson's disease, non-alcoholic fatty liver disease (NAFLD), and multiple sclerosis.

6. Aging

Aging is considered by some as the most important risk factor for human illnesses or disease. So, reducing aging is the logical step to minimize these risk factors of disease.

Good news extending from the technical description of the ketosis process presented earlier shows the increased energy of youth as a result. Because of the usage of fat as a fuel source, the body can go through a process where it can misinterpret signs so that the mTOR signal is suppressed, and a lack of glucose is evident. Therefore, it is reported that aging may be slowed down.

Until now, multiple studies have noted that caloric restriction can aid to slowing aging and even increase a lifespan. With the ketogenic diet it is possible to have an effect on anti-aging without reducing carories. An intermittent fasting method used with the keto diet can also have an effect on vascular aging.

When a person fasts intermittently or when on the keto diet, BHB or Beta-hydroxybutyrate is produced, which is believed to induce anti-aging effects.

To be fair, the ketogenic diets, which are very low in carbohydrates and usually high in fats and/or proteins, are used effectively in weight loss during treatment of obesity and cardiovascular diseases. This was reported in the article of US National Library of Medicine National Institutes of Health, called "Effects of Ketogenic Diets on Cardiovascular Risk Factors" in May 2017.

However, an important note in the article was that "Results regarding the impact of such diets on cardiovascular risk factors are controversial" and "Moreover, these diets are not totally safe and can be associated with some adverse events."

Keto For Sportsmen

Ketogenic diets are not just for losing weight. Many endurance athletes also turn to these very low-carb, high-fat diets to boost their performance. But athletes involved in high-intensity, short-duration sports might see drops in performance while on a ketogenic diet, suggests new research.

Researchers from Saint Louis University tested the anaerobic exercise performance of 16 men and women following either a low-carbohydrate ketogenic diet or a high-carbohydrate diet for four days.

People on the ketogenic diet performed more poorly at anaerobic exercise tasks than those eating more carbs. Depending on the task, their performance was 4 to 15 percent lower than the high-carbohydrate group.

The study was published in the Journal of Sports Medicine and Physical Fitness. Its author Edward Weiss, PhD, associate professor of nutrition and dietetics at Saint Louis University, said that the results could make a big difference to athletes involved in sports that depend on short-burst anaerobic activities.

This includes sprint-type activities that occur in soccer and basketball and also short, intense activities like the 100-meter sprint and the triple jump.

Weiss added that the study "probably also applies to many aerobic activities, as other studies have demonstrated that high-intensity aerobic exercise performance may be compromised by low-carb diets — including keto."

In light of these results, he advised athletes to avoid this diets unless they have "compelling reasons for following a low-carb diet." While this is a small study and people were on the two diets for only a few days, a 2017 Trusted Source review of previous research found similar early onset fatigue during short-duration activities while on a ketogenic diet.

Weiss said that additional studies will provide more insight into the pros and cons of ketogenic diets for athletic performance. For now, he suggests that athletes "err on the cautious side."

Carbs or low carbs for energy

Endurance athletes, such as marathon runners and long-distance cyclists, might fare better on a ketogenic diet than players who use short bursts of energy.

Dr. Clifton Page, an assistant professor of orthopaedics and family medicine at the University of Miami Miller School of Medicine, said: "ketogenic diets appear to be beneficial for endurance athletes after a period of adaptation."

Also, he said it can take several months on a ketogenic diet for the body to switch from using carbohydrates as its main energy source to using fats — the "adaptation period."

Zach Bitter, an ultra-marathoner and holder of the 100-mile American record and 12-hour world record, said "fat is always the primary macronutrient in my diet. It can reach as high as 70 percent when I am recovering from a big race or workout."

But this doesn't mean ketogenic diets are high-protein diets

In fact, eating too much protein can interfere with the production of ketones. These ketones are by-products from the breakdown of fats and can be used as an alternative fuel source for the body when there isn't much glucose.

Also, continuing to carb-load — such as with energy drinks and gels — can inhibit the body's switch to using ketones for energy.

"Metabolically, a high-carbohydrate diet locks an athlete into a dependence on glucose as the dominant fuel for exercise," said Jeff Volek, PhD, professor of human sciences and a registered dietitian at The Ohio State University and a leading researcher of carb-restricted diets.

The body stores some glucose for later as glycogen. But Volek has mentioned that the body has only enough glycogen to last about one day, or for just a few hours of hard exercise. So, athletes on a high-carb diet need a steady intake of carbohydrates "to prevent this small carb fuel tank from running dry," he said.

Bitter assured that since he switched to a ketogenic diet, he has been able to cut his in-race fueling by over 50 percent. In addition, he is quick to point out, though, that he doesn't "demonize carbs." But he tends to favor "low-glycemic sources of carbs in my meals when I do have them during peak training."

One diet fits all athletes?

For endurance athletes, long-term use of ketogenic diets may boost not only performance, but also overall health.

"Keto-adaptation has enabled endurance athletes to set course and national records," said Volek. "And a growing number of military personnel are using ketosis to improve physical and cognitive performance and manage obesity, metabolic health, oxygen toxicity symptoms, and post-traumatic stress disorder."

Research — including a recent study by Volek — found that ketogenic diets may reduce body fat, type 2 diabetes, and metabolic syndrome. The last one is a group of conditions that includes high blood sugar and abnormal cholesterol levels.

"More than half of adults have prediabetes or diabetes in the US, including athletes," said Volek. "A well-formulated ketogenic diet reverses the insulin-resistance phenotype more potently than any drug or lifestyle therapy."

Bitter said he was attracted to a ketogenic diet not for the performance boost, but because during his training he would "wake up multiple times a night, experience big energy shifts throughout the day, and would get noticeable swelling in my legs and ankles after big workouts and races."

The ketogenic diet helped with these symptoms.

Not everyone thinks ketogenic diets are for every athlete

"In many cases, you can still perform well at your chosen sport on very few carbs. But you are unlikely to perform at as high a level as you're accustomed to, and you're certainly not likely to perform your best," said Mike Israetel, PhD, head science consultant at Renaissance Periodization.

He added that your recovery after exercise will also be "significantly hampered, which will of course interfere with both performance and rates of improvement from training."

Page warned that research shows that "without long-term adaption to the ketogenic diet, an athlete could experience adverse effects including reduced muscle glycogen, hypoglycemia, and impaired athletic performance."

If you do opt for a ketogenic diet, it's important to follow a plan designed by a nutritionist — or even work directly with someone experienced with these diets.

While a lot of research focuses on the benefits of ketogenic diets for competitive athletes, weekend warriors and others may also benefit.

"Recreational athletes tend to see more consistent benefits from adopting a ketogenic diet," said Volek. "In part because, on average, they have a greater emphasis on weight loss, metabolic, and health benefits."

Keto For Diabetes

Special diets for type 2 diabetes often focus on weight loss, so it might seem crazy that a high-fat diet is an option. The ketogenic (keto) diet, high in fat and low in carbs, can potentially change the way your body stores and uses energy, easing diabetes symptoms.

With this nutrition system, your body converts fat, instead of sugar, into energy. The diet was created in 1924 as a treatment for epilepsy, but the effects of this eating pattern are also being studied for type 2 diabetes.

The ketogenic diet may improve blood glucose (sugar) levels while also reducing the need for insulin. However, the diet does come with risks. Be sure to discuss it with your doctor before making drastic dietary changes.

Understanding "High-Fat" In The Ketogenic Diet

Many people with type 2 diabetes are overweight, so a high-fat diet can seem unhelpful.

The goal of the ketogenic diet is to have the body use fat for energy instead of carbohydrates or glucose. On the keto diet, you get most of your energy from fat, with very little of the diet coming from carbohydrates.

This doesn't mean you should load up on saturated fats, though. Heart-healthy fats are the key to sustaining overall health. Some healthy foods that are commonly eaten in the ketogenic diet include: eggs, fish such as salmon, cottage cheese, avocado, olives and olive oil, nuts and nut butters, seeds.

Effects On Blood Glucose

The ketogenic diet has the potential to decrease blood glucose levels. Managing carbohydrate intake is often recommended for people with type 2 diabetes because carbohydrates turn to sugar and, in large quantities, can cause blood sugar spikes.

However, carb counts should be determined on an individual basis with the help of your doctor. If you already have high blood glucose, eating too many carbs can be dangerous. By switching the focus to fat, some people experience reduced blood sugar.

The Atkins Diet And Diabetes

The Atkins diet is one of the most famous low-carb, high-protein diets that's often associated with the keto diet. However, the two diets have some major differences.

Dr. Robert C. Atkins created the Atkins diet in the 1970s. It's often promoted as a way to lose weight that also controls numerous health issues, including type 2 diabetes.

While cutting excess carbs is a healthy step, it's not clear if this diet alone can help diabetes. Weight loss of any kind is beneficial for diabetes and high blood sugar levels, whether it's from the Atkins diet or another program.

Unlike the keto diet, the Atkins diet doesn't necessarily advocate increased fat consumption. Still, you might increase your fat intake by limiting carbohydrates and eating more animal protein.

The potential drawbacks are similar. Aside from a high saturated fat intake, there's the possibility of low blood sugar, or hypoglycemia, from restricting carbs too much. This is especially true if you take medications that increase insulin levels in the body and don't change your dosage.

Cutting carbs on the Atkins diet can potentially aid weight loss and help you control diabetes symptoms. However, there aren't enough studies to suggest that Atkins and diabetes control go hand-in-hand.

Potential dangers

Changing your body's primary energy source from carbohydrates to fat causes an increase in ketones in the blood. This "dietary ketosis" is different from ketoacidosis, which is an extremely dangerous condition.

When you have too many ketones, you may be at risk for developing diabetic ketoacidosis (DKA). This is most prevalent in type 1 diabetes when blood glucose is too high and can arise from a lack of insulin. Although rare, DKA is possible in type 2 diabetes if ketones are too high. Being ill while on a low-carb diet may also increase your risk for DKA.

If you're on the ketogenic diet, be sure to test blood sugar levels throughout the day to make sure they are within their target range. Also, consider testing ketone levels to make sure you're not at risk for DKA.

The American Diabetes Association recommends testing for ketones if your blood sugar is higher than 240 mg/dL. You can test at home with urine strips.

DKA is a medical emergency. If you're experiencing the symptoms of DKA, see your doctor immediately. Complications can cause diabetic coma.

The warning signs of DKA include: consistently high blood sugar, dry mouth, frequent urination, nausea, breath that has a fruit-like odor, breathing difficulties.

Monitoring Your Diabetes

The ketogenic diet seems straightforward. Unlike a typical low-calorie diet, however, a high-fat diet requires careful monitoring. In fact, you may start the diet in a hospital.

Your doctor needs to monitor both blood glucose and ketone levels to make sure that the diet isn't causing any negative effects. Once your body adjusts to the diet, you may still need to see your doctor once or twice a month for testing and medication adjustments.

Even if your symptoms improve, it's still important to keep up with regular blood glucose monitoring. For type 2 diabetes, testing frequency varies. Be sure to check with your doctor and determine the best testing schedule for your situation.

Research, The Keto Diet, And Diabetes

In 2008, researchers conducted a 24-week study to determine the effects of a low-carbohydrate diet on people with type 2 diabetes and obesity.

At the end of the study, participants who followed the ketogenic diet saw greater improvements in glycemic control and medication reduction compared to those who followed a low-glycemic diet.

A 2013 review reported that a ketogenic diet can lead to more significant improvements in blood sugar control, A1c, weight loss, and discontinued insulin requirements than other diets.

A 2017 study also found the ketogenic diet outperformed a conventional, low-fat diabetes diet over 32 weeks regarding weight loss and A1c.

Other beneficial diets

There's research that supports the ketogenic diet for diabetes management, while other research seems to recommend opposing dietary treatments like a plant-based diet.

A 2017 study found that people with diabetes who followed a plant-based diet experienced significant improvements in blood sugars and A1c, cardiovascular disease risk factors, gut bacteria that is responsible for insulin sensitivity, and inflammatory markers like C-reactive protein.

Outlook

The ketogenic diet may offer hope to people with type 2 diabetes who have difficulty controlling their symptoms. Not only do many people feel better with fewer diabetic symptoms, but they may also be less dependent on medications.

Still, not everyone has success on this diet. Some may find the restrictions too difficult to follow over the long-term.

Yo-yo dieting can be dangerous for diabetes, so you should only start the ketogenic diet if you're sure you can commit to it. A plant-based diet may be more beneficial for you both short and long term. Your dietician and doctor can help you determine the best diet choice for managing your condition.

While you may be tempted to self-treat with a more "natural" route through dietary changes, be sure to discuss the keto diet with your doctor first. The diet may throw off your blood sugar levels, causing further issues, especially if you're on medications for diabetes.

Keto For Children

Why The Keto Diet Is Not Recommended For Children And Teens

The keto diet is not recommended for weight loss in children because it seriously limits carbohydrates, and children need carbs to be mentally and physically active.

Children on a healthy, well-balanced diet should typically eat about 130 grams of carbohydrates a day (approximately 45-65% of their calories), whereas the keto diet limits carbohydrates to approximately 20-30 grams a day.

Foods high in a carbohydrate called fiber help promote feeling full and aid in weight control or weight loss. Fiber found in vegetables, fruits, and whole grains helps maintain steady blood sugars and prevent constipation as well.

"Carbohydrates provide us with energy and important nutrients," explains Fossier. "Children need carbohydrates for growth and development, to do homework, to read books and to go outside and play."

Side Effects Of Keto Diet For Children

When the body goes through ketosis, children (and adults) might feel some initial side effects, including constipation, diarrhea, fatigue, irritability, nausea, vomiting.

"The side effects happen because the body literally thinks it's starving," explains Fossier.

Additionally, the keto diet may affect focus and concentration, cause nutritional deficiencies. Also, it can lead to high levels of cholesterol and triglycerides, weak bones, and kidney stones.

Healthy Weight Loss Options Instead Of Keto For Kids

For children and teens who need to achieve a healthy weight, dietitians from Children's Health recommend establishing healthy habits over specific fad diets. Fossier recommends seven tips:

1. Eat a healthy, well-balanced diet

To provide children with a wide variety of nutritious foods, refer to MyPlate guidelines. "If you make a plate like that at every meal, you're doing a great job," says Fossier. "Whether a child's weight is high or low, at least you know you're providing all the nutrients your child needs to grow and thrive."

2. Limit processed foods and foods with added sugar

These foods include soda, sweetened drinks, cookies, candy, chips, desserts and baked goods.

3. Choose nutritious snacks

Make sure kids are snacking only when truly hungry, and choose healthy options. Encourage small portions that incorporate one or two food groups. For example, try half a peanut butter sandwich on whole grain bread, sliced veggies with hummus or bean dip, or unsweetened yogurt with fruit.

4. Stay positive and give your child the facts

Explain to your child that it's most important to eat the right foods to support healthy growth and maintain energy throughout the day. For example, tell them, "You want to eat fruits and vegetables because they help you concentrate at school, give you energy to play and make you feel better overall."

5. Don't focus on the number on the scale

"Children come in all shapes and sizes. What's important is how our body functions, how we feel, and how healthy a child is," says Fossier.

6. Offer new foods repeatedly

Even if a child didn't like certain nutritious foods a year ago, offer them again. Children's tastes change as they grow.

7. Encourage children and teens to pick an activity they love

Walk, run, ride a bike. If your child likes video games, download a game that requires them to be active. Find a favorite sport. Turn on music and dance. If they enjoy the movement, go for it.

Conclusion

Keto has a number of benefits and many virtues. But everyone will find their own. We've looked at the main features of the keto diet for women, men, kids, and athletes. We examined the features of the diet for people 40/50/60 years old, as well as for diabetics.

The ketogenic diet has been shown to be beneficial when used as a complementary treatment method for certain types of cancer alongside traditional medications. I am very glad if you found this information useful for yourself.

Next, I propose to move on to probably the most interesting chapter of this book, namely keto for weight loss.

CHAPTER 7.
KETO AND WEIGHT LOSS

About Weight Loss With Keto

Weight loss! Wow! But more importantly, how a ketogenic diet will help to achieve that? We shall be having a brief on what exactly brings about weight loss, the more common principles for successful weight loss, and also some useful, actionable tips at the end as well.

Most experts agree that, if nothing else, the keto diet will help you lose weight (and relatively fast). In fact, one study concluded that those on a keto diet can lose up to 2.2 times more weight than those on a calorie-restricted or low-fat diet. During the same study, both triglyceride and HDL cholesterol levels also improved.

While a standard or high-protein keto diet will help you lose weight and theoretically keep you full in the process, that doesn't mean it's critic-proof. On the contrary, some health experts describe keto as nothing more than a fad and a faulty one at that. For starters, strict carb abstinence is very difficult to maintain over extended periods of time. That means you might experience rapid weight loss and then gain the weight back as soon as you relapse.

When your body is in a state where calorie input is lesser than what it needs to function daily, it will seek to get energy from stores of energy within your body. Most of the time, these would be from the stores of glucose found in the liver as well as from your muscle.

The other major energy store located in our body would be the fats that we carry on our frame. It is where the difficulty arises. If your body isn't conditioned for burning fats, it will quickly use up the glucose stores, and that is when the feeling of hunger will come into potentially derail you from your weight loss mission.

Being mindful of hunger

As we said earlier, keeping hunger pangs at bay is one of the most important ways to ensure your weight loss regime is on track.

The other spiffy thing about going on the keto diet is the resultant leveling of your insulin levels. Insulin is known to induce the feeling of hunger, and when ketosis kicks in, you no longer have those roller-coaster ups and downs that are associated with the consumption of carbs and with that stability means your hunger pangs are held mostly at bay due to the reduction of insulin produced by your body.

Now, you will eat when your body truly feels hungry, and that is quite liberating. Not to mention that because of this removal of hunger pangs from the overall equation, your weight loss journey will become much, much more straightforward.

Quicker recovery from exercise

While we engage in strength training in our bid to lose weight and get in shape, our bodies need time to recover from the physical activity. Practitioners of the keto diet will find that their recovery time will be somewhat quicker than of the others.

With the more stable energy levels achieved due to fewer fluctuations in the blood sugar levels, again due to the diet switch, this then allows you to work out without feeling faintish or light-headed. These are typical symptoms of hypoglycemia or just a simple lack of glucose in the bloodstream because you are burning fats and producing ketones as a more stable energy source!

More motivation from quicker results

Quick question, which would you prefer, a weight-loss method that requires you to toil consistently at it for up to six months a pop, and having a loss of four or five pounds to show for it, or a ketogenic diet that can see weight loss come in the range of twenty to thirty pounds within six to seven weeks?

If you are like me, then the choice would be the latter. Quicker results, especially in the area of weight loss, are almost always going to be a welcome morale booster. When you see how much weight you have lost within those short weeks, it gives you that confidence that this method works, and you gain that conviction and strength to keep going.

Low-Carbohydrate Diets Weight Loss

Great weight loss on a low-carb diet is evident because of the fact that carbs hold water in the muscles at a ratio of 1:3. As carb intake decreases then so, too, does water retention. Much water flushes as a result of lack of glycogen to hold water molecules. Moreover, by increasing protein intake, excess nitrogen flushes with even more water since the kidneys use water to dilute the concentration of nitrogen. Once leaving a low-carb diet and the muscles refill with glycogen, fluid concentrations increase and the dieter regains some of the weight.

Low calorie diets of 400-600 calories that consist primarily of protein have the same problems as fasting and low-carbohydrate diets: proteins are used for energy and weight loss comes largely from water. Low-cal diets must be supervised properly by a medical professional and only as a last resort for those who cannot seem to lose weight by other methods. However, even those individuals tend to regain most of their weight back once they return to a balanced diet.

High-Protein Diets for Weight Loss

The use of high-protein diets have intermittently come under immense criticisms from a lot of nutrition experts. Despite these criticisms, the use of these diets have continued to receive a lot of increased interest from weight loss seekers.

High-protein diets are essentially diets in which about 20% or more of the total daily calorie consumption comes from proteins. These diets attempt to reduce the amount of consumed carbohydrate while making increased protein consumption the mainstay of the diet.

However, nutrition experts are of the opinion that although eating a high-protein diet may actually reduce food intake. It's due to the fact that they make people become quickly satiated and for longer while also increasing the thermic effect of food temporarily, the long-term health risks such as kidney problems, bone mineral loss, and other risk factor outweigh the benefits.

Notwithstanding the above, especially the issue of high-protein diets not being really sustainable for long, these diets can, however, become very effective and sustainable diet plans. So, how exactly does a high-protein diet really affect weight loss?

Proteins are fundamentally made from amino acids and for the most part are not stored in the body because the resultant amino acids are metabolized or split apart by enzymes within hours. While the resulting nitrogen is excreted by the kidney in urine, the remaining amino acids are either converted into glucose to be used for energy or stored as glycogen. However, protein is generally regarded as an inefficient source of energy fuel partly due to the fact that it is the hardest and slowest to be metabolized of the three macronutrients.

Naturally, the muscle cells and brain are designed to run exclusively on glucose which is a faster burning energy as it's quite rapidly processed from carbohydrate foods. The brain is also known to consume about 80% of our calories while we are at rest.

High-protein, low-carbohydrate diets, however, result in a significant reduction in available blood glucose causing decreased energy. The low glucose level triggers the release of a hormone called glucagon, which causes two different but interrelated processes (glycogenolysis and lipolysis) to take place.

In response to the low blood sugar level, the pancreas secretes glucagon. It triggers the process of glycogenolysis through signaling cells in the liver and muscle to release glycogen, which is subsequently converted back into glucose for use by the body. Additionally, glucagon triggers the process of lipolysis - the release of fat from fat cells for use as energy fuel.

Glucagon, therefore, has the opposite effect of insulin on blood sugar level. Insulin is known as a store-and-save hormone that removes glucose from the bloodstream for storage as glycogen in liver and muscle cells and as fat in fat cells (adipose tissues). Glucagon, on the other hand, does just the opposite as it causes the release and conversion of stored glycogen back into glucose and also releases stored body fat from fat cells for energy production.

The process of using stored glycogen causes a drastic weight loss occasioned by a major loss of water from body cells. This loss of water is drastic because a stored glycogen molecule is comprised of about 75% water and 25% glucose. Additional body water loss is occasioned by the increased need to flush out nitrogenous wastes resulting from protein metabolism. The combination of both of these processes result in a lot of body water loss.

However, when glycogen stores become significantly depleted, the body is forced to further increase the rate of lipolysis (fat burning) to meet its energy demands. The increased lipolysis leads to a condition known as ketosis - whereby there is an increased accumulation of ketone bodies in the bloodstream due to the increased metabolism (burning) of stored body fat for energy. Forcing the body to get to the point of moving into the secondary stage of lipolysis (ketosis) is actually the ultimate aim of a high-protein, low-carbohydrate diet.

One of the unfortunate side effects of ketosis is the increased build-up of ketone bodies in the bloodstream. Ketones are the by-products of the break down of fat into fatty acids. Although under normal circumstances they are quickly oxidized to water and carbon dioxide, the production of ketones in a state of ketosis is much higher than the rate at which they are capable of being oxidized by body tissues. This consequently leads to acidosis - a state of abnormal increase in blood acidity. In order to effectively rid itself of the accumulated ketones in the blood, the body subsequently increases its urinary output leading to further body water loss.

Therefore, the use of a high-protein and low-carbohydrate diet results in a significant loss of body water through at least three mechanisms which include the: release and conversion of glycogen into glucose; flushing out of nitrogenous wastes resulting from protein metabolism; and flushing out of ketones from the body.

Besides the above body water loss effects, which normally occur during the first phase of about two weeks of using a high-protein, low-carbohydrate diet, there are other weight loss effects, which can be caused by increased protein intake. These diets have the ability to cause early satiety thereby making people eat less while staying fuller for much longer time. Also, the high thermic effect of protein-containing foods plays another significant part.

The thermic effect of foods refers to the number of daily calories that is utilized in eating, digesting, and absorbing food. This energy accounts for about 10% of all our daily calorie expenditure. However, about 20-30% of the calories derived from protein-containing foods are used up in metabolizing them compared to the 6-8% and 2-3% used for carbohydrates and fats, respectively. Therefore, proteins do not just make you feel fuller but it is equally harder to metabolize and therefore burns more calories.

Nevertheless, the real weight loss effect of using a high-protein, low-carbohydrate diet comes from the effect of the induced state of ketosis. The increased fat burning experienced in this condition causes one of the most significant and rapid weight loss effect possible.

Most high-protein and low-carbohydrate diets start with very low amounts of carbohydrate intake aimed primarily at inducing the state of ketosis during the initial phase of the diet. However, subsequent phases, which can be up to three or more, allow the dieter to gradually start increasing the amount of consumed carbohydrate until he or she achieves his or her weight loss goal and neither loses nor adds weight.

The major drawback of most low-carbohydrate diets has always been the reported issue of them not being sustainable due to the reduced energy levels a lot of people experience. This can, however, be overcome by following through with the prescribed phases or stages of the diet and modifying the final phases to achieve and maintain your desired bodyweight.

Foods You Can Eat on a Ketogenic Diet for Weight Loss

While on a ketogenic diet, it is very important to ensure that one eats within the restrictions of the diet. This is vital so as for the individual to be able to remain in a state of ketosis.

Going out of ketosis can be as simple as eating one or two meals that are not recommended on the diet.

However, coming back into ketosis is another different story entirely. This can often takes days or weeks depending on how strict you become when you get back on the diet.

Meals in a ketogenic diet comprise of three basic food types. These are:

- Berries or vegetables
- Protein-rich food
- Fat source.

Fats

Ketogenic diets by nature involve the consumption of increased amounts of fats in the diet. They can come in as part of the cooking process or as sauces and dressings.

The best types of fats are those medium-chain triglycerides (MCTs). These include both MCT oil and coconut oil. Medium-chain triglycerides are easily metabolized to produce ketones. Some other equally good fats for ketosis include:

- Omega-3 and Omega-6 fatty acids
- Salmon, Shellfish, Trout, Tuna
- Monounsaturated and Saturated fats
- Olive oil, Avocado, Butter, Cheese, Red palm oil, Egg yolks
- Non-hydrogenated oils (when cooking)
- Coconut oil, Beef tallow, Non-hydrogenated lards
- High oleic
- Sunflower oils.

Other fat sources:

Chicken skin, Coconut butter, Peanut butter, Fat on meats.

Proteins

When buying your protein foods, always try to choose grass-fed, organic, and humanely raised meat and wild-caught seafood. Apart from offering more nutrients, they have not been exposed to added hormones, antibiotics, and other potential toxins.

Meat

The ketogenic diet accepts basically any type of meat. There is no discrimination about the type of cut or preparation.

Beef, Goat, Lamb, Pork, Veal, Venison.

Poultry

Any type of poultry is also allowed by the diet. You can improve the content of the meal by leaving the skin on. However, breading and batter should not be used in the preparation of poultry as they are usually high in carbohydrates. Other than that, you can prepare your poultry to your liking.

Chicken, Duck, Game hen, Goose, Ostrich, Partridge, Pheasant, Quail, Squab, Turkey.

Seafood

Another great source of protein is seafood. Seafood is a great source of omega-3 fatty acids. They also have high amounts of minerals and vitamins to help keep you well-nourished and healthy.

Clams, Crab, Lobster, Mussels, Oysters, Prawns, Scallops, Shrimp, Snails.

Fish

Fish have good amounts of omega-3 fatty acids. You should go for fish that are caught in the wild and also in mercury-free areas.

Ahi, Catfish, Cod, Flounder, Halibut, Herring, Lobster, Mackerel, Mahi mahi, Mussel, Salmon, Sardines, Scallops, Snapper, Squid, Swordfish, Trout, Tuna, Walleye.

Carbohydrates

Vegetables are the primary source of carbohydrate on a ketogenic diet. When you are buying them, always opt for the organically grown ones. Also, the dark leafy vegetables contain the least amount of carbohydrates with good nutritional value.

Arugula, Asparagus, Bok choy, Broccoli, Cabbage, Cauliflower, Celery, Collard greens, Endive, Garlic, Kale, Kelp, Lettuce, Mushrooms, Onions, Peppers, Radishes, Seaweed, Spinach, Swiss chard, Watercress.

Milk and Dairy Products

These are very essential in a ketogenic diet. Grass-fed and organic source are more preferable. The full fat variety is better suited for the ketogenic diet than the fat-free and low-fat verities.

Butter, Cheddar, Crème fraîche, Heavy cream, Mozzarella, Sour cream, Cream cheese, Mascarpone cheese, Cheeses, Hard cheeses.

Nuts

Moderate amounts of nuts and seed are allowed on the ketogenic diet. Nuts and seed are rich in protein, fats, and carbohydrates. The total nutrients content of the nut varieties should be checked and added to the total daily calorie calculation.

Roasted nuts and seeds are the best. Anything that may cause harm or interfere with ketosis in the body has been removed from them through the roasting process. Nuts should be used mostly as a snack.

Almonds, Macadamia, and Walnuts are some of the best.

Some nuts have high content of omega-6 fatty acid, which can cause inflammation in the body. However, they can hold some people back from their goals. If your weight loss is purely your purpose of using the ketogenic diet, then it would be advisable to remove nuts and seeds to improve your results.

Almonds, Brazil nuts, Hazelnuts, Pine nuts, Macadamia nuts, Pecans, Pili nuts, Pumpkin seeds, Sesame seeds, Sunflower seeds, Walnuts.

Herbs and Spices

After some time on the ketogenic diet, the foods may start to become boring. However, adding spices to your meals can help to spice things up. You can add fresh and dry spices to your meals and even beverages so that they become more enticing and exciting to the palate.

Spices and fresh herbs are some of the most nutrient-dense foods on the planet you can eat. Adding condiments to your meal doesn't only add more flavors to the meals but also offer a lot of various health benefits to your body.

Spices contain carbohydrates thus you should ensure to add them to your daily carbohydrate count. Also, endeavor to check the labels of pre-made spice mixes for their accurate carbohydrate content as they usually contain added sugars.

Salt also enhances flavors. It is best you chose high quality sea salt instead of traditional table salt. Unprocessed salts such as Celtic or Himalayan sea salt provide you with more than eight trace minerals that your body need to perform optimally.

Anise, Annatto, Basil, Bay leaf, Black pepper, Caraway Cardamom, Cayenne pepper, Celery seed, Chervil, Chili pepper, Chives, Cilantro, Cinnamon, Cloves, Coriander, Cumin, Curry, Dill, Fenugreek, Galangal, Garlic, Ginger, Lemongrass, Licorice, Mace, Marjoram, Mint, Mustard seeds, Oregano, Paprika, Parsley, Peppermint, Rosemary, Saffron, Sage, Spearmint, Star anise, Tarragon, Thyme, Turmeric, Vanilla beans.

Sweeteners

Adding keto-friendly sweeteners to your meals can help in curbing cravings for carbohydrates and sweets. Sweeteners help a lot of people to be able to adhere to the ketogenic diet. However, natural sweeteners, such as honey, maple syrup, and agave raise blood sugar levels. It does not only cause inflammation, but can also kick you out of ketosis.

Always go for the liquid form of sweeteners as they do not have binders like dextrose and maltodextrin. Dextrose is an anti-caking agent and is a form of sugar. Maltodextrin, on the other hand, is a bulking agent which has higher glycemic index than table sugar.

The following is a list of recommended sweeteners which have little effect on blood sugar:

Stevia, Liquid Stevia, Erythritol, Allulose, Monk fruit, Sucralose, Xylitol.

Beverages

Using a low carbohydrate diet like the ketogenic diet has a diuretic effect on the body. Carbohydrates draw water to them, which causes water retention in the body. However, the reduced carbohydrate intake in a ketogenic diet leads to a lot water loss as less water is retained in the body and more is excreted.

This diuretic effect can easily lead to dehydration. Therefore, you need to drink a lot of water - well above the recommended intake of 8 glasses - when you are on a ketogenic diet. This will help you to reduce the risk of bladder pain and urinary tract infections.

Besides water, you can add other types of beverages like coffee and teas to help keep your hydrated throughout the day. Both of these do not significantly affect the ketosis state.

However, the added substances like sugar and milk might affect the ketosis state. As a result, it would be best to avoid the sugar completely and use either full cream or keto-friendly sweeteners together with your coffee or tea.

Another way to increase your beverage intake is to make vegetable juice by combining varieties of the approved vegetable types. You can also use a power smoothies or protein shakes instead of a fruit smoothies as the fruits contain sugars (fructose) that can kick you out of ketosis.

Below are some additional beverages you can consume to help keep you hydrated:

Unsweetened almond milk, Unsweetened coconut milk, Unsweetened hemp milk, Green tea, Herbal tea, Organic caffè Americano (espresso with water), Mineral water.

Using another approach: keto with intermitting fasting

The keto diet and intermittent fasting are two of the hottest current health trends. Many health-conscious people use these methods to drop weight and control certain health conditions.

While both have solid research backing their purported benefits, many people wonder if it's safe and effective to combine the two.

What Is Intermittent Fasting?

It is an eating method that cycles between calorie restriction — or fasting — and normal food consumption during a specific time period. There are many different types of intermittent fasting routines, including the 5:2 method, the warrior diet and alternate-day fasting.

Perhaps the most popular kind of intermittent fasting is the 16/8 method, which involves eating during an eight-hour timeframe before fasting for 16.

Intermittent fasting is mainly used as a weight loss technique. However, studies found that it may benefit health in many other ways. For example, intermittent fasting has been shown to reduce inflammation and improve brain function and blood sugar control.

Potential Benefits of Practicing Both

If you commit to the ketogenic diet while at the same time doing intermittent fasting, it could offer the following benefits:

1. May smooth your path to ketosis

Intermittent fasting may help your body reach ketosis quicker than the keto diet alone. That's because your body, when fasting, maintains its energy balance by shifting its fuel source from carbs to fats — the exact premise of the keto diet.

During fasting, insulin levels and glycogen stores decrease, leading your body to naturally start burning fat for fuel.

For anyone who struggles to reach ketosis while on a keto diet, adding intermittent fasting may effectively jumpstart your process.

2. May lead to more fat loss

Combining the diet and the fast may help you burn more fat than the diet alone. Because intermittent fasting boosts metabolism by promoting thermogenesis, or heat production, your body may start utilizing stubborn fat stores.

Several studies reveal that intermittent fasting can powerfully and safely drop excess body fat. In an eight-week study in 34 resistance-trained men, those who practiced the 16/8 method of intermittent fasting lost nearly 14% more body fat than those following a normal eating pattern.

Similarly, a review of 28 studies noted that people who used intermittent fasting lost an average of 7.3 pounds (3.3 kg) more fat mass than those following very low-calorie diets. Plus, intermittent fasting may preserve muscle mass during weight loss and improve energy levels, which may be helpful for keto dieters looking to improve athletic performance and drop body fat.

Additionally, studies underscore that intermittent fasting can reduce hunger and promote feelings of fullness, which may aid weight loss.

Should You Combine Them?

Combining the ketogenic diet with intermittent fasting is likely safe for most people. However, pregnant or breastfeeding women and those with a history of disordered eating should avoid intermittent fasting. People with certain health conditions, such as diabetes or heart disease, should consult with a doctor before trying intermittent fasting on the keto diet.

Though some people may find merging the practices helpful, it's important to note that it may not work for everyone. Some people may find that fasting on the keto diet is too difficult, or they may experience adverse reactions, such as overeating on non-fasting days, irritability, and fatigue.

Keep in mind that intermittent fasting is not necessary to reach ketosis, even though it can be used as a tool to do so quickly. Simply following a healthy, well-rounded keto diet is enough for anyone looking to improve health by cutting down on carbs.

Other information for weight loss with keto

The Side Effects of Using a Ketogenic Diet for Weight Loss

The ketogenic diet, colloquially called the keto diet, is a popular diet containing high amounts of fats, adequate protein and low carbohydrate. It is also referred to as a low carb-high fat (LCHF) diet and a low carbohydrate diet.

Ketogenic diets are designed to force the body to enter into a state called ketosis. The body generally makes use of carbohydrate as its primary source of energy. This owes to the fact that carbohydrates are the easiest for the body to absorb. However, should the body run out of carbohydrates, it reverts to making use of fats and protein for its energy production.

Ketosis effectively alters your body's natural equation from burning glucose to rather start burning fat as fuel. This alteration of the body's metabolism may come with some possible side effects as the body tries to adjust it functioning.

Changing to the ketogenic diet is not that easy to adapt to especially at the initial onset. However, remember that these side effects are temporary. Some of them can last for a few days while other can last for months.

Therefore, you need to give yourself time, both physically and mentally, to effectively make the switch. While making the switch to a ketogenic diet, there are two physical changes that you may experience. These are the keto flu (we have talked about it before) and keto breath.

Keto Breath

There are two possible reasons put forth why people on ketogenic diets experience this peculiar breath issue. The body does not store ketones and thus they must be excreted from the body. Ketones can be excreted through the urine as acetoacetate.

They can also be excreted through the breath in form of acetone. So, the more ketones you produce, the more acetone you pass out through your breath. Unfortunately, this can cause unpleasant-smelling breath when using a ketogenic diet.

On the other hand, increased protein ingestion can also cause keto breath. This is because the way the body digest fats and proteins is quite different. The digestion of proteins usually produces ammonia which the body excretes through the urine.

However, the increased consumption of proteins may result in the indigestible amounts remaining in your gut system and undergoes fermentation. This produces ammonia which is subsequently released through your breath.

Keto breath can last for about a week to just under a month. It mostly depends on how well your body adapts to ketosis.

Micronutrient Deficiencies

This may result from the strict restrictions on carbohydrate intake. A lot of carbohydrate-rich foods are equally rich in vitamins and minerals.

The severe restriction on carbohydrate intake may therefore cause deficiencies in some essential nutrients. Therefore, we should not only be focused on the micronutrient counting in terms of fat, proteins, and carbohydrates but should also remember the vitamin and mineral micronutrient contents as well.

This is often why supplements are mostly recommended when using a ketogenic diet. Supplementation will help to augment any micronutrient imbalance that might occur when using a ketogenic diet.

Most Important Principles For Weight Loss

A lot of people think that an all-meat diet is very appealing but remember that the ketogenic diet does not work this way. It is crucial that you watch what you put into your plate so that your body can maintain ketosis. But while knowing how much fat, protein, and carbs is essential, it is not enough to promote healthy weight loss. Thus, here are top tips on how to lose as much weight while following the ketogenic diet within the shortest possible time.

Weigh Your Every Food

Being accurate about your macros is very crucial to the success of the ketogenic diet. Make sure that you invest in the right food scale so that you can monitor your macro intake. So, avoid the guesswork and use a scale to measure your food. If you can, buy scales that you can connect to apps and websites.

To help with the process of losing the unwelcome weight from your body, here are some of the more common principles which are useful to base your weight loss strategies on.

Keep Hunger At Bay

Many folks start off on dieting to lose their excess weight and attempt to get healthy, but quite a number fail and fall by the wayside. In the end, these folks have to resort to medications and drugs to suppress the symptoms and conditions that accompany obesity. It is not a pretty sight, and it sometimes is quite depressing to see people consign themselves to such a fate when more efficient and healthier solutions are just around the corner.

They may have started strong and see results after some time, but invariably, the one thing that always put paid to these efforts would be the feeling of hunger that many of these diets entail. Take a straight calorie restriction diet plan. For example, if your daily requirement works out to be about 1,750 calories, just polishing off a bagel for a snack would set you back by 250 calories. That is like one-seventh of your total requirement. Imagine eating seven bagels for the whole day, would that be enough?

The trick, of course, is to get onto a diet and lifestyle change where you can feel full and keep the hunger pangs at bay and yet get your body to lose weight. Know of any diet that does just that?

Be Sustainable All The Time

There are many ways to lose weight, that is for sure. Getting on the latest fad diet, juicing, fasting, going the vegan way.

Fasting, for example, is an excellent way to let the body rebalance itself and to get rid of toxins that have built up over time. One of the side effects of fasting would be a loss of body weight. Not expect that a person to fast for a lifetime, without any consumption of food. For any method of efficient weight loss, it must be sustainable in practice to allow for continued shedding of the excess pounds and also to prevent the dreaded bounce back in weight that has plagued so many.

One of the benchmarks of sustainability for diets would be the ease of implementing it in everyday life. Imagine if you are on a diet that requires you to eat six to seven small meals a day, you would have to pack for those meals and also find the time to consume them during the workday.

Exercises

One of the essential principles for weight loss, exercise, especially strength training, can help to build muscles that burn more calories, not to mention getting you that ripped figure. Yes, it was always good to dream that there was some magic pill in the market that could get you whipped into shape without any effort, but alas, it remains a dream.

Strength training, done through weights at home or by hitting the gym, is one of the surest ways that weight can be lost. Better to have a schedule for the days that your workout to concentrate on specific muscle groups. This targeted training helps to speed muscle development, leading to higher calorie usage and hence weight loss.

There will be loads of resources online on how to work out a proper strength training routine. The most important thing is to have the discipline to keep plugging at it until you see or feel the results. It will be worth it.

Reduce Your Stress

Stress can affect your hormone levels by causing your blood sugar level to rise, thus increasing your cravings. Have you ever noticed why you often crave sweets when you are stressed out? That's your hormone talking. While you cannot control the stress that comes your way, find ways on how to mitigate it. You can practice yoga, mindfulness, and breathing exercises to take away your stress.

Choose Quality Carbs

Some of you may say that carb is carb no matter what form they exist in. Remember, not all carbs are created equally. Some carbs are nutrient-rich and are found in non-starchy vegetables and some fruits. So, when making a meal plan, make sure that you use good quality carbs.

Stay Away from Diet Soda

Just because it comes with the word "diet" with it does not mean that it is right for you. Diet soda uses a wide variety of sugar substitutes that tells your body that is has an overload of sugar, thereby shutting the metabolism down. So, if you need to quench your thirst, drink sparkling water instead.

Get Enough Sleep

If you lose weight (fast), sleeping is crucial and necessary. Remember that the lack of sleep causes stress to the body. Stress, as I have discussed earlier, can affect the hormone levels in your body, thus increasing your cravings to snack on food frequently. So, make sure that you get at least 6 to 8 hours of sleep daily.

Be Attentive With Sport

What is healthier and more effective for getting rid of excess weight: the keto diet or intensive exercise in conjunction with the usual high-carbohydrate diet? One group for ten weeks followed the keto diet: its participants consumed no more than 30 grams of carbohydrates per day, without doing any physical exercise.

Participants in the second group followed the so-called "standard American diet," i.e., They ate the high-carbohydrate food habitual for themselves, also without doing any physical exercise.

And in the third group, participants ate ordinary high-carb foods, doing sports for 30 minutes 3-5 times a week.

Researchers measured some indicators of participants at the beginning and end of the research, incl. body mass index, triglyceride level in the blood, a percentage of fatty tissues, glycated hemoglobin level (HgA1c), and ketone level in the blood.

Participants in the group following ketogenic low-carbohydrate diet were in diet ketosis - i.e., in a state where the primary source of energy for the body is not glucose, but unique molecules - ketones, produced by the liver from fat.

The results of analyzes showed that, as might be expected, sports or physical activities are useful but not enough to neutralize the negative consequences of malnutrition and reverse metabolic syndrome. However, following the ketogenic diet led to the most significant improvement in almost all indicators of metabolic health and weight loss.

Also, the members of the keto group significantly increased the level of basal metabolism (speed), in which the body "burns" fat at resting state - more than ten times compared with two groups of "standard" nutrition.

The authors of the research stated, "Physiological ketosis has the clinical capabilities to prevent, weaken and heal the metabolic syndrome and the obesity, prediabetes, and diabetes that it causes, and is, therefore, a worthy alternative treatment."

Conclusion

Indeed, the all-meat diet is very interesting. After all, it helps to lose a lot of weight over short distances. But now you know and will understand that the ketogenic diet does not work that way. It is critical to keep track of what you put on your plate so that your body can maintain ketosis.

You already know how much fat, protein, and carbohydrates you need to eat on a keto diet, and that it's not enough for healthy weight loss.

Remember the basic principles: weigh each meal; keep hunger at bay; always be steady; do exercise, but be careful in sports; reduce stress; choose quality carbohydrates; stay away from diet sodas; get enough sleep.

We now know pretty much everything about losing weight with the keto diet:

- Basic principles and laws
- Using other methods
- An extended list of what you can and cannot eat
- Other useful information.

I am sure that this will help you, as it helped me in due time. Remember - the main thing is practice, belief in success. And if you make mistakes, then don't give up. You will definitely succeed.

But the next chapter will help you to avoid the main mistakes in the keto diet, in which we will discuss the main ones.

CHAPTER 8.
KETO MISTAKES AND HOW TO AVOID THEM

Fear of Eating Too Much Fat

People often not eat enough fat when they start keto because our society has been conditioned to believe that fats will make you fat.

Since you're limiting carb intake on keto, it's important that you're replacing those calories with calories from fats. If you aren't getting enough calories, it can impair your hormone function and metabolism in the long term. You'll also feel more lethargic because you aren't providing your body enough micro and macronutrients.

In addition, your body needs increased dietary fat to prime your metabolism to burn fats as a main source of energy, also known as ketosis. If you're a beginner to keto, you'll need to consume more fats than experienced keto-ers as this will help your body get used to using ketones as a new fuel source.

Not Eating the RIGHT Fats

Eating enough fats is half the battle. The other half is eating the heathy types. Fats are not created equal, and because fats are the foundation of the ketogenic diet, it's crucial that you're consuming the right fat sources.

Healthy fats to eat on keto include:

- Animal fats, preferably from pastured or grass-fed animals
- Olive oil
- Monounsaturated fats, like from avocado
- Coconut oil.

Avoid these unhealthy fats: Cotton seed oil, Grapeseed oil, Safflower oil, Margarine, Canola oil, Processed vegetable oils, Any trans fats.

Not Drinking Enough Water

Staying hydrated should be a top priority no matter what diet you are following. But when your body is adjusting to burning fats for fuel, water intake should be increased. This is because carbohydrates are responsible for storing water in the body. When you limit your carb intake, water is excreted along with electrolytes, which means they must be replenished.

The general rule of thumb is to drink 0.5 oz to 1 oz of water per pound of bodyweight. Others like to gauge their hydration levels by urine color. If it's a darker yellow, drink more water. If it's clear, you're in the clear.

Not Consuming Enough Sodium

Sodium is excreted along with water when your body is running on ketones for energy.

If you don't replace your sodium on keto, you may fall victim to the dreaded keto flu, which is the main cause of not replacing your electrolytes. To prevent this, increase your sodium intake by salting every meal, adding pink Himalayan sea salt to your water, and sipping on it throughout the day, as well as drinking broth from bouillon cubes.

Too Much Dairy

While dairy may seem like the perfect low-carb and high-fat food source, it can be extremely easy to overeat. If you aren't tracking the amount of dairy you consume, you may end up going over your calorie goal for the day.

In addition, dairy contains a certain type of protein that can lead to unwanted insulin spikes. When this happens, you may get kicked out of ketosis. To add fuel to the fire, many dairy products also contain sugar, so it's important to always check the nutrition label when purchasing dairy products.

Too Much Snacking

If you're following a properly formulated ketogenic diet, you shouldn't have to snack. The keto diet has satiating effects, which means that if you're in ketosis, your cravings for snacks should be nonexistent. We suggest incorporating intermittent fasting into your keto diet, as this can provide a synergistic effect.

Too much snacking has a tendency to increase your blood sugar levels, which can knock you out of ketosis. If you feel the need to snack, it usually means your meals weren't nutritious enough, and you may need to increase your meal size to get enough calories in throughout the day.

Having Cheat Meals

A part of you might be telling yourself to go and grab a burger after a week of dieting because you deserve a reward. But let me tell you that having a cheat day can kick your body out of ketosis, which is something that you worked hard for in such a long time. It is a counterproductive move for your diet.

Not Sleeping Enough

If you aren't getting enough sleep, your body can't repair itself fully, which prevents you from functioning optimally. Lack of sleep has been shown to increase sugar cravings and stress levels, which directly affect ketone production.

Try getting at least seven to eight hours of sleep every night. Limit screen use one to two hours before bed so that your body can perform at its best.

Worrying Too Much About the Scale

Although the ketogenic diet is known for its tremendous weight loss benefits, the scale doesn't always depict an accurate reading.

When you first start keto, you'll experience water weight loss during the first few days. But once your body has adjusted to this new way of eating, it will retain some water.

Checking your weight multiple times a day will only discourage you from sticking with the ketogenic diet because weights naturally fluctuate.

A better metric to measure is your overall body composition and body fat levels. If you're slowly gaining muscle and losing body fat over time, then you're on the right track, even if your scale says otherwise.

Consuming Too Much Protein

You need to keep in mind: the primary goal of a low-carb ketogenic diet is to consume healthy fat and not protein, as we all know that protein is a crucial macronutrient that can improve satiety while increasing fat burning. With this belief, more protein should lead to weight loss and drastically enhance your body composition. Still, the problem is that low-carb dieters, who consume lean animal proteins, will end up overeating it.

When you eat more protein than your body needs, your body will convert the excess into glucose, and this will prevent your body from getting into the "ketosis" phase. Your body will not burn sufficient fat to cause you to lose weight until it enters the ketosis phase. Thus you need to limit your protein consumption to 15% or less of your total diet. An ideal formulated ketogenic diet should be low-carb with high-fat and moderate-protein.

Consuming More Carbs Than Recommended Levels

Some people don't stick with the recommended <5% carb for the ketogenic diet. Some may be confused at what exactly constitutes a low-carb diet by estimating that anything less than 150g of carb a day is "low-carb." There may be no problem if you get 150g of carbs a day from unprocessed carbohydrate foods. Still, quick drinks, such as carbonated soft drinks and ripe fruits, can sharply increase your carb intake, causing you to take more than necessary. This can lead to an increase in blood glucose, with a resultant effect of an increase in insulin levels.

Not Being Patient

Low-carb ketogenic diet is not a "quick" weight loss program that will make you lose fat immediately. It takes some dedication and consistency to make it work for you. People often get into stumbling blocks when they expect too much within a short period. There is one thing you need to understand about ketogenic diets. First, your body was designed to preferentially burn carbs instead of fat, especially when carbs are available. So, if you always make carbs available, that is what your body will burn. If you drastically reduce your carb intake, your body will automatically shift to another source of energy — in most cases, fats. The fat your body breaks down must come either from your diet or from the stored fats in your body.

Full adaptation of the body to low-carb ketogenic diet may take between a few days to weeks, but it will eventually yield results once your body has shifted focus to burning fat. You need to be patient to reap the full benefits of this nutrition system.

Eating Too Many Nuts

While nuts are great snacks for keto dieters, too many of them will kick you out of ketosis. Nuts contain high amounts of calories. For instance, 100 grams of almonds are equivalent to 700 kcal, and more than 70 grams of fat is too much for people who want to lose weight. That doesn't mean that you have to avoid consumption of nuts entirely. What you can do is to reduce your total intake to a few grams.

Eating Products that Are Labeled "Low-Carb"

It is effortless to be deceived, especially if the product comes with the label "low-carb." The thing is that products that are labeled as such contain a lot of additives that are not good for health.

Not Planning Your Meals

Not planning your diet can easily kick you out of ketosis. Planning your meals is helpful so that you avoid excessive snacking or getting involved in binging accidents. While it is impractical to keep track of your diet forever, you can do meal prepping so that it omits the need for you to eat anything randomly.

Not Getting Enough Exercise

Not getting enough exercise is counterproductive for the keto diet. Choose the right type of activity, depending on your goals. For you to reap the most health benefits of exercise, you can do light cardio exercises as it is suitable for both the mind and heart. Doing weight training and high-intensity workout can also build your muscles. On the other hand, post-workout nutrition is also critical to help you succeed with the ketogenic diet. Make sure that you avoid eating foods that are high in fat while exercising.

Not Dealing with Stress

Stress can affect your weight loss because it increases your cortisol levels. Due to the production of this hormone, the mechanism of fat burning in your body is disrupted; it also increases your cravings for sugary foods. There are many ways for you to deal with stress, and these include exercising, music therapy, or taking in supplements.

Conclusion

I'm sure that now you will eat only the right fats, drink enough water, consume enough sodium, plan your meals, be patient, and sleep enough.

Also, I'm sure that you will not eat too much dairy, too many snacks, too many nuts, and eat "low-carb" products.

I tried to point out here the most basic errors that I encountered myself - mistakes that prevent you from achieving results on a keto diet. Or those mistakes that you make, but think that this is absolutely normal.

Unfortunately, I cannot include every possible error here, but there is a reason for that. Many people learn only through practice, and each person can solve their own difficulties.

Now let's move on to the next, equally interesting chapter, in which I will talk about all kinds of tips and tricks of being on a keto diet.

CHAPTER 9.
KETO TIPS AND TRICKS

Keto On A Budget

The very low-carb, high-fat ketogenic diet has become increasingly popular, mainly as a tool to lose weight.

Following a keto diet involves limiting carbs to fewer than 50 grams per day and increasing your fat intake. As a result, the diet tends to be high in animal products, fats, and other low-carb foods like avocado and coconut.

These foods can be expensive, especially for individuals with a limited grocery budget. Still, there are ways to follow a keto diet in an affordable way.

Most meals on a keto diet consist of low-carb proteins, such as meat or eggs, oils, non-starchy vegetables, and high fat foods, such as avocados, coconut, or nuts.

Here are some tips for stocking up on these keto meal components when money is tight:

Buy in bulk. Purchasing foods in bulk can help you cut down on expenses. Things like nuts, seeds, and shredded coconut can be found in bulk containers at most stores. Cooking oils can be purchased online or at a discount store in large quantities.

Look for sales and stock up. If you have room in your freezer, stock up on meats, vegetables, and even avocados (you can freeze the flesh) when they're on sale. You can also take advantage of nonperishable goods like nuts, seeds, and oils at a discounted price and store them in your pantry.

Buy vegetables that are in season. Seasonal vegetables, as well as locally grown ones, tend to be less expensive than veggies that are out of season. Plan your meals around when certain non-starchy veggies are in season.

Go for frozen over fresh. Most frozen fruits and vegetables, like keto-friendly berries, cauliflower, and broccoli, are more affordable than their fresh counterparts. Plus, they last longer, so you don't have to worry about wasting money on produce that spoils if not eaten quickly.

Start a meal plan and prep routine. Making a plan for your meals before you head to the store can help you avoid unnecessary purchases. What's more, prepping a few meals or foods like boiled eggs and shredded chicken ahead of time will help you stick to your plan throughout the week and prevent expensive take-out orders.

Opt for cheaper proteins. Eggs are an incredibly affordable, keto-friendly food that you can use in a variety of meals to cut back on food costs. You can also save money by buying cooked whole chickens and using or freezing all parts. Get cheaper cuts of meat like pork, beef sirloin, ground chuck, and chicken thighs.

Skip the packaged keto-friendly foods. Keto ice creams and snack foods may sound tempting, but their price points can add up. Instead of stocking up on these foods, get your whole foods first and reserve these fancier options as a treat.

Keto Grocery List On A Budget

The following grocery list includes keto-friendly foods that won't break the bank.

Meats/proteins: eggs, canned tuna, whole chickens, chicken thighs, pork chops, frozen ground meats, discounted fresh meats to store in the freezer, cottage cheese, plain full-fat Greek yogurt.

Healthy fats: bulk amounts of shredded coconut, walnuts, almonds, pecans, sunflower seeds, hemp hearts, chia seeds, flax seeds, and nut butters; avocado and olive oils; avocados on sale (freeze the flesh for later); frozen coconut cubes and canned coconut milk; cheeses, butter, and ghee on sale.

Non-starchy vegetables (in-season, on sale, or frozen): zucchini, broccoli, cauliflower, asparagus, celery, green beans, spaghetti squash, cabbage, Brussels sprouts, cucumber, lettuce, spinach, arugula, eggplant, mushrooms, bell peppers.

Low carb fruits (in-season, on sale, or frozen): raspberries, strawberries, blackberries, blueberries.

In addition to sticking with these foods, shopping at Trader Joe's, Aldi, Costco, or discount grocery stores can help you find the most affordable prices.

Sample Meal Plan For Keto On A Budget

Here's a 7-day meal plan with affordable keto meals. The non-starchy vegetables, meats, and nuts or seeds on this menu can be swapped out with what's on sale or in season. Keep in mind that the ideal number of net carbs eaten on keto depends on the individual. These meals may or may not fit your specific needs.

Day 1

Breakfast: 3 egg and cheese omelet with spinach, side of frozen berries.

Lunch: chicken soup with shredded chicken, broth, celery, garlic, herbs, and topped with plain Greek yogurt.

Dinner: pork chops with sautéed green beans and almonds.

Day 2

Breakfast: cottage cheese with frozen strawberries and seeds.

Lunch: hard-boiled eggs mashed on cucumber slices, topped with hemp hearts and full fat salad dressing.

Dinner: lettuce cups with ground turkey, frozen non-starchy vegetable mix, and plain Greek yogurt.

Day 3

Breakfast: smoothie with frozen raspberries, nut butter, spinach, and coconut milk.

Lunch: tuna salad stuffed in red bell peppers.

Dinner: cauliflower "rice" (bought on sale or made in the food processor) stir fry with frozen broccoli, shredded chicken, sesame seeds, garlic, and ginger.

Day 4

Breakfast: fried eggs with sautéed spinach cooked in butter or oil.

Lunch: turkey roll-ups with plain Greek yogurt, sliced peppers, and cucumbers.

Dinner: bunless burger on a bed of greens topped with cheese, side of roasted Brussels sprouts.

Day 5

Breakfast: full-fat Greek yogurt with nuts.

Lunch: salad with hard-boiled eggs, cheese, sliced peppers, mushrooms, and lemon olive oil dressing.

Dinner: ground chuck meatballs served over spaghetti squash, tossed in avocado oil and Parmesan.

Day 6

Breakfast: bell pepper and mushroom omelet with shredded cheese.

Lunch: arugula salad with canned tuna, cucumbers, radishes, sunflower seeds, and olive oil dressing.

Dinner: chicken thighs with coconut cauliflower soup.

Day 7

Breakfast: nut and seed porridge made with canned coconut milk.

Lunch: egg salad made with plain Greek yogurt on celery sticks.

Dinner: pork tenderloin, eggplant, and zucchini cooked in butter and topped with cheese.

Keto Snack Options

Most keto meals are filling enough that you may not feel the need to snack. But if you get hungry between meals, try one of these budget-friendly keto snacks:

- sliced veggies with nut butter
- full-fat Greek yogurt with frozen berries
- a handful of nuts or seeds
- 1–2 hard-boiled eggs
- string cheese
- celery sticks with cottage cheese or pimento cheese
- 70% or more unsweetened dark chocolate (or Stevia-sweetened chocolate)
- homemade kale chips roasted with healthy oils.

Essential Tips To Keto Lifestyle

Remember To Limit Net Carbs Per Day

By "net carbs" we mean the total carbohydrate intake minus the amount of fiber. Yes, fiber is a type of carb. But fiber passes through the digestive system without being digested or used, so you don't need to count it toward your total carbs. So, just subtract the grams of fiber from the total grams of carbs.

This tip allows you to add more high-fiber vegetables to your diet without throwing off your ratio of fats to carbs and protein. It also allows you to feel fuller at the table while eating fewer calories. Not all vegetables are labeled for fiber content, but you get that info online at various nutrition-counting sites like SELF Nutrition Data.

Find The Calorie Level That's Right For You

Not everyone has the same rate of metabolism or the exact nutritional needs, so a little tinkering is usually necessary until you get things right.

You're shooting for just enough calories to satisfy your hunger and keep your energy levels up. Too few calories will leave you feeling tired, and too many will prevent you from losing as much weight.

But remember that anytime you make a significant change in your diet, it will throw your system off a bit at first, so you'll probably need to tinker with your calorie levels at first until your body adapts to the changes.

Clean The Refrigerator Of Old Food

Time to give your kitchen a makeover! Ridding your cupboards, fridge, and freezer of carbs, fruits, and sugars is the best beginner tip for starting the ketogenic diet. You're able to give yourself a clean slate and start fresh with new foods that work with your body to change how your organs process foods.

All the rest must go. If you feel guilty about throwing out perfectly good food, then call up a friend or family member and bring it over to them. You can donate canned beans and boxed pasta or grains to your local food bank as well.

Create a New Keto Grocery List

Along with cleaning out your kitchen, you'll want to throw out your old grocery shopping lists, too. Those lists probably include your former cupboard staples like sandwich bread, crackers, hot dog buns, and burger buns.

But, now you're going to creating a new keto diet-friendly grocery list.

Make Your Schedule

While you're planning out your meals, think of how the keto diet can realistically fit into your weekly schedule. You'll want easy morning recipes that are simple to make, work snacks and lunches you can pack and take to your job, simple dinners that don't take long to prepare after work, and a couple of sweet treats to give you some indulgence in the evening. All of this should be accomplished with keto ingredients, too.

You might also want to think about the times you get hungry during the day. Are you a desk snack? A TV-and-munchies eater? We're not trying to eliminate all of your secret snacking times drastically, but it is crucial to keep in mind that you're used to reaching for carb snacks like cookies, crackers, and chips.

You're going to want to replace those carb snacks with the keto diet ones, which are listed as part of the grocery store ingredients and in the recipes. Snack times do strike us all, and it helps to have keto fat bombs in the fridge as a pick-me-up. Oh, you don't know what a fat bomb is? You are in for a treat!

You're not only planning out your meals, but you're also planning out how to live without carbs! Make the keto diet work with your schedule so that you're not reaching for 'convenience carbs'. Instead, you're getting for 'fast fats'!

Stock Up For Your New Keto Kitchen

If you thought that many keto diet ingredients are expensive and hard to find, then think again. You'll mostly be purchasing produce, meats, dairy, and some condiments so that the price will be similar or perhaps even less than your current grocery bill. That's because the keto diet uses all-natural foods!

Plan Out Your First Time Meals

With your kitchen fully stocked with keto ingredients to make plenty of dishes, it's time to plan out your very first seven days of meals. Have you ever meal planned before? Many don't because it seems like just one more thing to add to your busy to-do list.

Meal plans might seem to be more work than you're worth, but they're the number one secret to not only getting started on a new diet but making it stick. Planning meals saves you money and time throughout the week, and, if you have a family and are cooking for more than just yourself, it answers that daily question, "What's for dinner?"

You might also want to add specific cooking notes and plan out how you're going to make the meals, too.

Focus on Eating What You Love

It can be all too easy and tempting to fall into the mindset that "diets equal deprivation." It's called a diet, so it must be hardcore, prevent you from eating your favorite foods, and be a way to torture yourself, right? This keto diet, in particular, sounds difficult because there are no carbs!

Well, not in this case! The keto diet doesn't have carbs, that's true, but carbs only make up a single portion of your diet. There's an entire supermarket of flavor waiting for you outside of the bakery section and the potato chip aisle.

Fill your kitchen with your favorite flavors and foods. You'll enjoy the cheeses, butter and oils, cream, milk, eggs, meats, fresh veggies, herbs and spices, and nuts that are included in this nutrition plan.

The more you focus on eating what you love, the better the overall experience be for you.

Try Different Flavor Combinations

The keto diet will work best for you if it tastes good! One of the little known secrets to becoming a great cook is to understand and work with different flavor combinations. Every cuisine on the planet has its specific group of flavors. After you purchase those ingredients, you can use those flavors to marinade meat, create a cheese or egg dish, and spice up fresh veggies.

Use The Keto Sticks or Khe Keto Strips

Since you measure ketosis on the keto diet, you want to have a scientific way to check that your liver is breaking down fat properly to produce ketones. You can find unique ketone strips or sticks on Amazon, at Walmart, and other major retailers. These sticks are meant for beginners and can be very helpful. They measure your urine.

When you get your keto sticks, open them up. Hold the keto stick in your urine stream for a few seconds and then set it on a clean paper towel. Within about 10-15 seconds, you'll see the strip change color. Ketone urine sticks are usually measured on the red spectrum. If it shows up light pink, that means you're low in ketone production. The darker the red, the more in ketosis you are! Deep ketosis is in the optimal weight loss range.

As you get more comfortable and familiar with the diet, you'll want to invest in measuring your ketones with special breath meters and the more expensive but very accurate blood meter.

Monitor Side Effects

People react differently to changes in diet. Symptoms might include dizziness, fatigue, quickening heart rate, and shortness of breath. If any of these symptoms occur, it's probably a good idea to avoid strenuous activity, though light exercise is perhaps adequate and might well help alleviate the symptoms. If these symptoms seem severe or if they persist for more than a few days, it's probably a good idea to talk to your doctor.

Monitoring side effects are especially significant for people with diabetes and other people with insulin problems who might be prone to ketoacidosis, a dangerous condition.

Compare The Ketone Levels

The main idea behind this diet is to raise the level of ketones in your bloodstream, ensuring that you're entering ketosis and burning fat instead of glucose. To keep track of this, you should test your ketone levels daily and compare them to what you ate that day. It will give you graphic evidence of what's going on in your body so that you can make the proper choices to regulate your diet. In particular, it will help in determining the ideal level of carbs you should be eating.

Decrease The Stress Factors In Your Life

A stressful lifestyle can cause you to gain weight and send false hunger signals to your body. If you're going to be making the change to a keto lifestyle, you must be in the right period of your life to make the changes with enthusiasm.

If you're going through a stressful patch, then maybe delay the diet until you feel more at calm with your life. If you still want to start the keto diet, that's great too, but be sure you are taking time to decompress from the stress of your day. Whether it's exercising, yoga, meditation, or ensuring you have a good night's sleep, you want to take some personal time to relax from a stressful lifestyle so your body can follow through on the demands of a keto diet.

Stay On The Keto - Stay Hydrated

Staying hydrated is an essential factor to overall health no matter what diet you are on. During a keto diet, it's even more critical at the start of your diet because your body first excretes water weight when you switch to a low carb lifestyle. To combat this, you must have a habit of drinking enough water to avoid dehydration. That number needs to be increased if the temperature is hotter or if you've been exercising. So, if you're going to start keto, it's a great idea to already adjust to drinking enough water. Keep a water bottle with you and keep it visible at all times to remind yourself to take a few sips.

Every Day Count Your Carbs

If you're serious about following a keto lifestyle, you will have to count your macros and your carbohydrates when you first begin, as you and your appetite get adjusted to what you can and cannot eat. To help yourself out, start counting carbohydrates in your routine diet to get an idea of just how much you will have to restrict yourself.

Don't forget those hidden carbs! Things like fruit, milk, and condiments also have carbs that should be counted. Look at the nutrition facts and be consciously aware of what you're eating. You want to calculate net carbs: Total carbs - fiber = net carbs. You want to try and naturally lower your carbohydrates so you can drop down even lower when you're on the keto diet. There are tons of apps you can download to help you!

Carbs Need To Be Removed

Look, the truth of the matter is, you're going to keep eating what you have access to. If you keep carbohydrates in stock, you're going to keep having them simply because they're there. So, to begin your keto diet, go ahead and clear out all the carbohydrates you have from your pantry. Bread, pasta, cereal, snacks, candy, rice, processed snacks. It sounds drastic, and you might be stunned at how much space you have! But that'space you can fill up with healthy ingredients that will make up your keto lifestyle.

Keep Keto-Friendly Snacks On Hand

It is a common pitfall for people who are embarking on the keto diet. They may meticulously plan out their keto-friendly meals, but if a craving hits, they satisfy it with an unhealthy snack. There goes your macro count for the day! To combat this, finish up all those unhealthy snacks in your pantry and fill it up with the healthy stuff! Try having more protein like bacon slices, beef jerky, and eggs. Fat bombs are also effortless recipes you can make to get a taste of what type of snacks you should be eating.

Get Ready To Eat Out

When you first start the keto diet, it can seem overwhelming when you're at a restaurant trying to decide what is keto-friendly and what isn't. But it gets more comfortable if you know what to ask for! Make sure you have your lists of approved keto foods and don't hesitate to ask for substitutes of sides in a meal.

For breakfast, eggs and bacon are a great meal and very filling! Say no to the pancakes or waffles and see if there's a healthy omelet with veggies you have can have instead. Lunch will always have a salad option for you. Be sure you ask for simple vinegar or olive oil dressing instead of one loaded with sugar! And for dinner, you can focus on protein by ordering a nice steak or salmon. For a side, order a serving of vegetables on the keto list like broccoli or cauliflower instead of potatoes or french fries.

Start Exercising

If you're not already living an active lifestyle, you must transition to one in order to see weight loss results on a keto lifestyle. Coupled with a healthy diet, you also need exercise to get rid of the glucose molecules your body has stored as fat. Try and go to the gym a few times a week or at least incorporate exercises like jogging or walking for a quick 15 to 20 minutes every day. You don't have to exercise every day. But a combination of strength training and aerobic workouts can induce weight loss much quicker than a sedentary lifestyle. Look up beginner workouts and incorporate a training schedule into your week! Grab a workout buddy to have extra motivation!

Cut The Soda And Sugar From Your Diet

Just like we mentioned above with carbohydrates, it's also vital that you're aware of how much sugar you're ingesting throughout the day. Whether it's just a spoon or two in your morning coffee, a sweet treat at lunch, or a handful of cookies before bed — all of that sugar you're going to cut from your lifestyle when you go keto. Start cutting back on that now. Diet soda is also detrimental to the keto diet because it uses sugar substitutes that send signals to your body as if sugar is entering your bloodstream. It increases your blood sugar levels and can produce different fat molecules. No more diet sodas! Try sparkling water instead.

Invest In A Food Scale Or Measuring Tools

As a keto beginner, weighing the food you eat and being aware of portion sizes is going to be critical. Buy a food scale. If you don't have one, you can't feel confident about portion sizes when trying new recipes. Also, make sure you have proper measuring spoons and cups. There's a big difference between one tablespoon of almond butter and two tablespoons - that's an extra 200 calories and as much as seven carbohydrates you'd be gaining that you don't need! Spoons/cups and food scales are relatively inexpensive, and you should find a handy space for them in your kitchen since you will frequently be using them in the beginning as you get used to serving sizes.

Educate Yourself On A Keto Diet!

Last but not least, if you're going to be embarking on a keto lifestyle, it's crucial you know exactly what you're getting into. Taking the time to read the appropriate literature (like this book!) is a great start, as well as listening to podcasts or viewing videos of people who successfully live the keto lifestyle. Find a printable that shows which foods are on the keto-friendly list, so you become familiar when you are shopping or eating out. The more aware you are, the more confident you'll feel about your lifestyle choices.

Conclusion

If you haven't started the keto diet yet, now you have a simple meal plan to get you started. You also know the basic principles of budget keto.

Lets repeat it: buy in bulk; look for sales and stock up; buy vegetables that are in season; go for frozen over fresh; start a meal plan and prep routine; opt for cheaper proteins and skip the packaged keto-friendly foods.

Remember to limit net carbs per day, find the calorie level that's right for you, clean the refrigerator of old food, create a new keto grocery list. Moreover, focus on eating what you love, try different flavor combinations, monitor side effects, and compare the ketone levels. Stay on the keto - stay hydrated, every day count your carbs.

If you find it difficult, remember to reread this chapter.

Next, I will briefly introduce you to keto cooking. And of course, then we will move on to keto recipes so that your life would not be boring and monotonous on a keto diet.

CHAPTER 10.
KETO MEAL PREP

What Is Meal Prepping?

Meal prepping does not have to be something that you dread each week. You can make it fun and involve the whole family. It always helps to have an extra hand along to keep up with everything. If you start eating the proper meals at the appropriate times, you are going to see the other benefits of eating healthy when you start losing weight and just feeling better mentally about yourself.

Meal prepping is what the word says; it means that you prepare several meals or even all of them beforehand. Instead of eating ready-made meals which you would typically buy at a store, you can now prepare your own. They will be better suited to your taste, contain far fewer preservatives, and will be a lot healthier.

The core part of success for meal prepping is that you must have a PLAN. You will not succeed if you do not have it, I can most certainly promise you that.

How to Meal Prep in a Few Easy Steps?

Once you are on the road to becoming good at meal prepping, you will never look back. You will very likely continue moving forward onto the next great set of healthy meal prep recipes!

1. Buy In Bulk

Whenever you can, always buy food supplies for meal preps in bulk. It is going to be a lot cheaper to do so, and it will undoubtedly make it easier for you to decide on meals for the evening. You can meal prep some of it, then freeze the rest to use for another meal prep session; perhaps the following week.

2. Prioritize Your Meals

Do this especially when you do not have time to prepare all of them at once. You need to pick the most important meals to complete first. It is preferable to trying to do big meal prep when you are short of time.

3. Set Aside Time To Do Meal Prep

If you are cooking large batches, then you will need to put aside a day each week to get this done. Make sure that you are doing it when you do not feel rushed so that you can prepare the best meals possible.

4. Cook Large Batches Of Food That You Are Fond Of

You do not want to make a large batch of food only to find that it is not something that suits your taste. Try new recipes in small amounts before you decide to cook them in batches. Cook foods that you are familiar with at first in sets then eventually expand to other new foods.

5. Slowly Build Up Food Variety

You do not have to cook 20 different food options in your first week. You can always start by having one meal for dinner one day and have the leftovers for lunch the next day. It will take time to build up different options, so approach it in a slow manner; don't feel rushed.

6. Bake Veggies & Meat On The Same Tray

You can save yourself fewer things to wash up by cooking your veggies and meat on one big tray in the oven. The juices will create a nice sauce that you can use on the meat to prevent it from going dry when you reheat it.

7. Make Some Smoothie-Cubes

Add smoothie mixture to the ice-cube tray, allow them to freeze, then add them all to a freezer bag. You can fill the ice-cube tray back up, repeat until you have filled your freezer bag with smoothie-cubes.

8. Multitask

While you are cooking dinner, use the time that you are waiting for the food to finish cooking to chop up some veggies for your meals for the next few days. Once you get multitasking under your belt, you will find it much easier to get more things done within a shorter timeframe.

9. Spice Up Your Meals

Keep your meals full of flavor and interesting by adding spices to them. You can make your meal taste so much better just by adding some spices or allowing your meat to soak in a marinade.

10. Keep Prepping When You Can

Just keep in mind that anything that you do in the preparation of a meal ahead of time is considered meal prep. It includes chopping up veggies to cover you for the next few days.

Benefits Of Planning Meals

Weight Loss. Meal prepping is going to *help you lose weight.* Knowing what you are going to eat is very important if you want to lose weight.

Finish Cravings. *Cravings are going to stop* as you continue to meal prep. In just a few weeks, you will find that you no longer crave sugar or junk. Instead, you will be looking forward to the meals and snacks that you have prepared.

Stress Is A Killer. It can cause so many problems with your health, such as increasing your blood pressure. It can cause sleep issues, lower your immune system, and even cause digestive issues.

No More Indecision. You arrive home from work, exhausted and ravenous with hunger. You open the cupboards, rummaging around while you wait for inspiration, but nothing springs to mind.

No Worse Choices. Without a proper plan for your next meal, you may fall into the trap of going for the perceived 'easy option' of a takeaway or ready meal.

A More Balanced Diet. Take the time to think back on what exactly you have eaten the past week. You will probably realize that it was the same dish most of the time.

Much More Variety. Some people think that planning your meals ahead of time is tedious since you know what you are going to eat a few days in advance. It is far from the truth; planning encourages variety.

No Food Wastage While Saving Money. How often did you find wilted veggies in your refrigerator or had to throw away food that is past its expiry date? If you plan cleverly, making use of leftovers, using what is in your kitchen cupboards, freezing food in batches, minimal food items will end up in your trashcan.

Less Arduous Arguing. You feel like eating a vegetarian dish, your partner wants hamburgers, but the kids plead for pizzas. Does this sound familiar? Your family may end up arguing unnecessarily over their next meal.

Go for Seasonal. Be creative and plan your meals according to the season. Not only will you have the freshest ingredients, but you will also look after your purse, as new produce items are a lot less costly when in season.

Saving Money. It is a massive misconception that healthy eating equals heavy spending. It is simply not true. There are many reasons why advance prepping can help you save money.

Must-Have Kitchen Essentials

Below are some of the essential kitchen equipment items that you might want to keep handy.

Cutting Boards: Try to get boards that are made from solid materials like plastic, glass, rubber, or marble. These are mostly corrosion-resistant, and the non-porous surface makes it easier to clean them than wood.

Measuring Cups: Required to measure out liquids, spices, and condiments.

Spoons: Have several different-sized spoons allow you to measure out small amounts of spices and other ingredients.

Glass Bowls And Non-Metallic Containers: These are required for storing items as well as for mixing ingredients.

Paper Towels: These are required for draining food of excess oil and other liquids.

Cold Storage: Many fresh and cooked foods needs to be stored at 40 degrees Fahrenheit or below, so a refrigerator is required.

Knives: Knives should be used to slice meat, vegetables, fruit, and other food. While using the knife, you should keep the following in mind:

- Always use a sharp knife
- Always keep your knives visible
- Always cut down toward the cutting surface and away from your body
- Never allow children to have unattended access to knives
- Wash the knives often when cutting different types of food.

The Kitchen Scales: The kitchen scale provides accurate measurements of ingredients. This is ideal for people on a diet.

Internal Thermometer: A meat thermometer helps you to measure the internal temperature of foods to ensure that they are safe to eat.

Baking Sheet: These are flat, rectangular metal pans that are used in an oven, ideal for roasting, baking, and keeping items warm.

Colander: A colander is a kitchen utensil [bowl-shaped] with holes that allows you to drain food like pasta. These are also used to rinse vegetables.

Aluminum Foil: This is used to wrap up and cover food and line baking sheets.

Parchment Paper: This is used to line baking sheets to help prevent items from sticking.

Storage Containers: These are the beating heart of meal prepping, so try to keep as many containers as possible. However, when selecting containers [boxes], you may notice there are two types of containers: plastic and glass.

Both have their merits and drawbacks. The following points should help you choose between the two.

Glass: Glass containers are a bit more expensive but are ideal for long-term storage. Due to their heavyweight, glass containers are not suitable for "on-the-go" eating. They are easier to clean. If you are concerned about plastic safety, then these are the ones to go with.

Plastic: Easy to carry and lightweight, ideal for individuals who are always on the go. They are more convenient and come in a wide variety of sizes and shapes.

They Are Easy To Dispose

Asides from glass and plastic, you may also notice that there are steel containers. Steel containers are excellent if you want to keep meals in the freezer as they help to avoid freezer burn.

Amazing Meal Prep Ideas

Keep in mind that meal prep ideas are not set in stone. The following are just some of the dozens of different meal prep ideas that you are can find on the Internet.

Make a plan ahead of time: If you are reading this book, then you have probably decided to go on a clean eating diet journey.

Keep an adequate supply of Mason jars: They are terrific, not only for storing memories and canning foods but also for storing healthy salads.

Multiple seasonings in one pan: If your diet requires you to stick with lean meats like chicken, then seasoning them as needed can become somewhat of a chore.

Boil eggs in an oven instead of a pot: Now, this might sound a little bit odd at first, but it is highly effective.

Keep your prepared smoothies frozen in muffin tins: The muffin tins can be useful here as well.

Roast vegetables that require the same time in one batch: When you are preparing large sets of vegetables for roasting, go ahead and roast some extras at the same time.

Learn to use a skewer effectively: When you think of skewers, you automatically think of kabobs.

Keep an adequate supply of sectioned plastic containers: Sectioned containers are an absolute necessity for meal-prepping severe savants.

Keep track of your accomplishments: This is perhaps the essential aspect of a meal prepping routine.

The Common Mistakes Made By Meal Prepping Beginners

As a beginner in meal planning, you want to make sure that you are using your time wisely. You don't want to waste ingredients, waste time, or do other things that take away from the benefits that come with this kind of prep. Common mistakes that you need to avoid as a beginner include:

Not building a balanced meal

Overeating of one food and not enough of another can mess up the day. The recipes below will help you to get the right balance between the carbs, protein, and fats that you need on the ketogenic diet.

But if you are choosing from other sources, make sure that you are balancing out the meals so that your macronutrients are still in place.

Preparing it all in one day

It may be tempting to prepare all the food in one day, but have you ever tasted chicken, or other meat, after it has been in the fridge for a week? These often taste poorly, and you will not want to eat it. You can choose a few options.

Some people make meals for a few days at a time and call that good. If you need to make a lot of meals at once, consider freezing them to keep everything fresh for when you need it.

Never mixing it up

Eating the same things or similar things can get boring. It is essential to think about the meals that you are preparing and that you pick out a variety of meals that will taste good.

Eating chicken every day for a month is going to get boring, but mixing up the meals to include some fish, some beef, some turkey, and even some vegetarian options can make things easier.

Not stocking up the kitchen

It is impossible to cook up these healthy meals without planning a bit.

If you are working on a recipe and you don't have the ingredients, you may reach for a substitute that is not that healthy. Always plan and know what you need for all of your recipes to make things easier.

Not storing properly

The containers that you store the meals in can affect how much food you are going to make and eat. If you are picking out huge boxes, your portion sizes are going to be large as well.

Pick out portion-controlled containers or ones that are only as big as the amount of food that your family will eat. You may find that some of the meals can be divided in two, saving you even more money.

Picking out complicated cooking methods

You do not need to pick out meals that are going to take hours to put together and need the most complicated cooking method possible. It is OK to keep things simple, especially when it comes to your meal planning.

For example, there is nothing wrong with doing a few recipes each time that uses the slow cooker. You need to throw the ingredients in the slow cooker, and the meal is done. You can always mix it up with different cooking methods but making it simple is the name of the game with meal planning.

Tips And Tricks For Making Meal Prep Easy

What is great about these tips is that they are going to work for you, whether you are prepping your food just for you or for your entire family.

What many people love about meal prep is that there is a huge community of people online that are sharing all of the recipes that they use, so there is no shortage of options.

Keep staples on hand. Even if you are not prepping all of your meals, it is best to keep staples such as boiled eggs or shredded chicken on hand.

Make sure that your containers of functional. Your containers [boxes] are going to determine how successful you are at meal prepping.

Don't feel like you have to go on Pinterest and create the most complicated meals because this is only going to lead to a bunch of Pinterest fails.

Practice makes perfect when it comes to many things in life, including meal prepping.

Get to know your vegetables. Not all vegetables are going to keep in the fridge for one week after they have been chopped.

Make sure that you plan your snacks and never leave the house without your water, snack, and meal if you are going to be gone for long.

Make prepping a party. Meal prep does take time; however, it is not a waste of time and should never be seen that way.

Cook all of the same foods at once. One of the great things about meal prepping is that you can cook once and create several meals.

Purchase containers that are of proper proportion.

After prepping all of your meals, no one wants to spend even more time cleaning up. You can also clean as you go. If you spill something on the stove, wipe it up instead of letting it dry on and struggling to get it off later.

Purchase bags of frozen produce when possible.

Make more than you will eat and then freeze the extra.

When you are first starting, choose your trigger meal to prep.

If you are prepping all of your meals, don't forget to give yourself some variety.

Cook multiple foods at the same time.

There are so many ways for you to ensure your success as you are meal prepping, but the best tip that I can give you is to just keep at it.

Meal prepping is not supposed to feel like a burden or another task that you have to complete, but instead, it is supposed to help you simplify your life while saving time and energy.

Volume measurements conversion:

Cups	Tablespoons	Teaspoons	Milliliters	Fluid Ounces
	1/3 tbsp.	1 tsp.	5 ml	1/6 oz.
1/16 cup	1 tbsp.	3 tsp.	15 ml	1/2 oz.
1/8 cup	2 tbsp.	6 tsp.	30 ml	1 oz.
1/4 cup	4 tbsp.	12 tsp.	60 ml	2 oz.
1/3 cup	5 1/3 tbsp.	16 tsp.	80 ml	2 2/3 oz.
1/2 cup	8 tbsp.	24 tsp.	120 ml	4 oz.
2/3 cup	10 2/3 tbsp.	32 tsp.	160 ml	5 1/3 oz.
3/4 cup	12 tbsp.	36 tsp.	180 ml	6 oz.
1 cup	16 tbsp.	48 tsp.	240 ml	8 oz.

Gallon	Quart	Pint	Cup	Fluid Ounces
1/16 gal	1/4 qt.	1/2 pt.	1 cup	8 oz.
1/8 gal	1/2 qt.	1 pt.	2 cup	16 oz.
1/4 gal	1 qt.	2 pt.	4 cup	32 oz.
1/2 gal	2 qt.	4 pt.	8 cup	64 oz.
1 gal	4 qt.	8 pt.	16 cup	128 oz.

Temperature measurements conversion:

Gas Mark	º F	º C
1 Cool	275º F	140º C
2	300º F	150º C
3 Very Moderate	325º F	165º C
4 Moderate	350º F	180º C
5	375º F	190º C
6 Moderately Hot	400º F	200º C
7 Hot	425º F	220º C
8	450º F	230º C
9 Very Hot	475º F	240º C

About Recipes

Take the nutrition facts from recipes as rough estimates. Always check the nutrient content on the manufacturer's label. To accurately calculate nutritional facts, always weigh the food you are preparing. Calculate nutritional facts only from the food you cook.

For example, different coconut or almond flour producers will have different protein, fat, and carbohydrate content. It will also differ from one cheese or meat producer to another. Butter or cream of various degrees of fat content will also contain different amounts of fat and, accordingly, calories.

Therefore, if you clearly monitor the number of calories you consume and strictly observe the keto proportions in fats, proteins, and carbohydrates, you should do it yourself (of course, you can use the applications or calculators mentioned in the book)

The calculations are made based on the exact energy value, where there are 9.3 calories in 1 gram of fat, 4.1 calories in 1 gram of protein or carbohydrates. The energy value of dietary fiber is not taken into account.

CHAPTER 11.
KETO RECIPES AND 21-DAY MEAL PLAN

21-DAY MEAL PLAN

Meal Plan. Week 1

	Breakfast	Lunch	Dinner
Monday	Smooth Coconut Porridge	Chicken Jalapeno Fritters	Chicken Caprese
Tuesday	Keto Mushroom Omelet	Chipotle Beef Chili	Skillet Lasagna
Wednesday	Keto Coconut Pancakes	Chicken Enchilada Soup	Cheese Stuffed Meatballs
Thursday	Baked Cheesy Egg Muffins	Salmon Avocado Devilled Egg	Garlic Chicken
Friday	Savory Breakfast Cookies	Chicken Paprika Meatballs	Low Carb Pasta
Saturday	Lettuce Sandwich	Zucchini Noodle Soup	Yakitori Chicken
Sunday	Cream Cheese Pancakes	Keto Cheesy Cauliflower	Garlic Butter Salmon

Meal Plan. Week 2

	BREAKFAST	LUNCH	DINNER
MONDAY	Vibrant Scrambled Eggs	Salsa Chicken	Cauliflower And Broccoli Casserole
TUESDAY	Keto Cereal	White Chicken Chili Soup	Lamb Kofta
WEDNESDAY	Keto Tuna Salad	Mexican Ground Beef With Veggies	Cabbage Casserole
THURSDAY	Keto Pancake Bites	Salmon With Pesto	Bacon Wrapped Chicken
FRIDAY	Beefy Baked Eggs	Mushroom Soup	Buttery Chicken With Broccoli
SATURDAY	Egg Salad	Bread Rolls	Roasted Pork Belly
SUNDAY	Keto Porridge	Lamb Chops	Butter Poached Shrimp

Meal Plan. Week 3

	BREAKFAST	LUNCH	DINNER
MONDAY	Avocado And Egg Delight	Butter Chicken	Garlic Chicken
TUESDAY	Scrambled Tofu	Chicken Fajita Soup	Lamb With Kale
WEDNESDAY	Peanut Butter Cupcakes	Keto Bread Sandwich	Stuffed Avocado
THURSDAY	Classic Bacon And Eggs	Tuna Steak	Chicken Adobo
FRIDAY	Keto Smoked Salmon And Egg Butter	Zucchini And Basil Soup	Garlic Butter Salmon
SATURDAY	Coffee And Chia Pudding	Keto Pepperoni Pizza	Keto Meatloaf
SUNDAY	Asparagus And Poached Eggs	Keto Fried Chicken	Salmon With Spinach

Recipes Part 1
KETO SWEET BREAKFAST

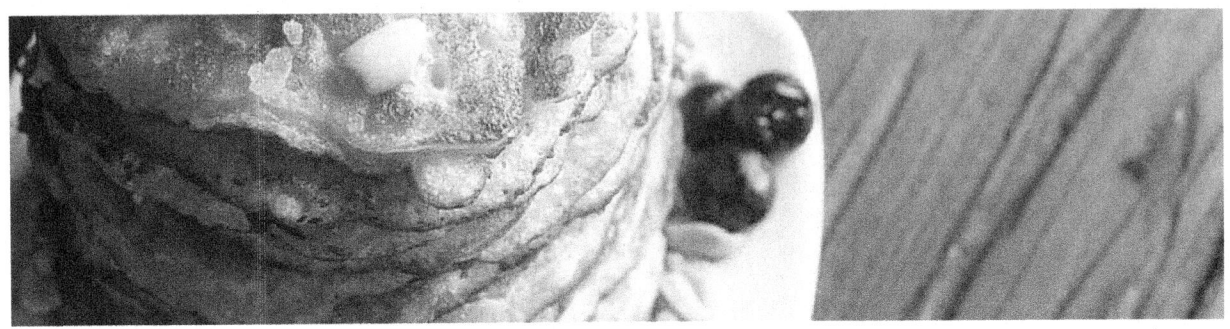

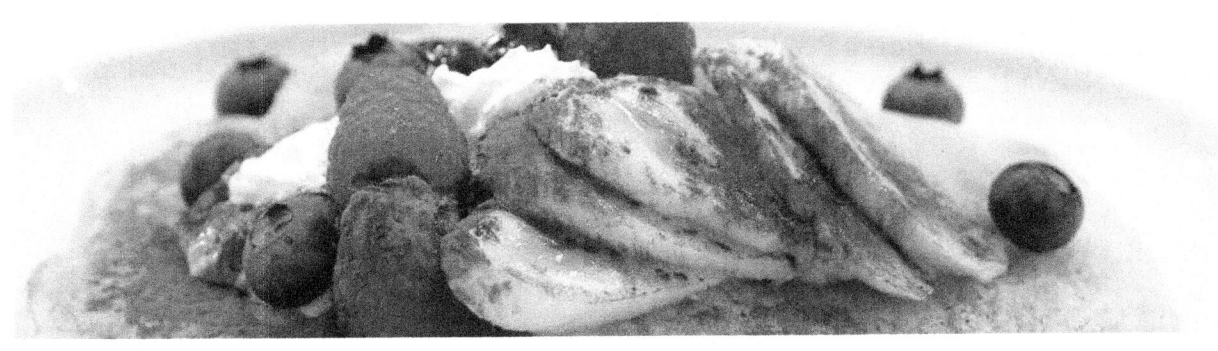

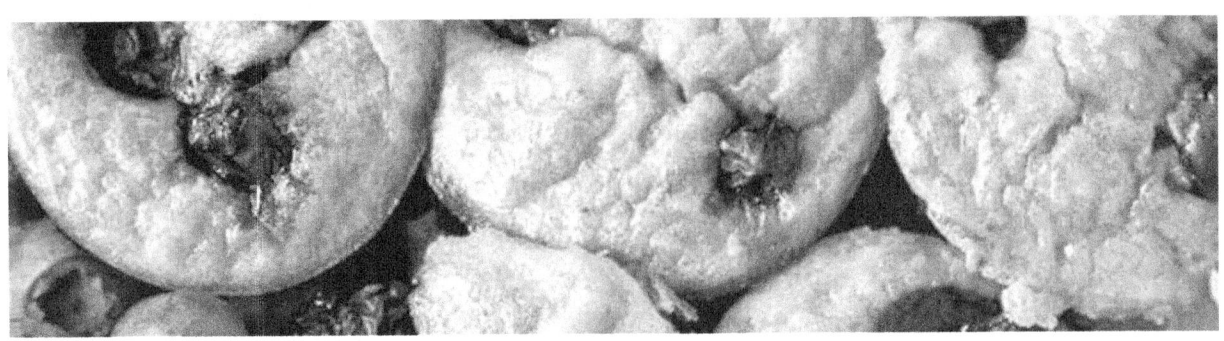

Smooth Coconut Porridge

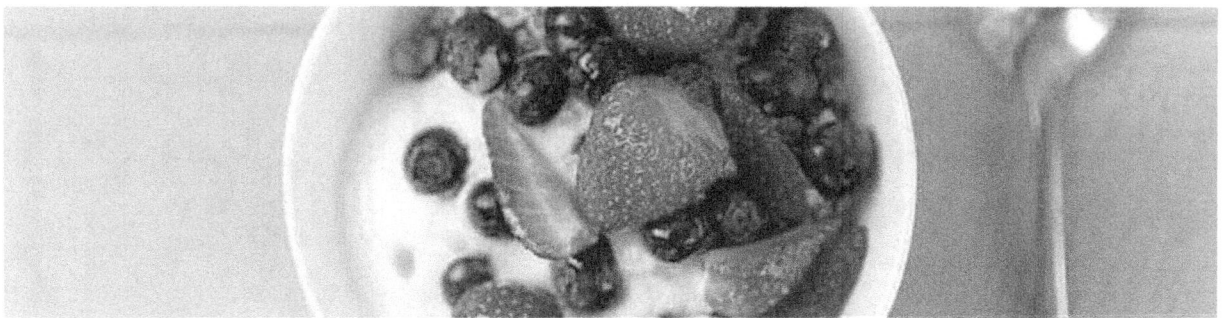

If you don't feel like eating an egg, make this warm, creamy, and smooth coconut porridge to satisfy your tummy.

Serving quantity: 1

Ingredients:

- 1 tbsp. coconut flour
- 1 beaten egg
- 1 pinch of psyllium husk powder
- 1 ounce of coconut oil
- 4 tbsp. coconut cream
- 1 pinch of salt

Directions:

Prep 5 min. | Cook 10 min. | Ready in 15 min.

- Combine coconut flour, egg, psyllium husk, and salt in a bowl.
- Melt the coconut cream and butter over low heat in a saucepan. Add the egg mixture slowly while whisking continuously. Mix until it is thick and creamy.
- Top it with unsweetened coconut milk and berries.

Nutrition facts:

Per Serving: 509 calories | 49 g fat | 9 g protein | 4 g carbs

Keto Coconut Pancakes

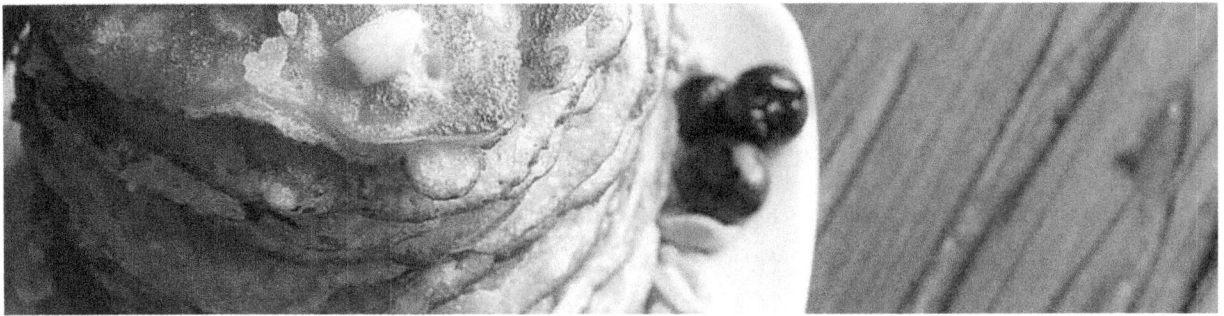

You don't have to let go of pancakes to be on a keto diet. These low-carb coconut pancakes are such a delight, especially when topped with butter and berries.

Serving quantity: 4

Ingredients:

- 6 eggs
- a pinch of salt
- 2 tbsp. coconut oil
- 1/2 cup coconut flour
- 3/4 cup coconut milk
- 1 tsp. baking powder
- butter for frying

Directions:

Prep 25 min. | Cook 15 min. | Ready in 40 min.

- Separate yolks from egg whites.
- Add a pinch of salt in egg whites and whisk until it's fluffy.
- Whisk the egg yolks, coconut milk, and oil in a separate bowl.
- Then add baking powder and coconut flour and make a smooth batter.
- Gently mix the egg whites into the batter and let it rest for 5 minutes.
- Spread butter in a pan and pour some mixture.
- Cook both sides on medium heat until they are golden.

Nutrition facts:

Per Serving: 285 calories | 24 g fat | 12 g protein | 3 g carbs

Keto Cereal

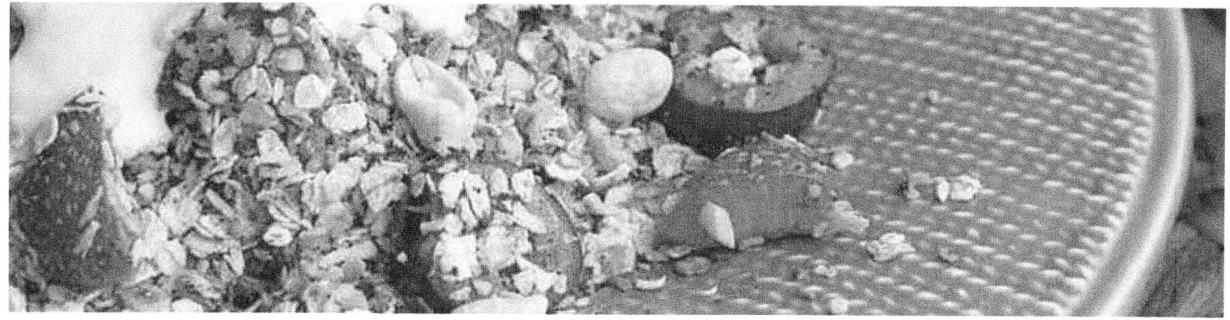

The ingredients in this recipe very healthy and packed with energy. It only takes three to four steps to make, and you will have three cups of this yummy cereal to eat all week long. Delicious and easy for your daily breakfast.

Serving quantity: 3 cups

Ingredients:

- 1 egg white
- 1 cup chopped walnuts
- 1 cup chopped almonds
- ¼ cup coconut oil
- 1 cup coconut flakes, unsweetened
- ¼ cup sesame seeds
- 1 ½ tsp. ground cinnamon
- ½ tsp. salt
- 1 tsp. vanilla extract
- ½ tsp. ground clove
- 2 tbsp. flax seeds
- 2 tbsp. chia seeds
- cooking spray

Directions:

Prep 10 min. | Cook 25 min. | Ready in 35 min.

- Preheat the oven at 350° F. Use the cooking spray to grease the baking sheet.
- Add walnuts, almonds, coconut flakes, sesame seeds, cinnamon, salt, vanilla extract, clove, flax, and chia seeds in a separate bowl and mix properly.
- Beat the egg whites in a bowl till foamy.
- Add it in the granola mixture and mix.
- Add coconut oil and mix again thoroughly.
- Spread the mixture on the sheet and bake for 20 to 25 minutes.
- Let it become golden and stir it gently halfway. Let it cool completely.

Nutrition facts:

Per serving: 347 calories | 32 g fat | 6 g protein | 6 g carbs

Nut & Coconut Porridge

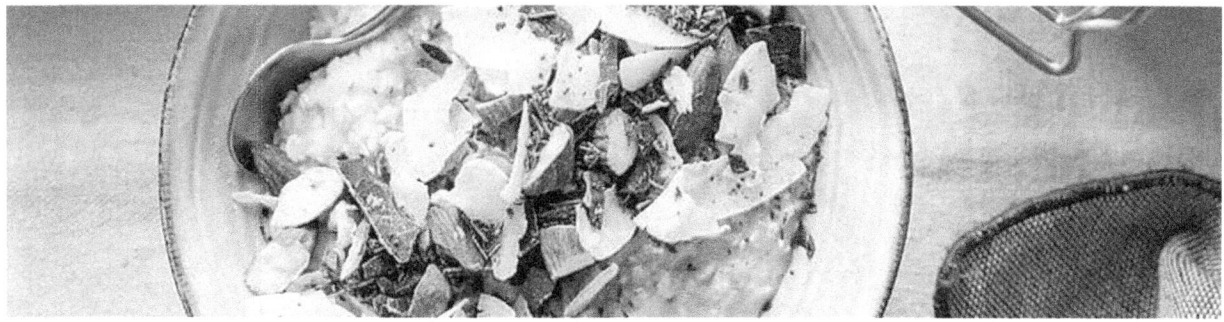

Do you want hot porridge for breakfast? Try this hearty keto dish that leaves a pleasantly satiated belly warmth. Really yummy! If you still have coconut milk after making your porridge, make a smoothie or smoothie out of it. Then the drink will become a little thicker in consistency and tastier.

Serving quantity: 1

Ingredients:

- 2 eggs
- 1 tbsp. coconut flour
- 1/2 cup chopped almonds
- 1/2 cup chopped walnuts
- 2 tbsp. of butter
- 4 tbsp. whipped cream (full fat)
- salt, to taste
- keto-friendly sweetener, to taste

Directions:

Prep 5 min. | Cook 5 min. | Ready in 5 min.

- In a small bowl, stir together the egg and coconut flour.
- Melt the butter and whipped cream over low heat. Then slowly pour them into the egg mixture, stirring constantly.
- Beat the mixture until the consistency of thick sour cream.
- Add salt and keto-friendly sweetener.
- Add the almonds and walnuts to the porridge.
- Enjoy your meal!

Nutrition facts:

Per serving: 846 calories | 76 g fat | 22 g protein | 12 g carbs

Sweet or Savory Breakfast Cookies

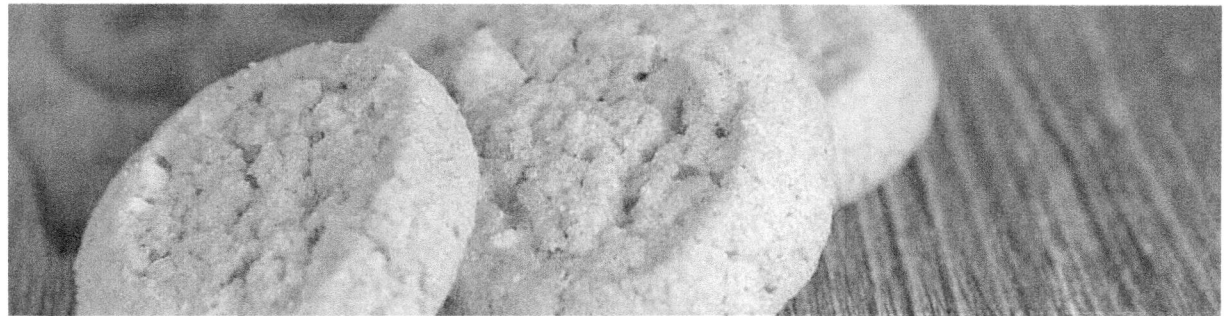

If you want a quick sweet or savory bite for breakfast on a busy morning, this is it for you. It's easy and delicious at the same time. You can even add your twist by using cooked ground beef or some kind of oily canned fish to add a meaty flavor to these cookies. Or can add some sweetener and enjoy a completely different taste

Serving quantity: 12

Ingredients:

- 1 ½ cups almond flour
- 1 cup shredded cheese (cheddar or cream cheese)
- 3 eggs
- 1 tsp. baking powder
- ½ tsp. salt
- black pepper, to taste
- keto-friendly sweetener, to taste

Directions:

Prep 5 min. | Cook 15 min. | Ready in 20 min.

- Preheat oven to 350° F.
- Line a baking tray with butter paper.
- Mix all the ingredients in a bowl. You can even add cooked ground beef or canned fish if you like. Or if you want some sweet – add stevia.
- Rub a little oil on your hands and shape the batter into cookies.
- Then place them on the baking tray.
- Bake for 15 minutes and check if they are done.
- Remove when cookies are done.
- Let them cool for 5 minutes and store in an airtight jar.

Nutrition facts:

Per Serving: 179 calories | 14 g fat | 8 g protein | 4 g carbs

Cream Cheese Pancakes

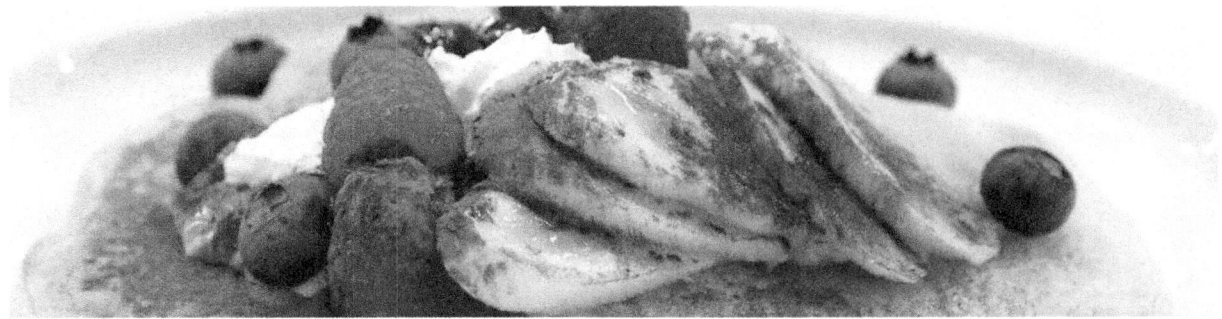

Sometimes you get tired of eggs. You want a delicious but healthy keto breakfast. These pancakes are cheesy goodness with low carbs and an excellent taste.

Serving quantity: 2

Ingredients:

- 2 eggs
- 2 ounces cream cheese
- 1/4 tsp. cinnamon
- keto-friendly sweetener, to taste

Directions:

Prep 3 min. | Cook 9 min. | Ready in 12 min.

- Blend all the ingredients until smooth.
- Let it rest for 2 minutes to let the bubbles out.
- Grease the pan with oil or butter. Pour 1/4 cup mixture in the pan.
- Cook for 2 minutes, flip and cook the other side for 1 minute.
- Repeat the procedure with other pancakes.
- Serve with syrup and butter. Add fresh berries as needed.

Nutrition facts:

Per serving: 352 calories | 29 g fat | 17 g proteins | 3 g carbs

Keto Pancake Bites

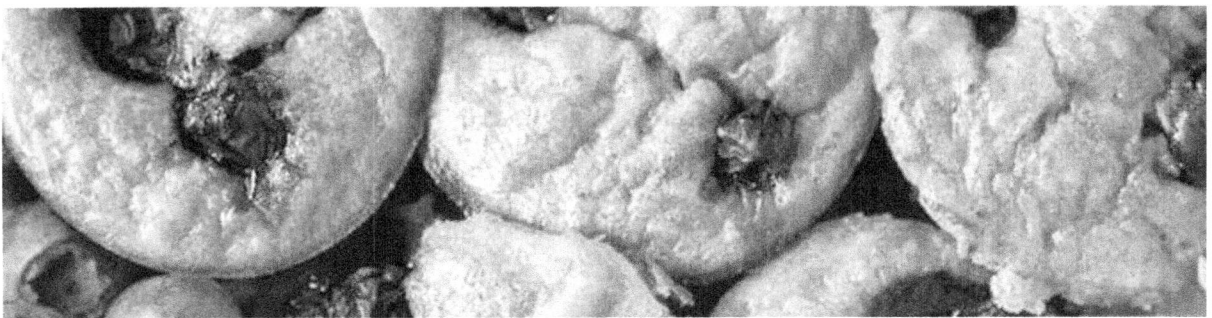

This recipe is keto-friendly, and children absolutely love it. The smell is mouthwatering, and they taste so heavenly. You will fall in love with these little pancake bites once you try them.

Serving quantity: 6

Ingredients:

- 4 eggs
- ½ cup coconut flour
- keto-friendly sweetener
- ½ cup water
- ¼ cup melted butter
- ½ cup frozen blueberries
- ½ tsp. salt
- 1 tsp. baking powder
- ¼ tsp. cinnamon
- ½ tsp. vanilla extract

Directions:

Prep 15 min. | Bake 25 min. | Ready in 40 min.

- Preheat the oven at 325°F and grease the muffin tin of 24 cavities.
- Grease them with butter and then coconut oil.
- Blend eggs, vanilla extract, and sweetener until smooth.
- Add coconut flour, salt, cinnamon, melted butter, and baking powder and blend well.
- Let it rest for a while so it can thicken considerably.
- Add 1/3 cup of water and blend again.
- If it is still thick, add more water to mix.
- Scoop it out of the blender and into the container.
- Add 4 to 5 blueberries in each bite and press them gently.
- Bake for 20 to 25 minutes until it is set.
- Let it cool and serve.

Nutrition facts:

Per serving: 188 calories | 14 g fat | 6 g protein | 8 g carbs

Keto Porridge

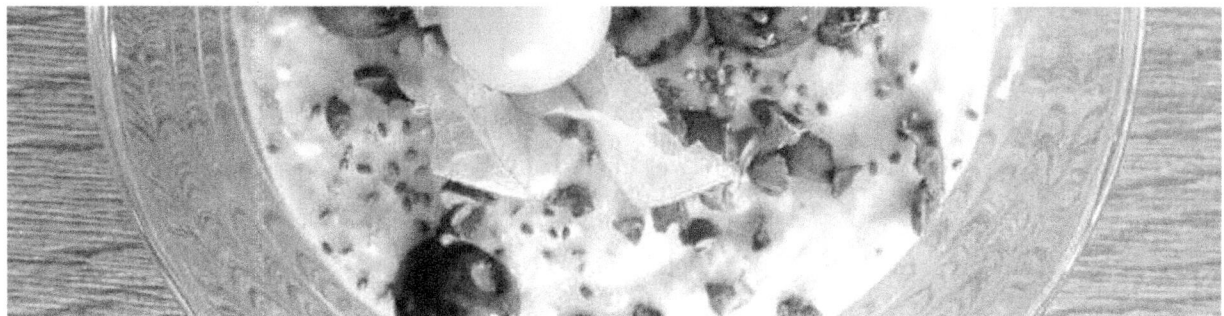

Porridge is equal to a complete meal. It is vegetarian (keto-friendly) and tasty with any kind of topping you like. Simple and an excellent alternative to the same old breakfast. Plus, the right amount of fiber for your keto diet.

Serving quantity: 1

Ingredients:

- 1 ½ cup almond milk, unsweetened
- 3 tbsp. golden flaxseed meal
- 2 tbsp. vanilla flavored vegan or keto protein powder
- 2 tbsp. coconut flour
- calorie-free sweetener, to taste

Directions:

Prep 5 min. | Cook 10 min. | Ready in 15 min.

- Take a bowl and mix golden flaxseed meal, protein powder, and coconut flour.
- Add these to a saucepan.
- Add almond milk and stir and cook on a medium flame.
- Let it thicken and add your favorite sweetener according to your taste.
- Add your favorite toppings and serve.

Nutrition facts:

Per serving: 219 calories | 13 g fat | 18 g protein | 6 g carbs

Peanut Butter Cupcakes

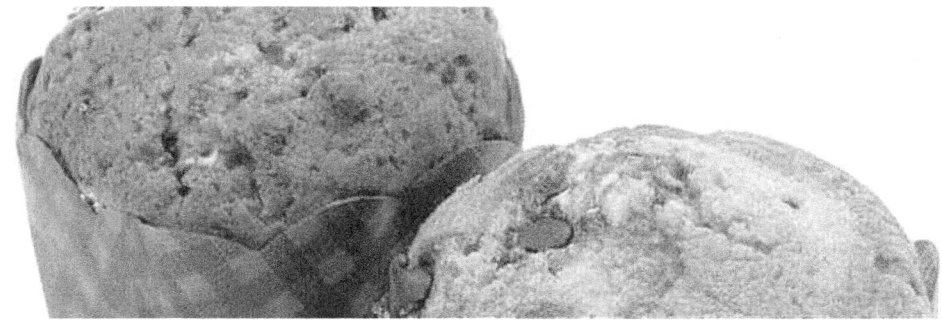

This delicious low-carb peanut butter cupcake will satisfy your sweet cravings and give a nice and lovely start to your day. The sugar-free dark chocolate chips will add a nice flavor to these cakes.

Serving quantity: 6

Ingredients:

- 1/3 cup peanut butter
- 2/3 cup almond flour
- 1/4 cup butter
- 2 eggs
- 2 tsp. baking powder
- keto-friendly sweetener, to taste
- 3 tbsp. sugar-free dark chocolate chips
- 1/2 tsp. vanilla extract
- 1/4 cup water

Directions:

Prep 5 min. | Cook 1 min. | Ready in 6 min.

- Melt butter and peanut butter in a microwave-safe bowl.
- Mix almond flour, baking powder, and sweetener in a separate bowl.
- Add peanut butter mixture, eggs, vanilla extract, and water.
- Mix well. Add the chocolate chips as well.
- Pour the mixture into six mugs or cupcake molds and microwave for 1 minute.

Nutrition facts:

Per Serving: 225 calories | 18 g fat | 7 g protein | 7 g carbs

Coffee And Chia Pudding

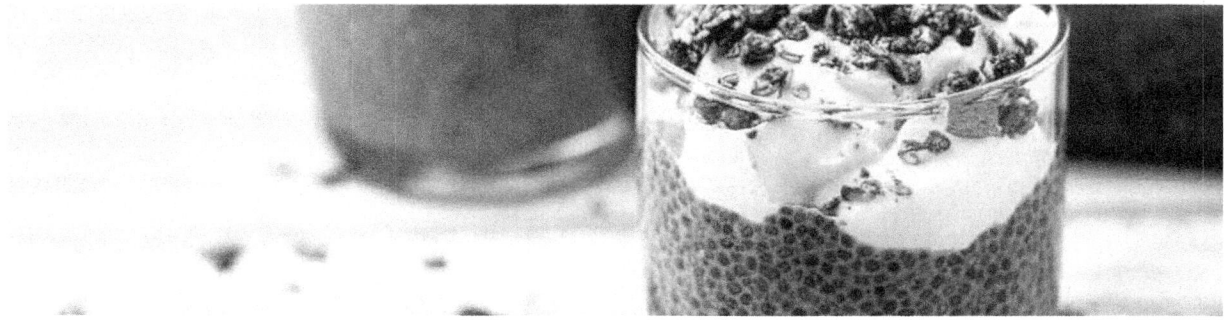

On a keto diet, you need variety, but something is filling and delicious too. With readily available ingredients, put it together to rest overnight and voila! All you need to do is eat it in the morning. It is also rich in fiber content.

Serving quantity: 2

Ingredients:

- 6 oz. full fat coconut milk (unsweetened)
- 6 oz. freshly brewed and cooled coffee
- 4 full tbsp. of chia seeds
- 1 tsp. vanilla paste
- ½ tsp. cinnamon
- keto-friendly sweetener, to taste
- 1 tbsp. almond butter

Directions:

Prep 3 min. | Ready in 3 min.

- Add all the ingredients in a bowl and mix.
- Cover it and put it to refrigerate overnight.
- Dress it with nuts and coconut milk or any dressing of your liking and serve.

Nutrition facts:

Per serving: 301 calories | 24 g fat | 6 g protein | 13 g carbs

Recipes Part 2
KETO BREAKFAST

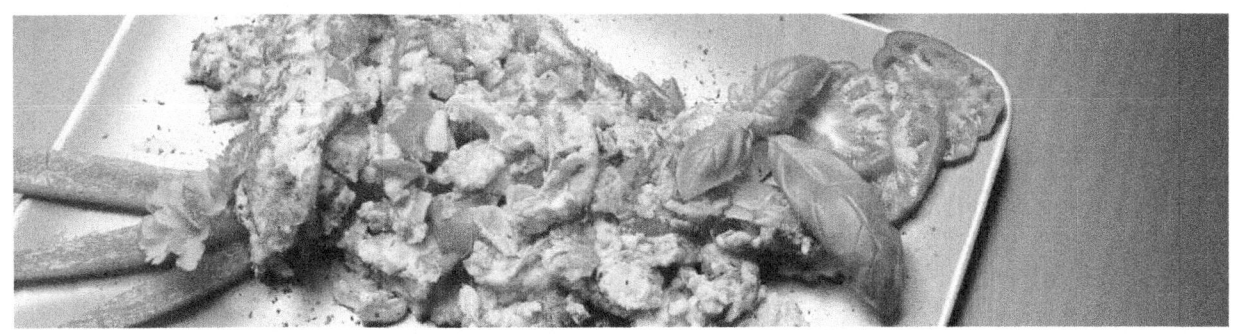

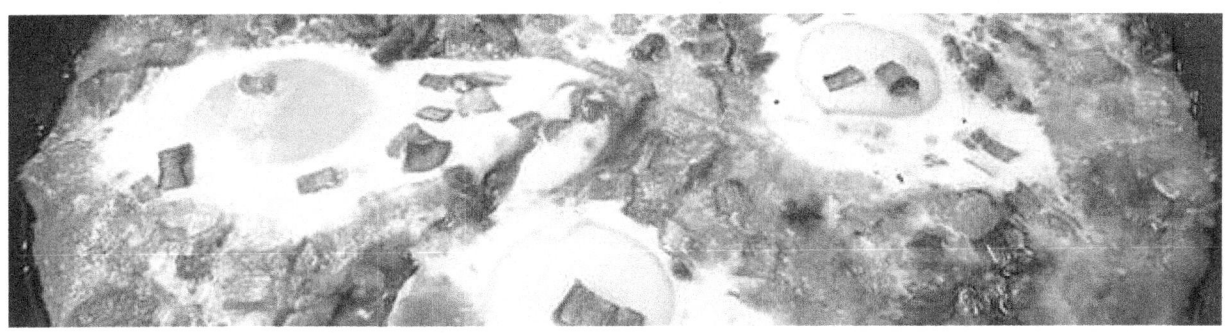

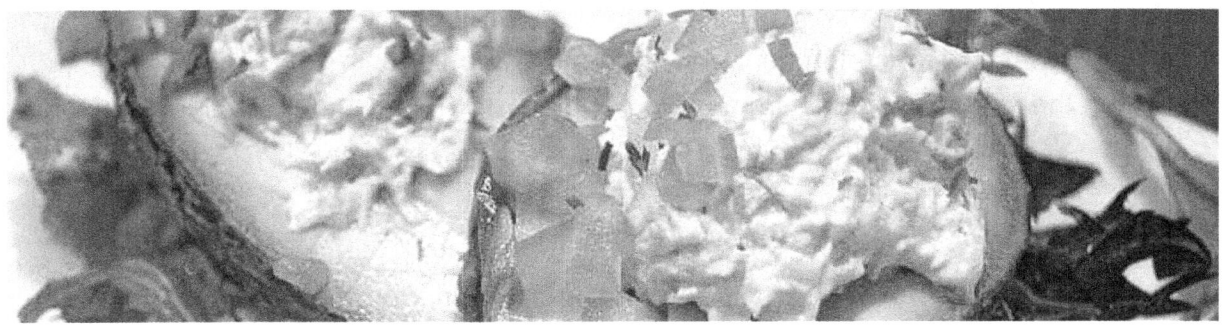

Keto Mushroom Omelet

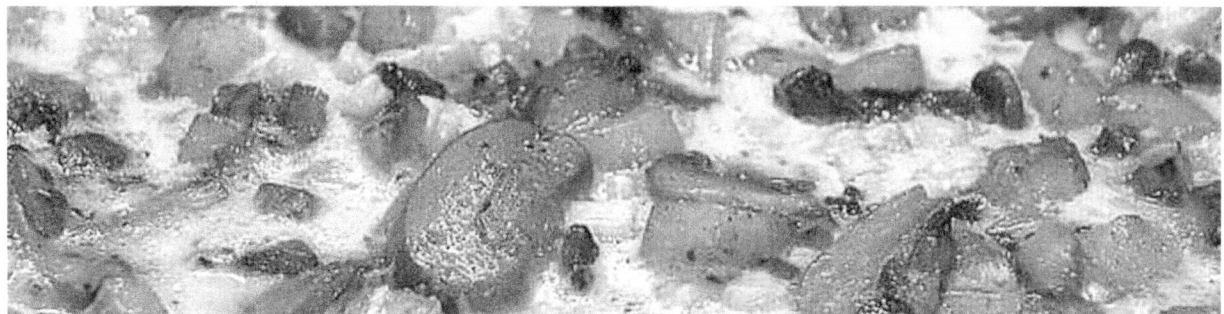

If you want to make a delicious, filling, and leisurely breakfast, this mushroom omelet is everything. It's healthy and takes a few minutes to complete.

Serving quantity: 1

Ingredients:

- 3 eggs
- 1 ounce of butter
- 1 ounce shredded cheese
- 4 mushrooms, sliced
- 1/4 chopped onion
- salt and pepper, to taste

Directions:

Prep 5 min. | Cook 10 min. | Ready in 15 min.

- Crack the eggs in a bowl with some salt and pepper and whisk well.
- Add butter in a pan and fry onions and mushrooms until they are soft.
- Then pour the eggs.
- When the eggs start setting but still raw on top, add the cheese.
- When the egg turns golden from underneath, gently fold it in half and slide onto your plate.

Nutrition facts:

Per Serving: 536 calories | 44 g fat | 26 g protein | 5 g carbs

Baked Cheesy Egg Muffins

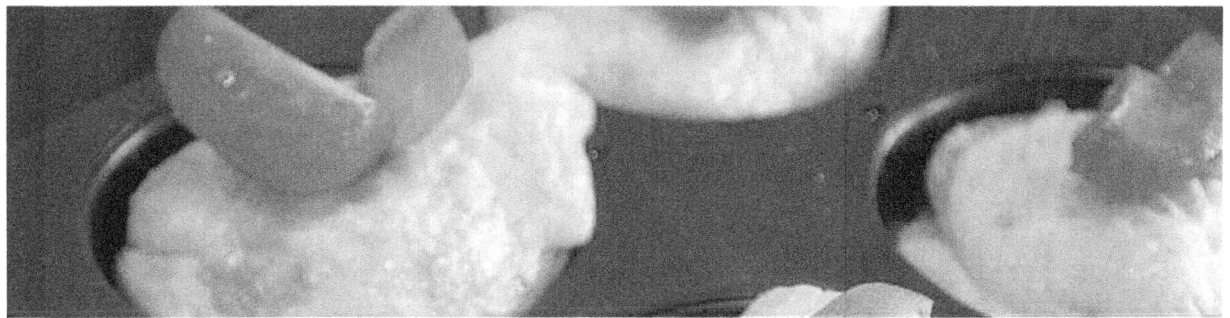

Making a yummy keto-friendly breakfast can become comfortable with this fantastic cheesy egg recipe. So, go for it and serve with a fresh green salad for a little extra boost.

Serving quantity: 6

Ingredients:

- cooking spray
- 12 eggs
- 2/3 cup shredded cheese
- salt and pepper, to taste

Directions:

Prep 5 min. | Cook 15 min. | Ready in 20 min.

- Preheat oven to 350°F.
- Take a muffin pan and use cooking spray.
- Crack your eggs in each cup in the muffin pan and sprinkle with one tablespoon of cheese.
- Bake for 15 minutes. If you want fully cooked yolks, bake for five more minutes.
- Remove the muffin pan from the oven when the eggs are cooked to your liking.
- Remove eggs carefully from the cups and season with a little salt and pepper.

Nutrition facts:

Per Serving: 204 calories | 14 g fat | 16 g protein | 2 g carbs

Vibrant Scrambled Eggs

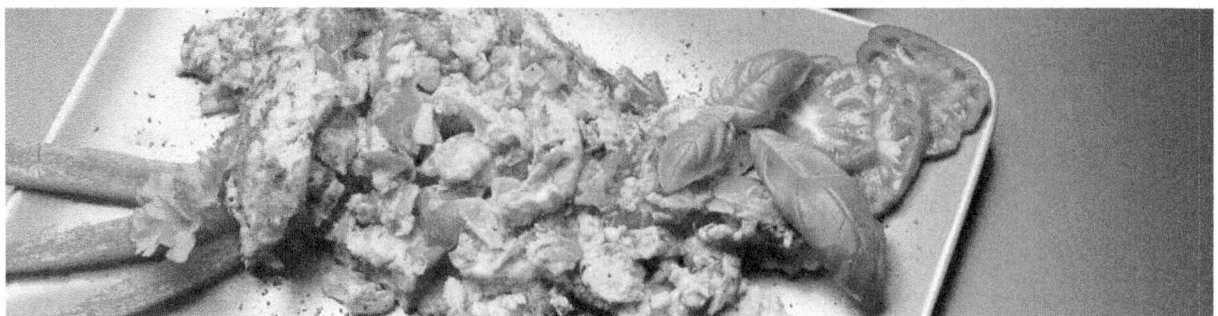

For those who love spice and a color pop in their breakfast, these vibrant scrambled eggs will make your day. Serve with avocado and a little green salad to make it even more popping.

Serving quantity: 4

Ingredients:

- 1 ounce butter
- 1 finely chopped tomato
- 2 pickled jalapenos, chopped
- 1 finely chopped scallion
- 3 ounces shredded cheese
- 6 eggs
- salt and pepper, to taste

Directions:

Prep 5 min. | Cook 10 min. | Ready in 15 min.

- Add butter, tomato, jalapenos, and scallions in a pan.
- Cook for 4 minutes.
- Beat the eggs and pour them into the pan.
- Scramble them for 2 minutes.
- Add cheese along with salt and pepper and mix them a little.
- The scrambled eggs are ready to serve.

Nutrition facts:

Per Serving: 233 calories | 18 g fat | 14 g protein | 2 g carbs

Lettuce Sandwich

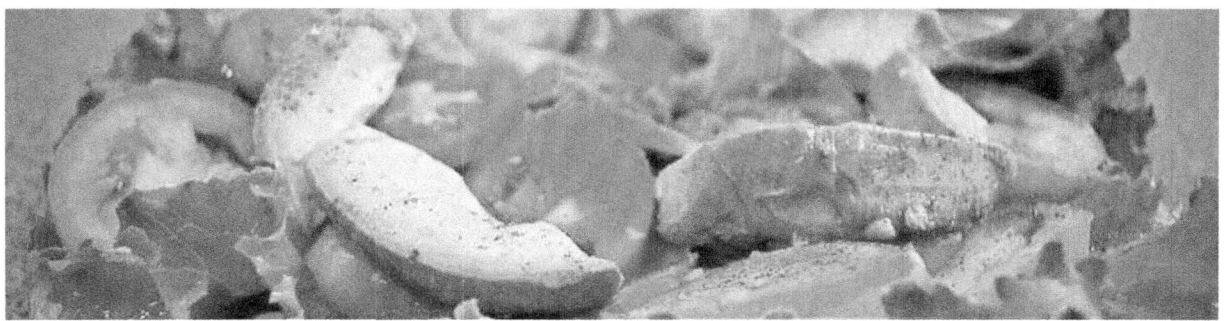

You can use lettuce to make great keto sandwiches. Try this recipe and even play around with other ingredients to make these sandwiches more fun to eat.

Serving quantity: 1

Ingredients:

- 2 ounces romaine lettuce
- 1 ounce butter
- 1 ounce cheese of your choice
- 4 sliced cherry tomatoes
- half sliced avocado

Directions:

Prep 5 min. | Cook 5 min. | Ready in 10 min.

- Wash the lettuce and sliced tomatoes and avocado.
- Spread butter on the lettuce leaves.
- Layer the cheese, tomatoes, and avocado on top.
- Serve like this, or you can even try tuna salad on these lettuce leaves.

Nutrition facts:

Per Serving: 411 calories | 34 g fat | 10 g protein | 5 g carbs

Beefy Baked Eggs

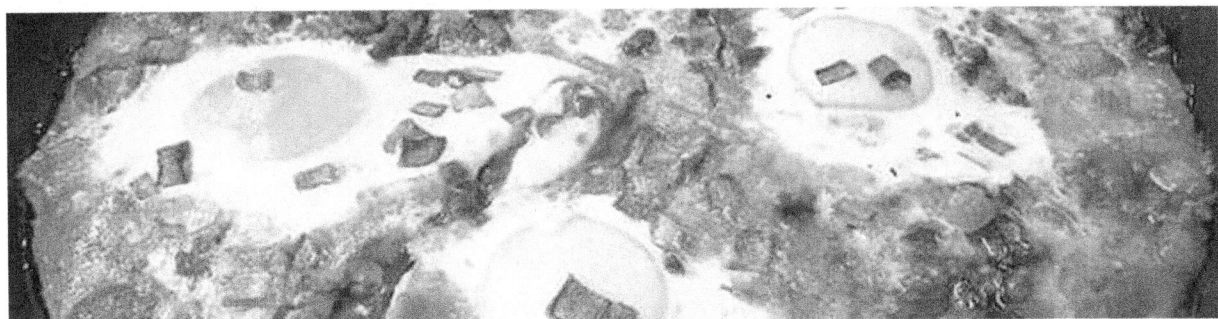

A perfect combination of cooked ground beef with baked eggs is delicious and also packs loads of energy. You can even use the leftover ground beef from dinner to make this mouthwatering and energy-packed breakfast.

Serving quantity: 1

Ingredients:

- 3 ounces cooked ground beef
- 2 eggs
- 2 ounces shredded cheese
- salt and pepper, to taste

Directions:

Prep 5 min. | Cook 10 min. | Ready in 15 min.

- Preheat oven to 400°F.
- Spread the cooked ground beef in a baking dish.
- Make two holes with a spoon and gently crack the eggs in these holes.
- Add cheese on top.
- Bake for 10 minutes or until the eggs are cooked to your liking.
- Serve with fresh salad, herbs, and avocado to enhance the flavor even more.

Nutrition facts:

Per Serving: 502 calories | 35 g fat | 41 g protein | 2 g carbs

Keto Tuna Salad

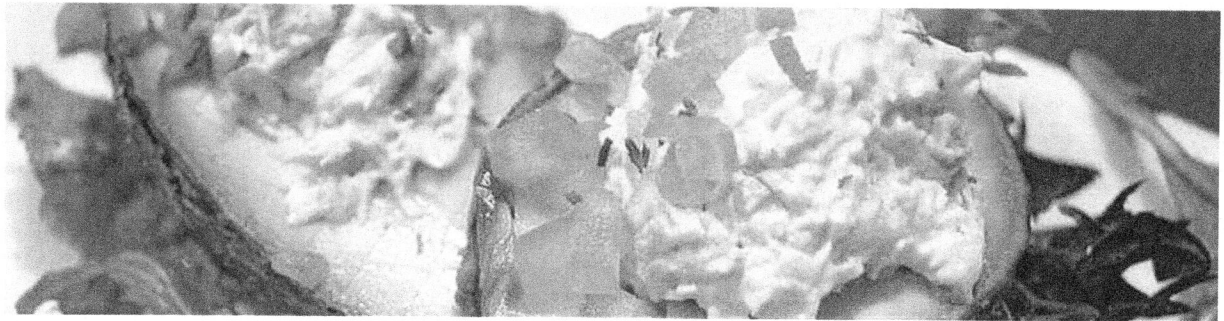

This classic tuna salad with some heat from chili flakes will brighten your mood. Serve on top of boiled eggs or avocado and enjoy this yummy tuna salad.

Serving quantity: 4

Ingredients:

- 4 ounces tuna preserved in olive oil
- 1/2 cup mayonnaise
- 2 tbsp. cream cheese
- finely chopped half leek
- 1 tbsp. capers
- ½ tsp. chili flakes
- salt and pepper, to taste

Directions:

Prep 5 min. | Cook 10 min. | Ready in 15 min.

- Drain the tuna.
- Mix all the ingredients in a bowl.
- Season with salt, pepper, and chili.
- Spread on top of boiled eggs or avocado and enjoy!

Nutrition facts:

Per Serving: 279 calories | 26 g fat | 8 g protein | 1 g carbs

Avocado And Egg Delight

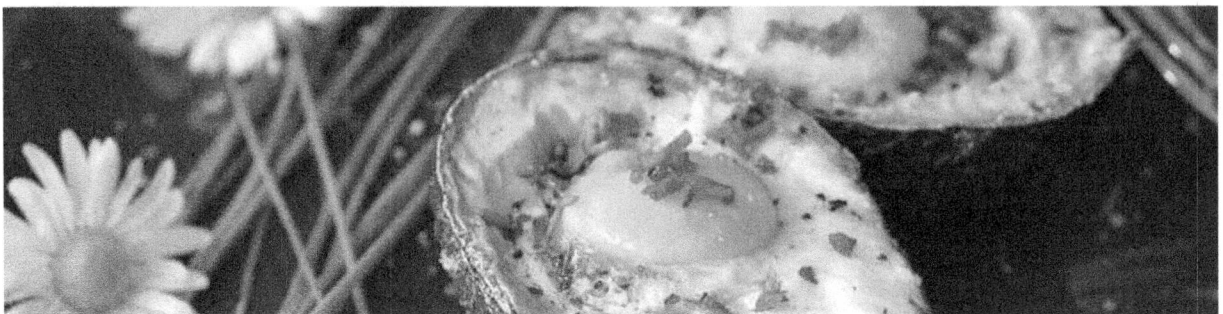

Avocados and eggs are a fantastic match for breakfast. Bake the eggs in avocados, and you are in for a yummy breakfast. Just make sure to use extra-large avocados.

Serving quantity: 4

Ingredients:

- 2 large avocados
- 4 eggs
- salt and pepper, to taste

Directions:

Prep 5 min. | Cook 20 min. | Ready in 25 min.

- Preheat oven to 400° F.
- Cut the avocados in half and take out the pits.
- Scoop out some of the flesh and keep it for later use.
- Arrange the avocados in a baking dish, sprinkle a little salt and pepper, and gently crack an egg inside each avocado.
- Season the egg with a bit more salt and pepper.
- You can even use fresh herbs and cheese for seasoning.
- Bake for 15-20 minutes.
- Remove from oven when eggs are cooked.
- Serve hot with creamy unsweetened coffee and enjoy.

Nutrition facts:

Per Serving: 268 calories | 20 g fat | 9 g protein | 11 g carbs

Egg Salad

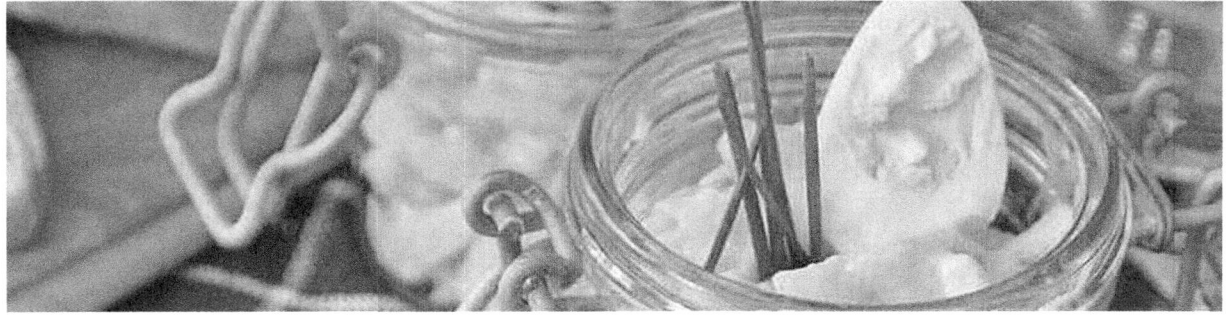

It is easy to make with the ingredients at hand. Simple, delicious, fresh, and filling at the same time.

Serving quantity: 1

Ingredients:

- 6 peeled and chopped hard-boiled eggs
- 1 cubed avocado
- 3 tbsp. mayonnaise
- 2 tsp. lemon juice
- 1 tbsp. chopped chives
- freshly ground pepper, to taste
- salt, to taste
- lettuce

Directions:

Prep time 15 min. | Ready in 25 min.

- Whisk mayonnaise, lemon juice, salt, and pepper in a bowl.
- Add eggs and avocado and mix properly.
- Serve it with lettuce and sprinkle fresh herbs.

Nutrition facts:

Per serving: 278 calories | 25 g fat | 9 g protein | 2 g carbs

Classic Bacon And Eggs

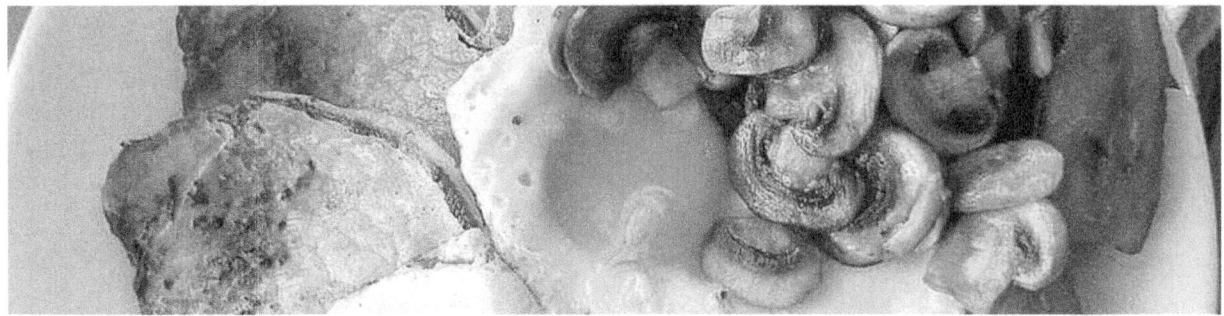

It is a classic, popular, and delicious breakfast made in a keto-friendly way. It uses simple ingredients and is easy to cook and smells heavenly when it is ready!

Serving quantity: 4

Ingredients:

- 8 eggs
- 5 ounces sliced bacon
- cherry tomatoes (optional)
- salt and pepper, to taste

Directions:

Prep 2 min. | Cook 8 min. | Ready in 10 min.

- Sauté the bacon on medium-high heat till it is crispy and golden.
- Set it aside on a plate.
- Use the bacon oil for cooking eggs.
- Cook eggs however you like.
- Add in cherry tomatoes to fry them at the same time.
- Add salt and pepper to taste.
- Serve on a plate along with anything you like, such as mushrooms.

Nutrition facts:

Per serving: 270 calories | 22 g fat | 15 g protein | 1 g carbs

Asparagus And Poached Eggs

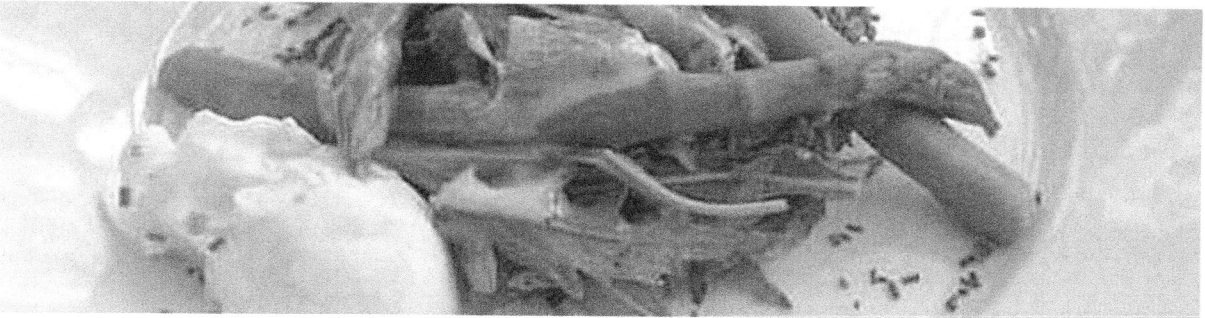

This recipe is simple but full of flavor. The poached eggs compliment the asparagus very well.

Serving quantity: 2

Ingredients:

- 2 eggs
- ½ cup boiling water, more for eggs
- 6 ounces asparagus
- 3 ounces butter
- a squeeze of lime
- salt and pepper, to taste

Directions:

Prep. 10 min. | Cook 20 min. | Ready in 30 min.

- Heat the frying pan at high heat and make sure it becomes scorching.
- Put the asparagus in the pan and cook one side till it changes color.
- Boil water in a separate large pot.
- When you turn over the asparagus, pour ½ cup of boiling water over it.
- Use the additional boiling water to poach your fresh eggs.
- Let the asparagus cook in the water till it evaporates.
- Add in a lump of butter and cook the asparagus for 30 seconds.
- Dish out your asparagus along with the butter from the pan and place the slightly soft-centered poached eggs on top after draining them.
- Season them with salt and pepper or lemon juice as you like.

Nutrition facts:

Per serving: 168 calories | 15 g fat | 4 g protein | 3 g carbs

Frittata With Spinach

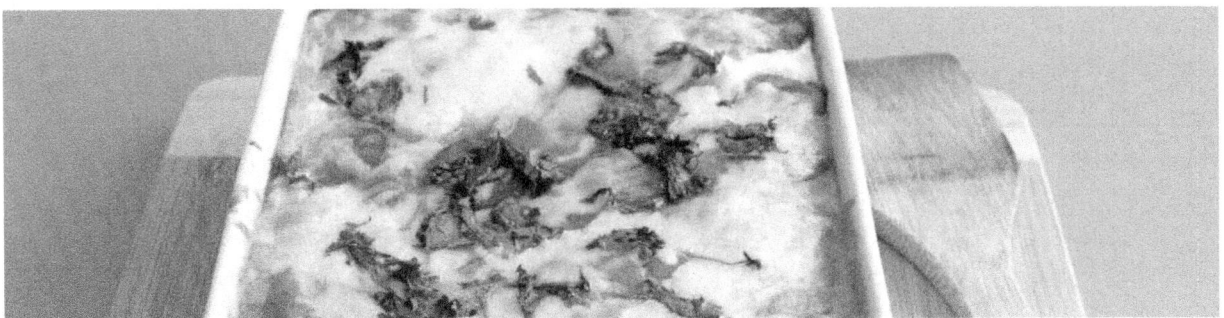

Combine eggs with healthy and fresh spinach, cream, cheese, and bacon. You would absolutely love it. This simple recipe is very delicious and comforting.

Serving quantity: 4

Ingredients:

- 8 eggs
- 5 ounces bacon, diced or chorizo
- 2 tbsp. butter
- 8 ounces fresh spinach
- 5 ounces cheese, shredded
- 1 cup heavy whipping cream
- salt and pepper, to taste

Directions:

Prep 10 min. | Cook 35 min. | Ready in 45 min.

- Preheat the oven at 350°F and grease a baking dish.
- Put butter in a frying pan and fry bacon on medium flame until crispy golden.
- Add spinach and cook till it sags.
- Set the pan aside.
- Crack the eggs in a separate bowl.
- Add cream and whisk them together.
- Add the egg mixture in the baking dish.
- Add the spinach, bacon, and cheese on top and put the dish in the oven.
- Bake for 25 to 30 minutes till it is golden brown on top and cooked in the middle.

Nutrition facts:

Per serving: 676 calories | 59 g fat | 27 g protein | 4 g carbs

Keto Bread

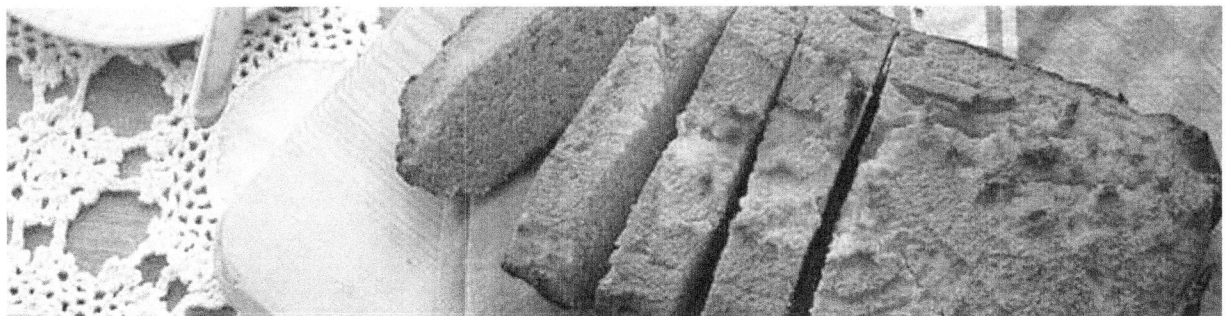

Keto diet is hard to maintain if you miss your bread but don't worry, this keto bread is made from almond flour. Besides, nothing is heartier than a healthy, homemade, delicious bread.

Serving quantity: 1 bread

Ingredients:

- 1 tbsp. baking powder
- 1/2 tsp. salt
- 6 eggs
- 1 ½ cup almond flour
- ¼ cup butter
- ½ tsp. cream of tartar

Directions:

Prep 10 min | Bake 30 min. | Ready in 1 hour 10 min.

- Preheat the oven at 375° F and put parchment paper in an 8 x 4 loaf pan.
- Separate the egg whites and yolks.
- Beat the egg whites and the cream of tartar in a separate bowl till it forms white peaks.
- Add egg yolks, almond flour, melted butter, baking powder, and salt and beat with the hand mixer until smooth.
- Fold in 1/3 of the egg white mixture first, mix, and fold in the remaining.
- Add the batter in the loaf pan and smooth the top.
- Let it cook for 30 minutes till golden crust forms.
- Let it cool for 30 minutes afterward.
- Cut into slices and serve warm and fresh.

Nutrition facts:

Per serving: 491 calories | 40 g fat | 19 g protein | 10 g carbs

Sausage And Cheese Casserole

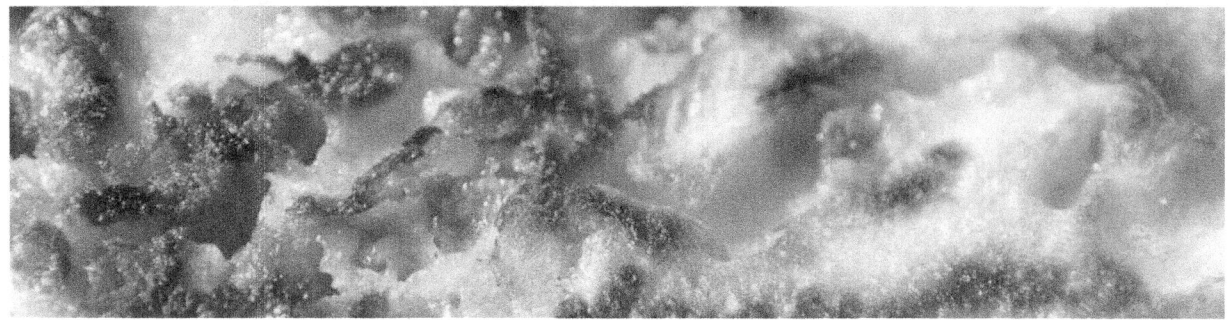

There are only four ingredients in this recipe, and it's so easy to make. The combination of cheese, sausage, and eggs are unusual, and you will be full for a long time.

Serving quantity: 8

Ingredients:

- 6 eggs
- 2 cups shredded cheddar cheese
- 1 pound breakfast sausage
- 1 can crescent rolls

Directions:

Prep 15 min. | Cook 30 min. | Ready in 45 min.

- Preheat oven to 350°F.
- Spray a baking dish with cooking spray.
- Fry sausage in a pan.
- Spread crescent rolls at the bottom of the dish.
- Arrange sausage, pour beaten eggs, and finally top with cheese.
- Bake for 30 minutes.

Nutrition facts:

Per Serving: 279 calories | 19 g fat | 12 g protein | 13 g carbs

Salmon And Asparagus Frittata

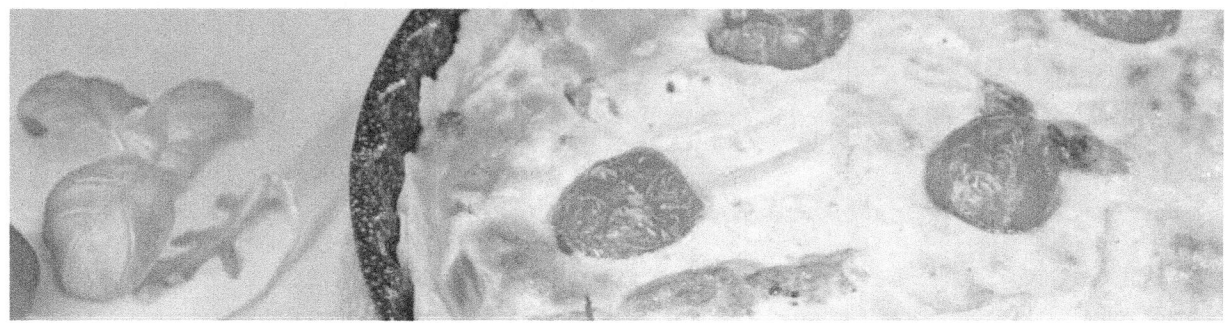

If you are looking forward to making a fantastic breakfast or brunch over the weekend, this salmon and asparagus frittata will impress your family. It's delicious, creamy, and fresh!

Serving quantity: 4

Ingredients:

- 3 ½ ounces smoked salmon
- 3 ½ ounces fresh asparagus
- 8 eggs
- 2 ounces shredded parmesan cheese
- 3 ½ ounces shredded mozzarella
- 1 cup heavy whipping cream
- ½ ounce butter
- salt and pepper, to taste
- 1 tbsp. dried dill

Directions:

Prep 10 min. | Cook 30 min. | Ready in 40 min.

- Preheat oven to 350°F.
- Beat eggs in a large bowl.
- Add the seasonings, cream, parmesan, and half of the mozzarella cheese.
- Grease an 8-inch baking dish with butter.
- Arrange the salmon in the dish.
- Then add chopped asparagus.
- Finally, add the egg mixture and cover it with the rest of the mozzarella.
- Bake for 30 minutes.

Nutrition facts:

Per Serving: 531 calories | 43 g fat | 29 g protein | 4 g carbs

Veggie Scramble

This veggie scramble is an excellent choice if you want a simple vegetarian breakfast.

Serving quantity: 1

Ingredients:

- 3 eggs
- 1 ounce sliced mushrooms
- half scallion, chopped
- 1 ounce diced red bell peppers
- 1 ounce shredded parmesan cheese
- 1 tbsp. butter
- salt and pepper, to taste

Directions:

Prep 5 min. | Cook 15 min. | Ready in 20 min.

- Melt butter in a large pan over medium heat.
- Add bell pepper, mushrooms, salt, and pepper.
- Cook until the veggies are tender.
- Add the eggs and mix well.
- Cook till the eggs are set but don't overcook them.
- Dress with scallions and cheese.

Nutrition facts:

Per Serving: 420 calories | 31 g fat | 28 g protein | 4 g carbs

Scrambled Tofu

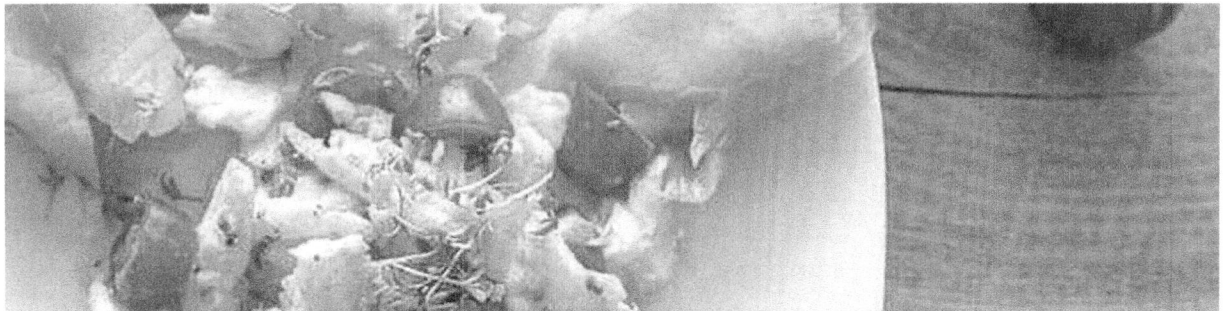

Go for scrambled tofu if you want something simple and full of flavor. The eggs can get boring sometimes so that this breakfast will give you that much-needed change along with extra proteins.

Serving quantity: 2

Ingredients:

- 13 ounces tofu
- 3/4 cup unsweetened almond milk
- 1 tbsp. yeast
- 1/4 tbsp. turmeric
- salt and pepper, to taste
- 1 tbsp. finely chopped chives

Directions:

Prep 5 min. | Cook 15 min. | Ready in 20 min.

- Start cooking tofu in a non-stick pan.
- Add yeast and turmeric and cook for 5 minutes.
- Pour the almond milk and let it simmer for 10 minutes.
- Season with salt and pepper and garnish with chives.

Nutrition facts:

Per Serving: 310 calories | 17 g fat | 35 g protein | 2 g carbs

Tomato And Spinach Muffins

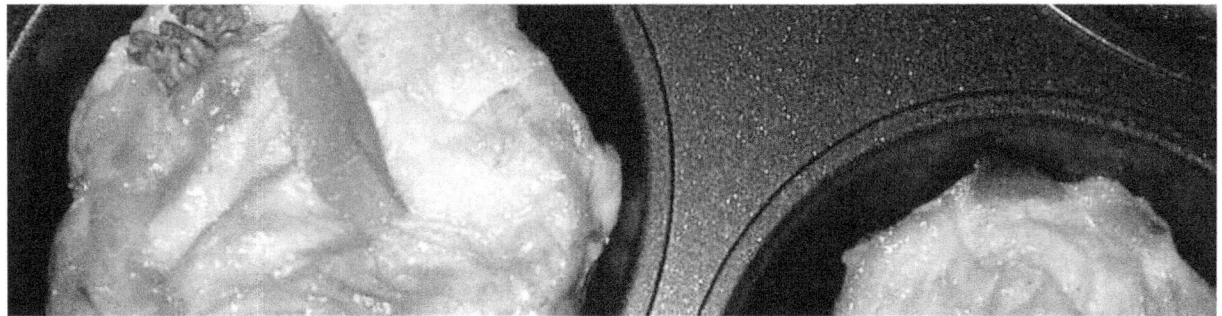

These cute little muffins pack the flavors from spinach, tomatoes, eggs, and cheese. You'll love them with coffee and even pack some for lunch.

Serving quantity: 6

Ingredients:

- 6 eggs
- 1/2 cup diced tomatoes
- 1/2 cup chopped baby spinach
- 1/4 cup diced onion
- ½ cup shredded cheddar cheese

Directions:

Prep 15 min. | Bake 25 min. | Ready in 40 min.

- Preheat oven to 350°F.
- Grease a muffin pan.
- Beat eggs in a large bowl, then add in the rest of the ingredients.
- Pour the egg mixture in 6 muffin cups.
- Bake for 25 minutes.
- Let them cool for 2 minutes and serve.

Nutrition facts:

Per Serving: 120 calories | 8 g fat | 8 g protein | 3 g carbs

Keto Smoked Salmon And Egg Butter

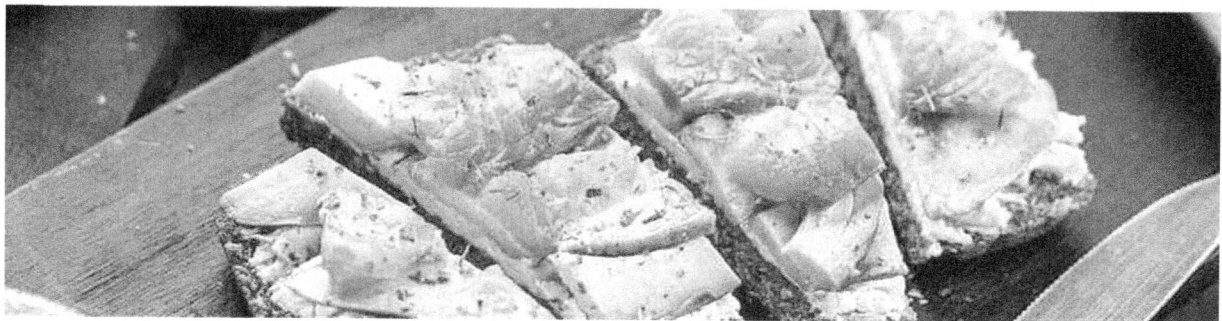

A healthy and nutritious meal capable of sustaining you for a long time and keto-friendly on top of that! It has eggs, avocado, and smoked salmon; very easy to put together and it's full of healthy fats and protein.

Serving quantity: 2

Ingredients:

- 4 eggs
- 2 avocados
- 4 ounces smoked salmon
- 5 ounces butter
- 2 tbsp. olive oil
- ½ tsp. of sea salt (or to taste)
- ¼ tsp. ground black pepper
- 1 tbsp. fresh parsley

Directions:

Prep 5 min. | Cook 15 min. | Ready in 20 min.

- Put the eggs in a pot and add cold water to cover the eggs.
- Let the water boil without the lid.
- Lower the flame and let the eggs simmer for 7 to 8 minutes.
- Drain the hot water and place them in ice-cold water to cool.
- Peel and cut them into pieces.
- Add butter and mix using a fork.
- Add salt and pepper per taste or any other seasoning of your preference.
- Toss the diced avocados in olive oil and finely chop the fresh parsley.
- Serve them along with the butter eggs and a few slices of smoked salmon.

Nutrition facts:

Per serving: 1169 calories | 112 g fats | 26 g protein | 5 g carbs

Keto Egg Casserole

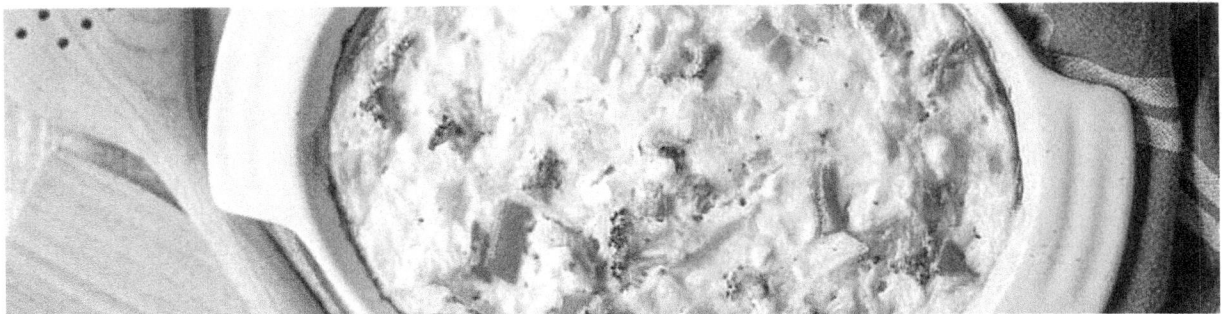

This version of egg casserole includes ham, ricotta cheese, and spinach. You can add a variety of things inside, and it will taste good anyway. It is an easy and filling breakfast meal.

Serving quantity: 15

Ingredients:

- 12 eggs
- ½ yellow onion
- 9 ounces spinach, well-drained
- 1 cup ricotta cheese
- ¼ cup heavy whipping cream
- 1 pound ham, diced
- ¼ tsp. salt
- ½ tbsp. garlic and herb seasoning

Directions:

Prep 10 min. | Cook 35 min. | Ready in 45 min.

- Preheat the oven up to 350°F first and then chop the yellow onion.
- Put four eggs, ricotta, cream, and onions in a blender and blend until smooth.
- Set it aside.
- Take a separate bowl and whisk together the rest of the eggs.
- Add the blended mixture and whisk it all together.
- Add the salt and seasoning and whisk again.
- Fold in the spinach and ham in the eggs.
- Spray a baking dish of 9x13 and pour the egg mixture into it.
- Let it cook for 30 to 35 minutes till a golden crust forms.

Nutrition facts:

Per serving: 153 calories | 9 g fats | 15 g protein | 2 g carbs

Breakfast Salad

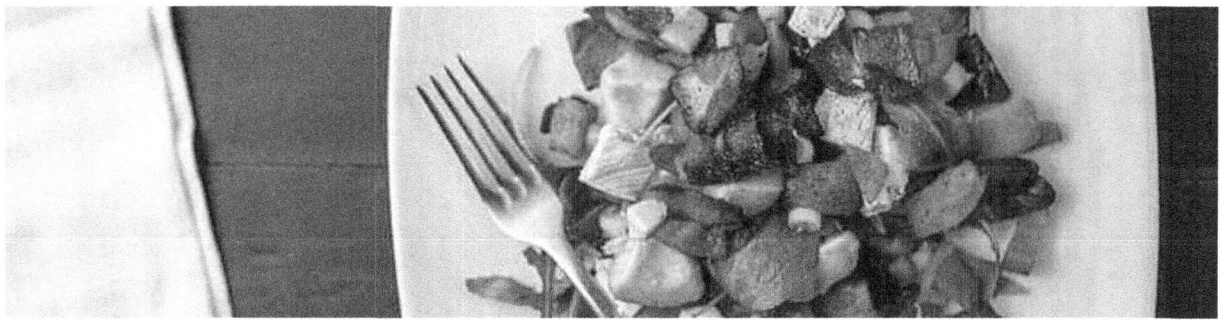

The salad is so fresh and so light, and it doesn't need much effort to prepare. It includes fruits, protein, and fiber, making it a very healthy and delicious keto breakfast.

Serving quantity: 6

Ingredients:

- 9 ounces cherry tomatoes
- 3 rashes of bacon, cut in half
- 6 cup wild rocket, rinsed and dried
- 1 peeled avocado, seed removed and thinly sliced
- a bunch of coarsely chopped chives
- ½ cup whole egg mayonnaise
- 1 bulb of garlic (to taste)
- 2 tbsp. olive oil & 2 tbsp. lemon juice

Directions:

Prep 15 min. | Cook 30 min. | Ready in 45 min.

- Preheat the oven at 475°F and place the cherry tomatoes in a tray.
- Put olive oil and season with salt and pepper.
- Cook for 7 to 8 minutes. Take them out and let them cool.
- Wrap garlic in a foil and place it in the oven for 20 minutes to cook.
- Take it out and cut it. Squeeze its pulp in a bowl and throw the skin away.
- Use the remaining oil to fry the bacon over medium-high heat in a nonstick pan.
- Cook for 2 to 3 minutes until golden and crispy from both sides.
- Remove and transfer on a plate.
- Add mayonnaise, lemon juice, and garlic in a food processor and blend until smooth paste forms. Add salt and pepper to taste.
- Mix avocado, bacon, tomatoes, and rocket in a bowl.
- Sprinkle chives, add the dressing, and serve.

Nutrition facts:

Per serving: 332 calories | 30 g fat | 7 g protein | 6 g carbs

Recipes PART 3
KETO SMOOTHIE

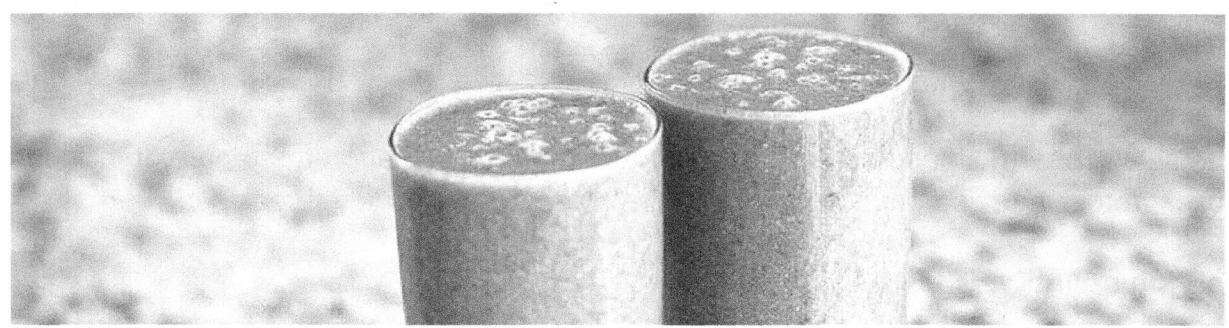

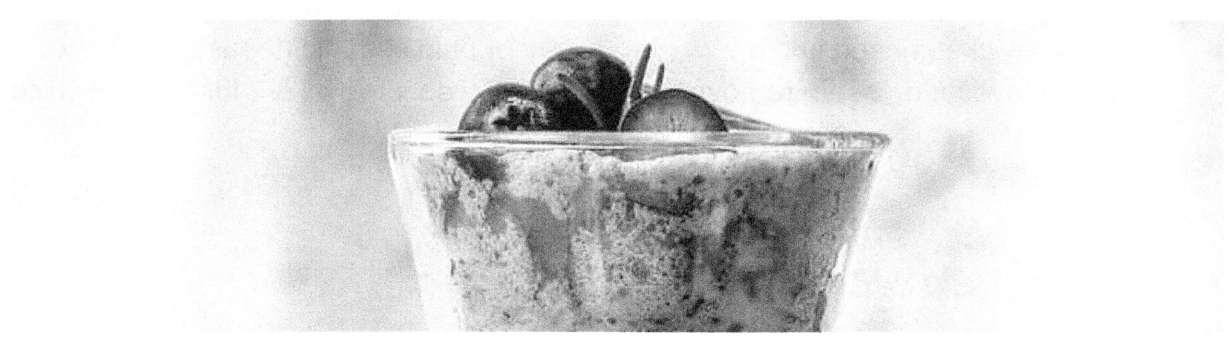

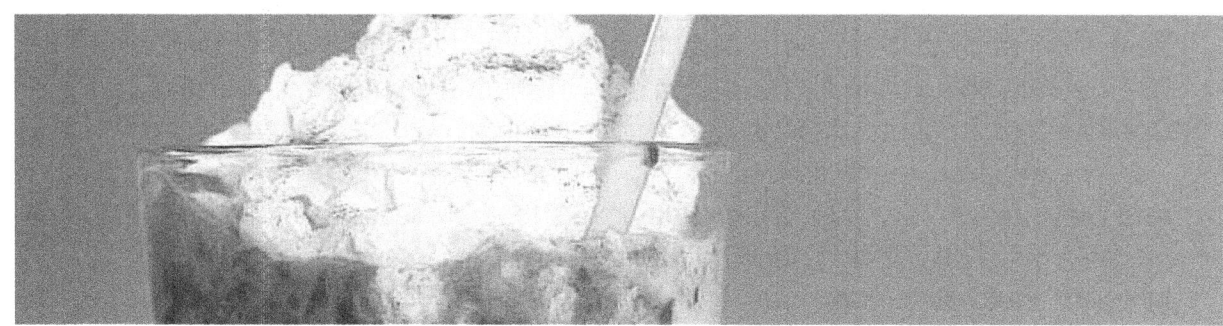

Spinach And Ginger Smoothie

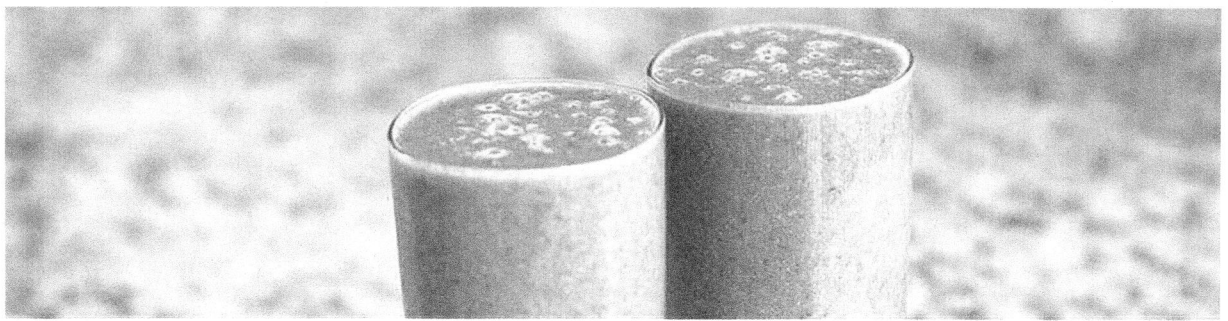

Smoothies are great for taking along with you when you are in a hurry. This low-carb green smoothie is full of nutrients, and it's also good for your stomach.

Serving quantity: 2

Ingredients:

- 1/3 cup unsweetened coconut milk
- 2 tbsp. lime juice
- 1 ounce frozen spinach
- 2 tsp. grated ginger
- 2/3 cup water

Directions:

Prep 5 min. | Blending 1 min. | Ready in 6 min.

- Add all ingredients to the blender, except lime juice.
- First, add 1 tablespoon of lime juice, then add more according to your taste.
- Blend until everything is smooth.
- Top with fresh ginger and enjoy the natural flavors.

Nutrition facts:

Per serving: 91 calories | 8 g fats | 1 g protein | 3 g carbs

Blueberry Smoothie

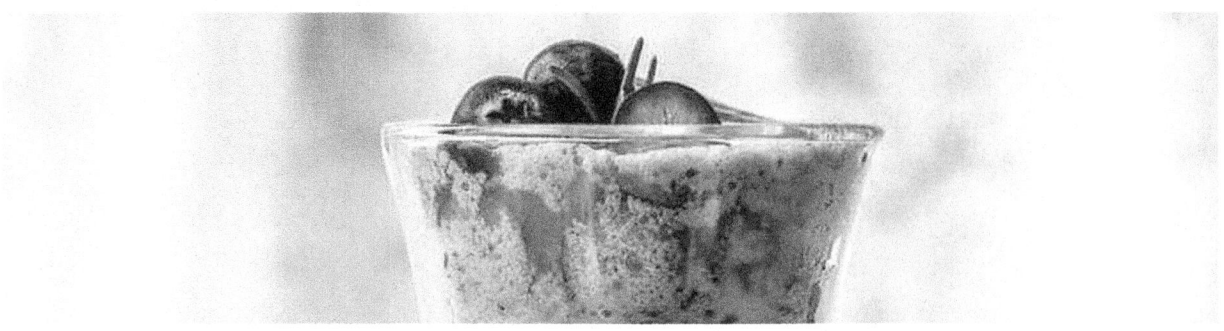

Fresh and flavorful! This blueberry smoothie combines the beautiful flavors of coconut milk, vanilla extract, lemon, coconut milk, and blueberries. You are going to love it!

Serving quantity: 2

Ingredients:

- 14 ounces unsweetened coconut milk
- 3 ounces of blueberries
- ½ tsp. vanilla extract
- 1 tbsp. lemon juice
- keto-friendly sweetener, to taste

Directions:

Prep 5 min. | Blending 1 min. | Ready in 6 min.

- Blend all the ingredients until smooth.
- Shake well and enjoy the fresh taste.

Nutrition facts:

Per serving: 457 calories | 43 g fats | 4 g protein | 10 g carbs

Keto Chocolate Smoothie

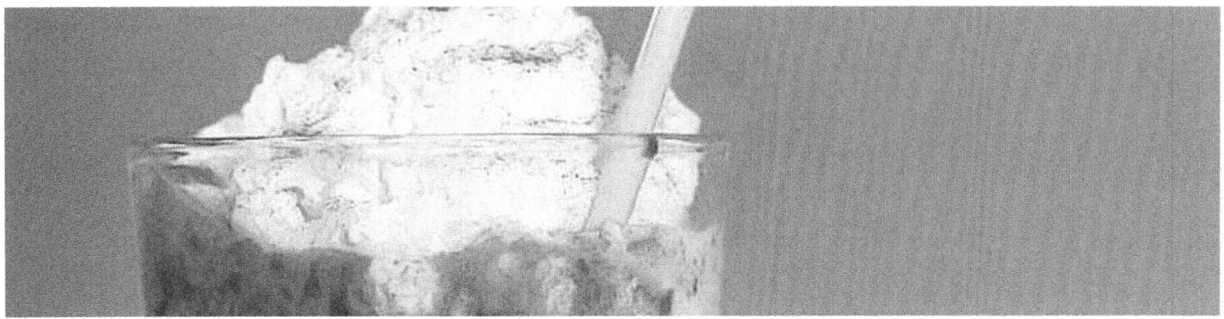

For a hasty morning, try this smoothie because it only takes five minutes. All you have to do is throw the ingredients in a blender and you will have a glass ready of the delicious drink.

Serving quantity: 1

Ingredients:

- 1 tbsp. cocoa powder, unsweetened
- 1 tbsp. flax meal
- 1 tbsp. almond butter
- 1 tsp. coconut oil
- ½ avocado
- 1¼ cup almond milk, unsweetened
- ¼ cups whipped cream
- liquid stevia or sweetener, to taste

Directions:

Prep 5 min. | Blend 5 min. | Ready in 10 min.

- Put the ingredients in a blender and puree until smooth.
- Pour it in a glass and top it with the whipped cream and cocoa nibs if you wish and serve.

Nutrition facts:

Per serving: 599 calories | 56 g fats | 11 g protein | 8 g carbs

Turmeric Keto Smoothie

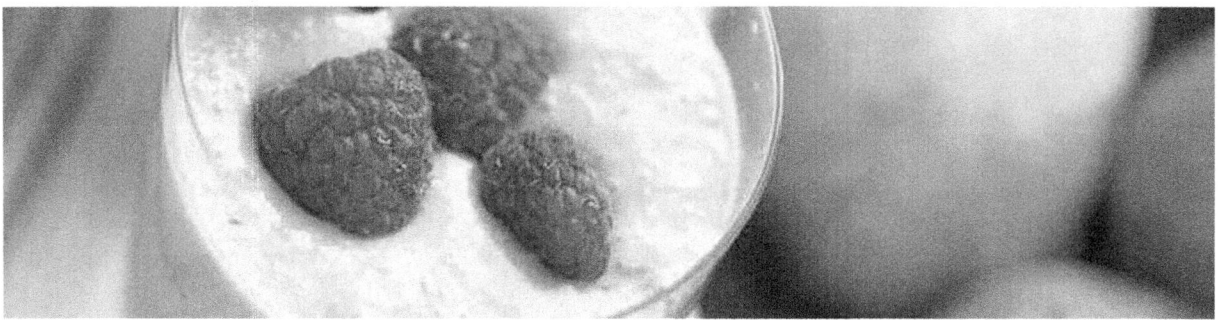

Turmeric is a healthy anti-inflammatory and antioxidant spice. Put it in a smoothie and boom! It is addicting to taste and attractive, looking for its bright yellow color.

Serving quantity: 1

Ingredients:

- 1 tbsp. ground turmeric
- 1 tbsp. ground ginger
- 1 tbsp. ground cinnamon
- 1 tbsp. chia seeds
- 1 tbsp. MCT oil, or coconut oil
- 1 cup almond milk, unsweetened
- 1 cup coconut milk, full fat
- keto-friendly sweetener, to taste

Directions:

Prep 2 min. | Blend 3 min. | Ready in 5 min.

- Put the ingredients and ice in the blender and blend until smooth.
- Sprinkle chia seeds as dressing and serve.

Nutritional facts:

Per serving: 602 calories | 56 g fats | 7 g protein | 6 g carbs

Avocado Smoothie

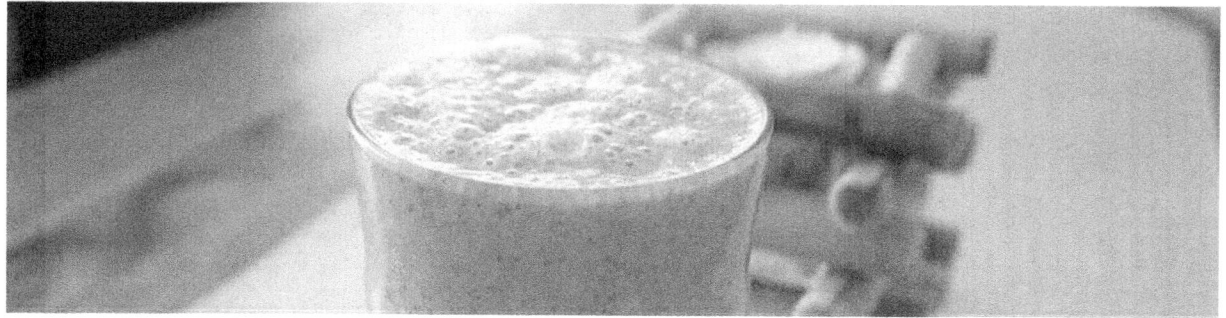

Avocado is an excellent fruit for keto dieters because of its healthy fats and nutrients. Mix it with some other healthy ingredients to make a keto-friendly smoothie you will love.

Serving quantity: 2

Ingredients:

- 1 avocado
- ½ of cucumber
- 1 cup spinach
- 1 celery stalk, chopped
- 1 tbsp. lime juice
- 1 cup of unsweetened coconut milk
- ¼ cup of water
- 2 tbsp. coconut oil
- ¼ tsp. turmeric
- salt, pepper, or sweetener, to taste

Directions:

Prep 5 min. | Blend 5 min. | Ready in 10 min.

- Blend all ingredients until smooth.
- Adjust the thickness by adding more water or coconut milk.
- Pour in glasses and enjoy.

Nutrition facts:

Per serving: 641 calories | 57 g fats | 6 g protein | 21 g carbs

Coffee Smoothie

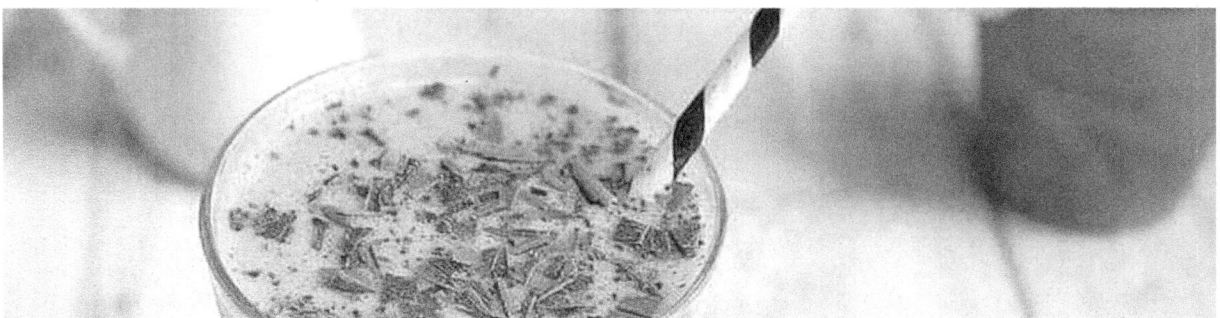

This coffee smoothie will definitely wake you up in the morning because it has the caffeine boost you need when you start your day. It is also delicious and easy to make.

Serving quantity: 1

Ingredients:

- ½ cup of chilled coffee
- ½ cup of coconut milk
- ¼ cup of frozen yogurt
- ¼ cup crushed ice
- 1 pinch ground cinnamon
- 1 tbsp. ground flaxseed

Directions:

Prep 5 min. | Blend 5 min. | Ready in 10 min.

- Blend all ingredients, pour in a glass
- Garnish with some ground cinnamon.

Nutrition facts:

Per serving: 361 calories | 26 g fats | 10 g protein | 19 g carbs

Spinach And Raspberry Smoothie

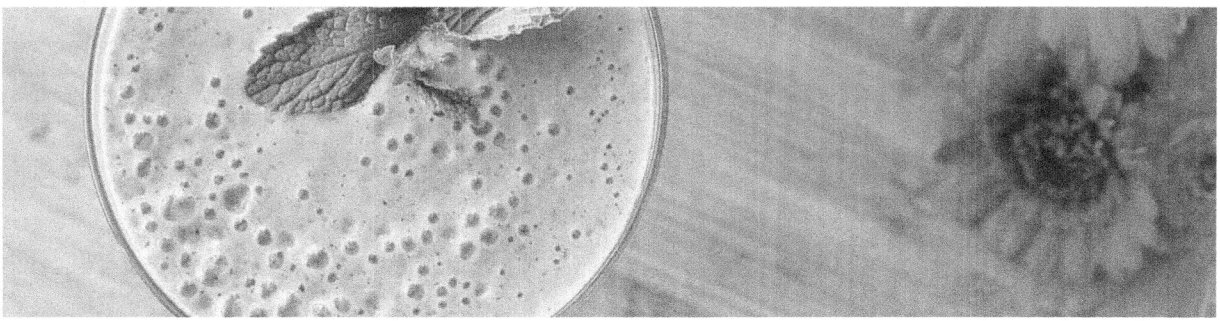

This smoothie is best for drinking after a workout not just because of the spinach and raspberries used in it but because it also gives you a protein boost.

Serving quantity: 1

Ingredients:

- 1 cup spinach
- ¾ cup raspberries
- 1 cup unsweetened almond milk (coconut milk)
- 1 scoop plant-based protein powder
- 2 tbsp. coconut oil
- Ice cubes
- salt, pepper, or sweetener, to taste

Directions:

Prep 5 min. | Blend 1 min. | Ready in 6 min.

- Pop all ingredients into the blender and blend for about a minute.
- Add ice cubes and pour into a bottle to take with you.

Nutrition facts:

Per serving: 420 calories | 31 g fats | 12 g protein | 20 g carbs

Chocolate Almond Smoothie

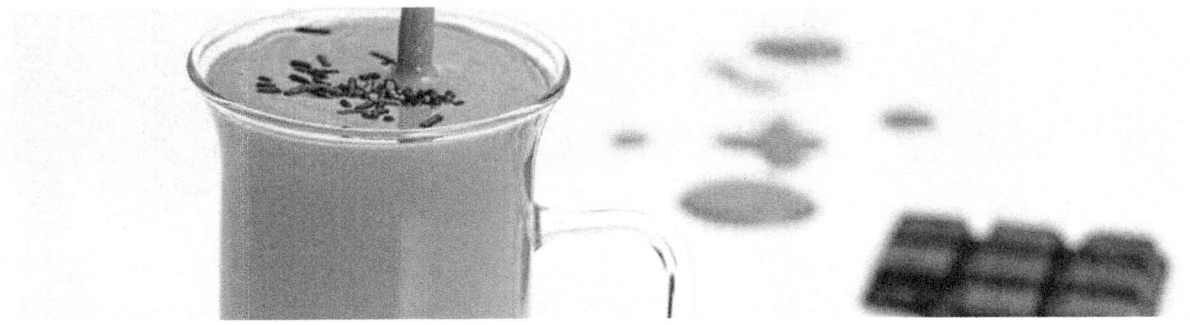

If you crave something sweet and chocolatey, this flavorful and energy-packed smoothie is what you should try to satisfy your craving without compromising on your diet.

Serving quantity: 1

Ingredients:

- 1 cup almond milk
- ¼ cup almond butter
- 2 tbsp. raw cacao powder
- 1 scoop of (vanilla) whey protein powder
- keto-friendly sweetener, to taste

Directions:

Prep 5 min. | Blend 2 min. | Ready in 7 min.

- Add all ingredients to a blender and blend for 2 minutes.
- Serve chilled and enjoy.

Nutrition facts:

Per serving: 535 calories | 39 g fats | 35 g protein | 7 g carbs

Avocado And Cucumber Smoothie

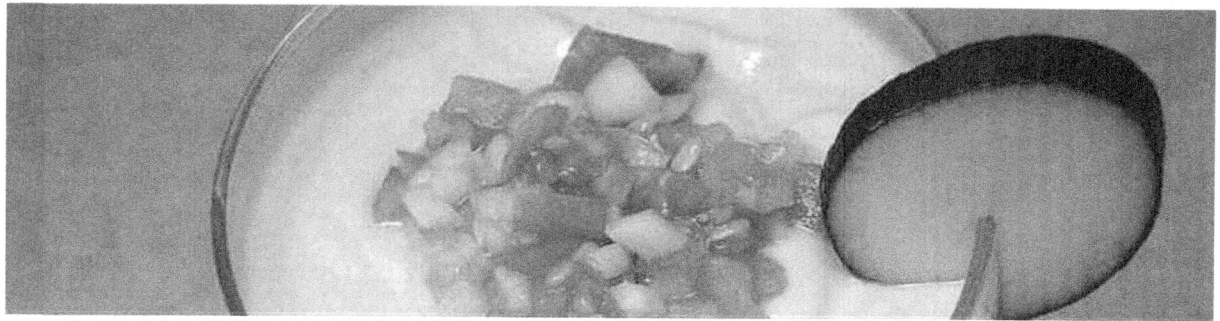

If you want something refreshing and low calorie during the day, this avocado and cucumber smoothie will freshen you up. Made with only 6 ingredients, you can easily make it any time and enjoy this amazing smoothie.

Serving quantity: 1

Ingredients:

- 1 avocado
- 1 cucumber
- 1 lime
- ½ cup cilantro
- 1 pinch of salt
- ½ cup water

Directions:

Prep 5 min. | Blend 2 min. | Ready in 7 min.

- Blend all the ingredients to make a smooth drink.
- Serve chilled.

Nutrition facts:

Per serving: 25 calories | 33 g fats | 5 g protein | 38 g carbs

Raspberry And Yoghurt Smoothie

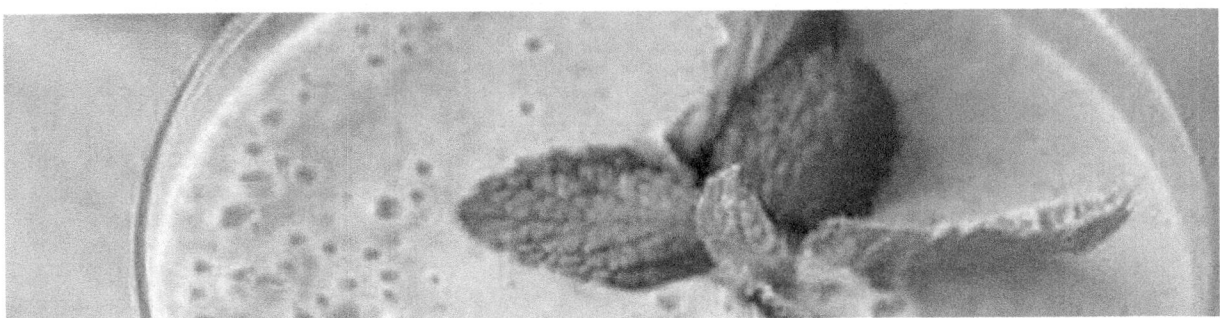

A smoothie so simple can taste really good. You can use any kind of full-fat yogurt or switch it with a non-dairy option like coconut yogurt. It's a good change from green smoothies, but it is still low-carb and will help you stay on your health goals.

Serving quantity: 4

Ingredients:

- 1 cup raspberries
- 6 oz. full-fat yogurt
- ¼ tsp. vanilla extract
- stevia or keto-friendly sweetener, to taste

Directions:

Prep 3 min. | Blend 2 min. | Ready in 5 min.

- Puree all ingredients in a blender.
- Serve chilled.

Nutrition facts:

Per serving: 112 calories | 9 g fats | 1 g protein | 6 g carbs

Recipes PART 4
KETO SALADS

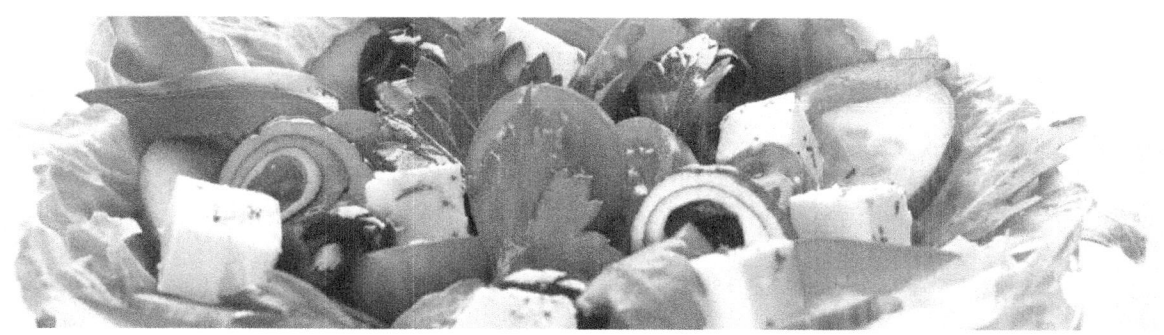

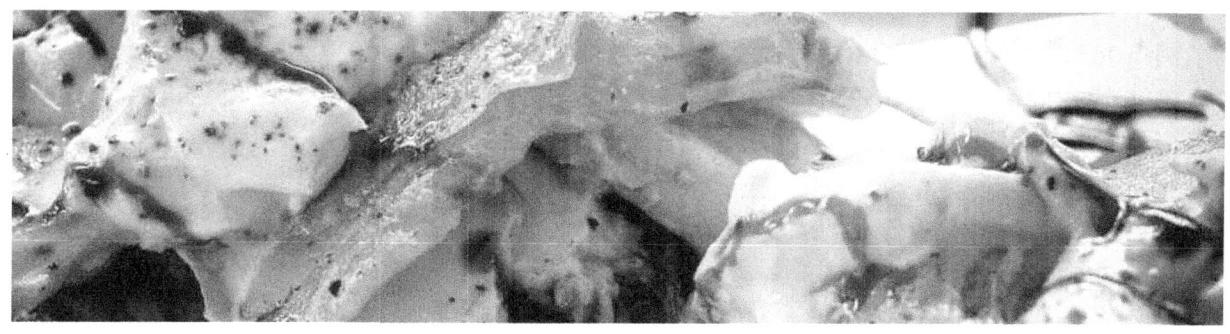

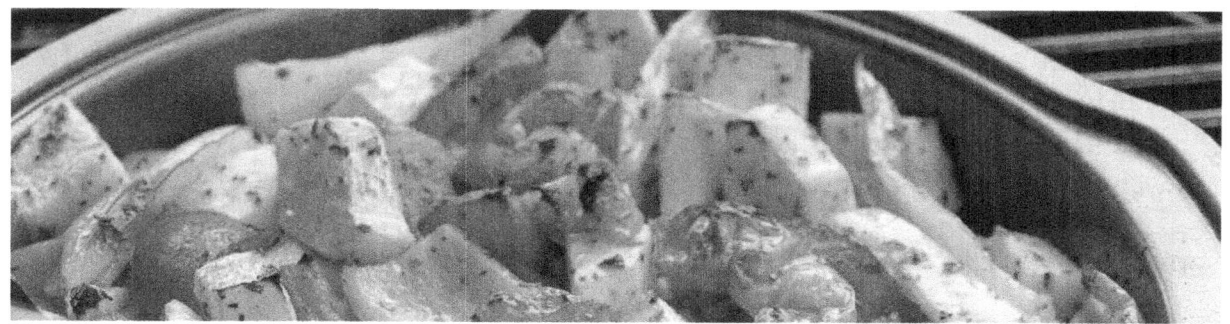

Salmon, avocado, and arugula salad

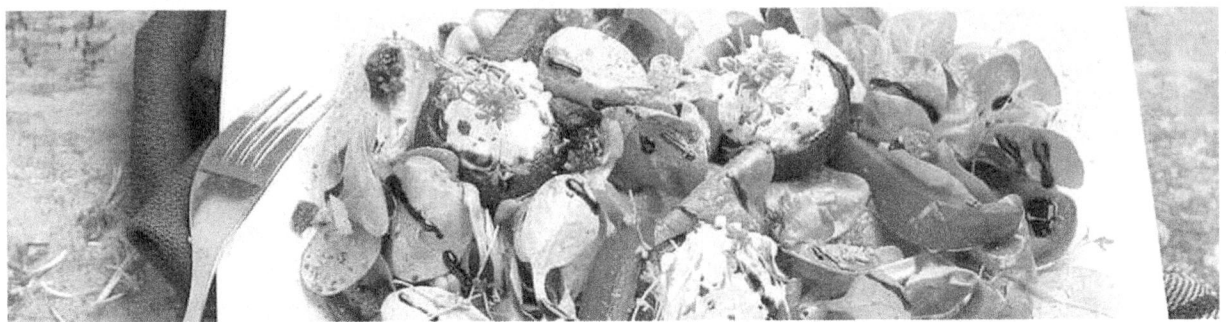

This recipe requires you to use salmon, avocado, lemon dressing, and arugula as its ingredients. Serve it either as dinner or an appetizer. Perfect for summer evenings!

Serving quantity: 2

Ingredients:

For salad

- 8 ounces cooked and smoked salmon fillet
- 3 ounces arugula
- 1 avocado

For lemon dressing

- 2 tbsp. lemon juice
- 1 tsp. white wine vinegar
- ¼ cup olive oil, extra virgin
- black pepper
- ½ tsp. mustard

Directions:

Prep 10 min. | Ready in 10 min.

- Combine all ingredients for the dressing together in a bowl and whisk it together until well mixed.
- Add diced avocado, cooked flaked salmon and arugula leaves to a serving bowl. Toss it all together gently.
- Add a bit of dressing over the salad and serve the dressing in a separate utensil along with the salad to add more if needed.

Nutrition facts:

Per serving: 575 calories | 49 g fat | 25 g protein | 4 g carbs

Green Bean Salad

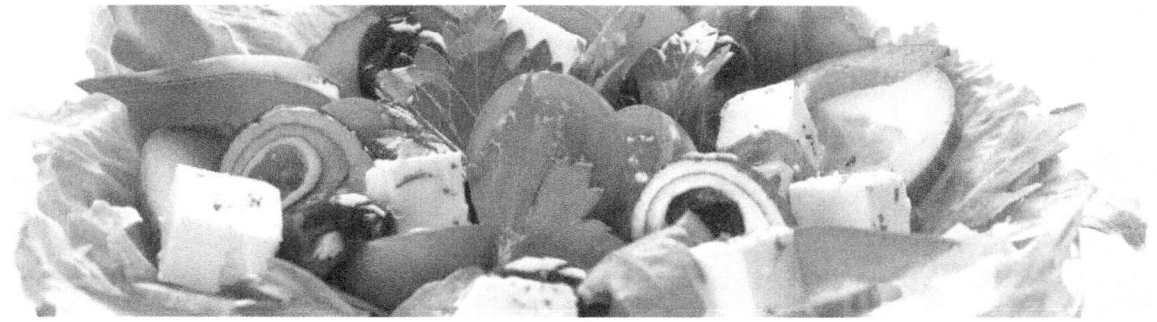

Make a green bean salad with tomatoes and feta cheese to make your meal or snack time more vibrant and healthy.

Serving quantity: 6

Ingredients:

Salad:

- 16 ounces green beans, cut into 1-inch pieces
- 1/2 cup cherry tomatoes, cut in half
- 4 slices chopped bacon
- 1/4 cup feta cheese, cut into cubes

Vinaigrette:

- 2 tbsp. olive oil
- 2 tbsp. apple cider vinegar
- 2 tsp. Dijon mustard
- 2 tsp. balsamic vinegar
- 1/2 tsp. Italian seasoning
- 1 minced garlic clove
- salt and pepper, to taste

Directions:

Prep 15 min. | Cook 10 min. | Ready in 25 min.

Salad:

Cook bacon over medium heat in a saucepan. Transfer to a plate when it is crispy. Add ice water to a large bowl. Fill a saucepan with water, place over medium heat, add salt, and let it boil. Cook green beans in the boiling water for 2 minutes and then transfer to the ice water. Drain the beans using a paper towel. Mix with tomatoes, feta cheese, and bacon.

Vinaigrette:

Add all ingredients of the vinaigrette in a jar. Seal the lid, and shake well. Pour it over the salad.

Nutrition facts:

Per Serving: 120 calories | 8 g fat | 5 g protein | 6 g carbs

Salmon And Avocado Salad

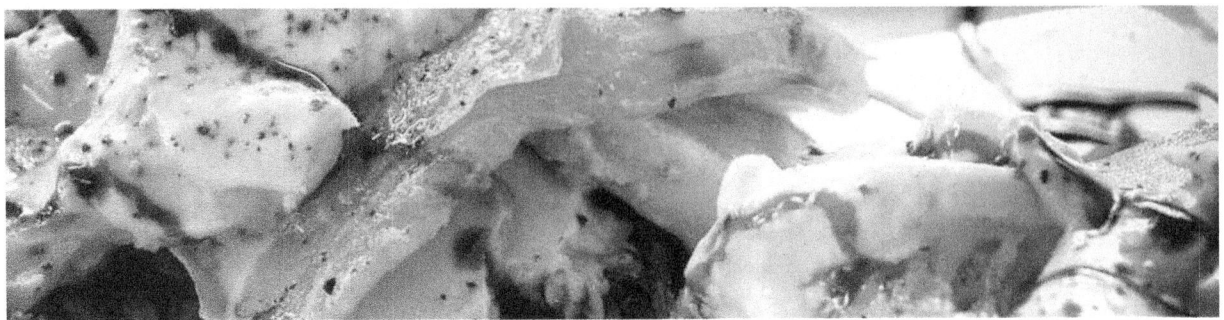

If you are up for a filling salad, make this oven-baked salmon and avocado salad. Top it off with a creamy dressing and enjoy!

Serving quantity: 4

Ingredients:

Salad:

- 16 ounces oven-baked salmon
- 1 sliced avocado
- 16 ounces baby spinach, washed and dried
- 2 slices onion rings
- 4 sliced radishes

Dressing:

- 2 tbsp. avocado oil
- 1/3 cup mayonnaise
- 1 tbsp. mustard
- 1 tbsp. apple cider vinegar
- 2 tbsp. freshly chopped dill
- 2 minced garlic cloves
- salt and pepper, to taste

Directions:

Prep 10 min. | Ready in 10 min.

Dressing:

- Add all ingredients into a jar and mix well.

Salad:

- Arrange salad in a big bowl or plate.
- Dress the salad or serve the dressing along with the salad.

Nutrition facts:

Per Serving: 464 calories | 34 g fat | 28 g protein | 8 g carbs

Grilled Vegetable Salad

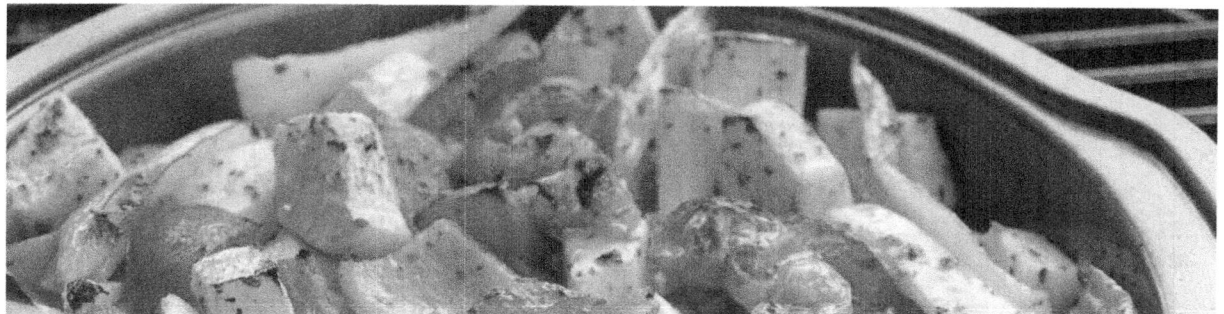

Grilled vegetables, dressed with olive oil, and topped with feta cheese; it's an amazing salad you can have on any occasion.

Serving quantity: 4

Ingredients:

- 1 sliced eggplant
- 1 red bell pepper, cut into strips
- 1 sliced zucchini
- 2 minced garlic cloves
- 3 tbsp. olive oil
- 3/4 tsp. salt
- ½ tsp. crushed black pepper
- ½ tsp. oregano
- ½ cup feta

Directions:

Prep 10 min. | Cook 10 min. | Ready in 20 min.

- Preheat grill to medium heat.
- Grill the sliced vegetables, 3 minutes each side.
- They should be nicely grilled and tender.
- Let the vegetables cool and chop into 1-inch pieces.
- Shift the vegetables in a large bowl and season with garlic, olive oil, oregano, salt, and pepper.
- Top with cheese and mix a little.

Nutrition facts:

Per Serving: 200 calories | 14 g fat | 5 g protein | 12 g carbs

Chicken Salad

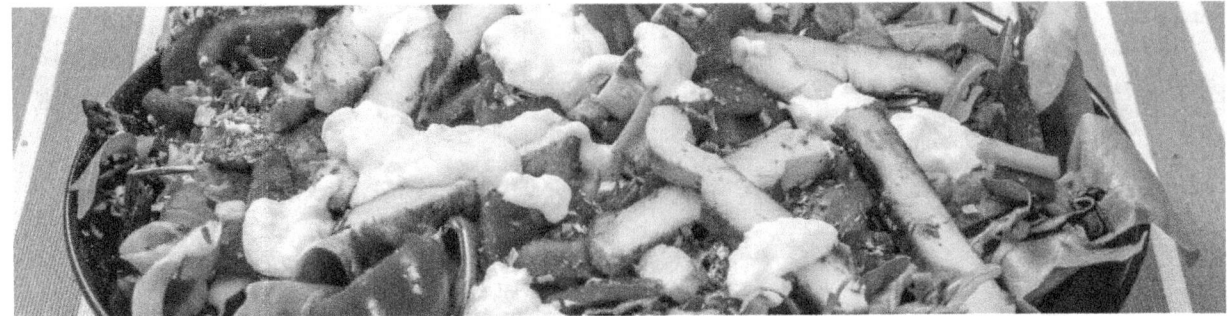

Grilled chicken with veggies is the ultimate mouthwatering salad with any meal. It's healthy and satisfying for both your taste buds and tummy.

Serving quantity: 4

Ingredients:

Salad:

- 20 ounces cooked boneless chicken
- 1 head diced romaine lettuce
- 1 diced tomato
- ¼ cup diced onion
- 2 cups diced cucumber
- 1/3 cup olives
- ½ cup feta

Dressing:

- ¼ cup olive oil
- ¼ cup vinegar
- 2 minced garlic cloves
- 1 tbsp. lemon juice
- 2 tsp. mustard
- salt and pepper, to taste

Directions:

Prep 20 min. | Ready in 20 min.

- Mix all salad ingredients in a bowl.
- Add all dressing ingredients in a jar, seal, and shake well.
- Serve along with the salad.

Nutrition facts:

Per Serving: 470 calories | 28 g fat | 42 g protein | 9 g carbs

Cheesy Bacon Mushroom Salad

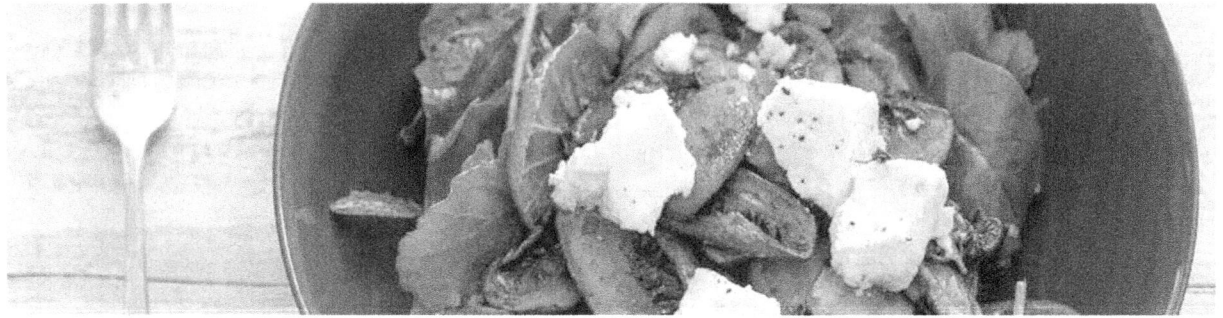

Greens spring mix, crumbled goat cheese, and cooked bacon will make a keto-friendly and really delicious salad. You can use a store-bought spring mix or mix together baby kale, some romaine lettuce, and spinach.

Serving quantity: 1

Ingredients:

- 4 ounces spring mix or mixed veggies
- 1 ounce crumbled goat cheese
- 2 ounces halved cremini mushrooms
- 1 tbsp. balsamic vinegar
- 1 tbsp. butter
- 1 ounce cooked, crumbled bacon
- 1 tbsp. olive oil
- salt and pepper, to taste

Directions:

Prep 15 min. I Cook 15 min. I Ready in 30 min.

- On medium heat, heat up the 1 tbsp. of butter in a pan.
- Add in the mushrooms and sauté till they turn golden brown and soften.
- Sprinkle in some salt and pepper. While the mushrooms are being cooked, put the spring mix vegetables in a bowl. If you're using baby kale, spinach, and romaine lettuce instead, chop them roughly beforehand and place them in the bowl.
- Top the salad greens with crumbled goat cheese and cooked bacon.
- When the mushrooms are sautéed, add them to the salad bowl and mix them with the other ingredients. In another bowl, mix the balsamic vinegar and olive oil together.
- Drizzle the balsamic vinegar dressing onto the salad to serve.

Nutrition facts:

Per Serving: 532 calories I 44 g fat I 20 g protein I 10 g carbs

Cauliflower Salad

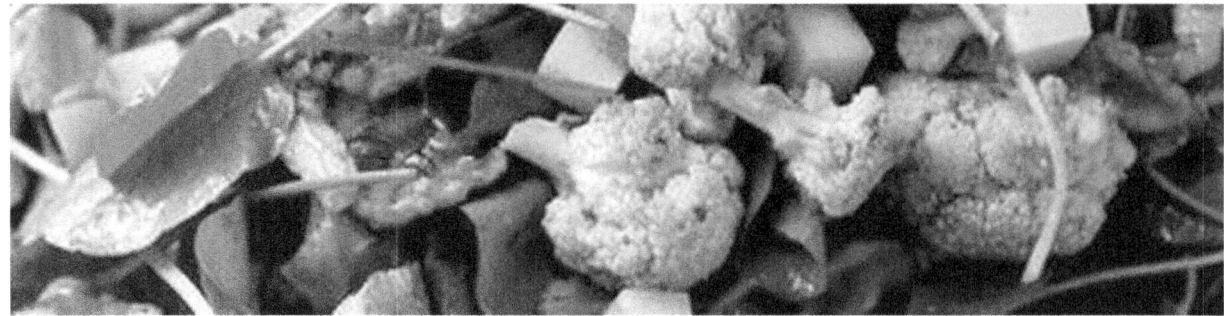

Make this creamy and tasty cauliflower salad to complement your meal and you will be really happy after tasting all the flavors of this salad.

Serving quantity: 8

Ingredients:

- 3 eggs
- 1 chopped cauliflower head
- 2 chopped celery stalks
- 6 chopped bacon slices
- 2 chopped green onions
- ½ cup mayonnaise
- 2 tbsp. mustard
- ¼ tsp. paprika
- salt and pepper, to taste

Directions:

Prep 15 min. | Cook 15 min. | Ready in 30 min.

- Hard boil eggs for 10 minutes.
- Fill another bowl with ice and water.
- Place boiled eggs in this ice bath for 10 minutes before peeling.
- Peel and chop the eggs.
- Boil cauliflower in a large pot until it becomes tender.
- Drain and let it cool.
- Combine cauliflower, eggs, bacon, celery, onions, paprika, mustard, and mayonnaise in a large bowl.
- Mix well and adjust the seasoning with salt and pepper.
- Transfer this salad into a serving bowl and serve.

Nutrition facts:

Per Serving: 243 calories | 20 g fat | 8 g protein | 6 g carbs

Strawberry Avocado Salad

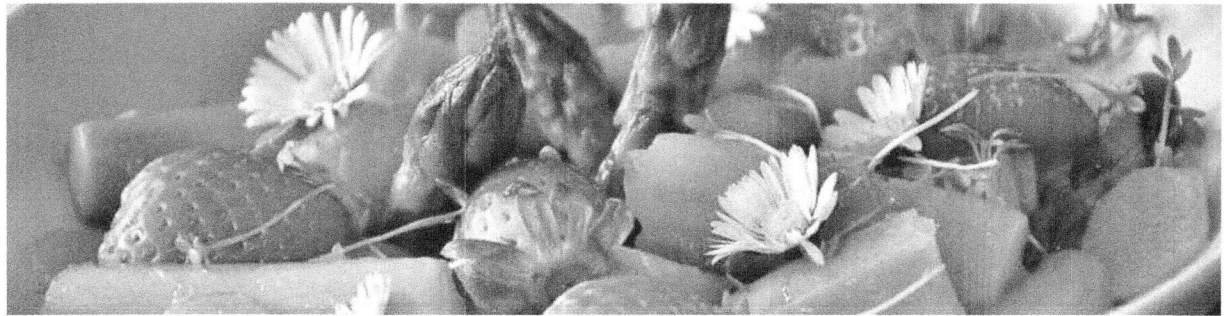

Enjoy the season of strawberry by making this amazing fresh strawberry and avocado salad. It has got so much going on with the punch of strawberries and tomatoes. Then combine the tastes and textures of avocado, fresh basil, and spinach. Dress it up with balsamic and you will love it!

Serving quantity: 4

Ingredients:

Salad:

- 1 cup strawberries, halved or cut into quarter pieces
- 1 chopped avocado
- 1 cup halved tomatoes
- ¼ cup freshly chopped basil
- 1 cup fresh small mozzarella balls
- 4 cups fresh spinach

Balsamic Dressing:

- 3 tbsp. olive oil
- 2 tbsp. vinegar
- 2 tbsp. balsamic vinegar
- 3 tbsp. mayonnaise
- ½ tsp. dried oregano
- 2 minced garlic cloves
- salt and pepper, to taste

Directions:

Prep 15 min. | Ready in 15 min.

- Mix all salad ingredients in a large bowl.
- Add all dressing ingredients in a jar, mix well, and dress the salad with this mixture.

Nutrition facts:

Per Serving: 339 calories | 29 g fat | 8 g protein | 9 g carbs

Fun Cucumber Salad

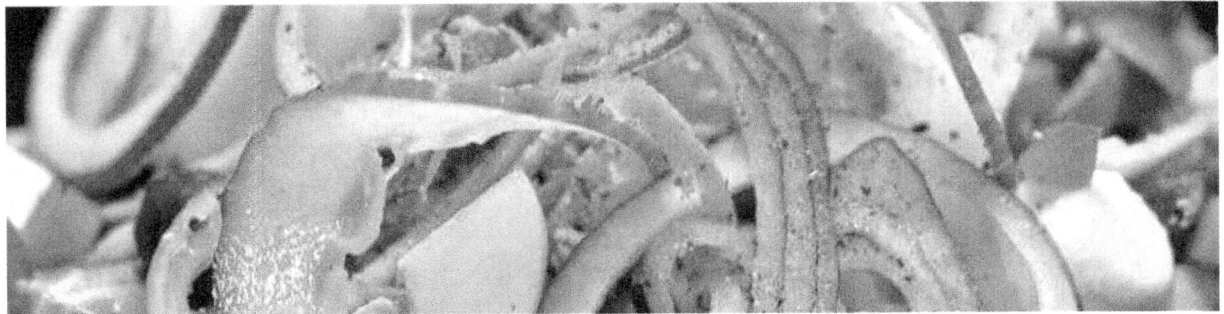

When you are in the mood for something light and refreshing with an added zing from Thai dressing, you are in for this cool low-carb salad.

Serving quantity: 4

Ingredients:

Salad:

- 2 cucumbers
- ½ cup freshly chopped cilantro
- ¼ cup toasted sesame seeds

Dressing:

- 2 tbsp. lime juice
- 1 tbsp. fish sauce
- 1 tbsp. apple cider vinegar
- 1 minced garlic clove
- 2 tbsp. sesame oil
- ¼ tsp. red pepper flakes
- ¼ tsp salt and pepper each

Directions:

Prep 10 min. | Ready in 10 min.

- Mix the ingredients of the dressing in a jar or bowl.
- Spiralize cucumbers using a spiralizer.
- Put the cucumbers in a bowl, mix with the dressing, and garnish with sesame seeds and cilantro.

Nutrition facts:

Per Serving: 124 calories | 8 g fat | 4 g protein | 8 g carbs

Broccoli And Kale Salad

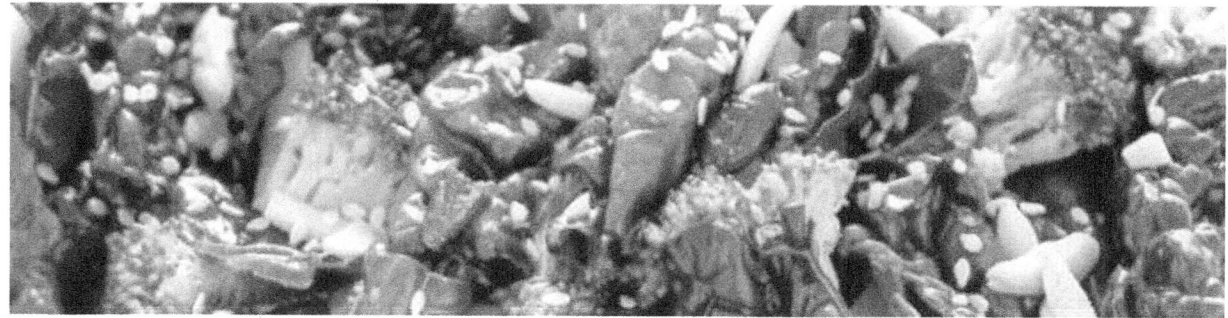

This broccoli and kale salad is a meal in itself. It's so filling and tasty! Wait till you try the hint of spices and the combination of amazing ingredients like broccoli, kale, and avocado. You'll love it so much!

Serving quantity: 2

Ingredients:

- 8 ounces broccoli
- 4 ounces kale
- 2 avocados
- 2 scallions
- 4 eggs
- ½ cup mayonnaise
- 1 tbsp. whole-grain mustard
- 2 tbsp. olive oil
- 2 cloves garlic
- ¼ tsp. chili flakes
- salt and pepper, to taste

Directions:

Prep 5 min. | Cook 15 min. | Ready in 20 min.

- Mix mustard and mayonnaise in a bowl and put aside.
- Boil eggs, peel and cut into halves. Cut the avocados in slices.
- Thinly slice the garlic and sauté in a frying pan till it turns golden.
- Let it cool and crisp on a paper towel. Chop kale and broccoli as you like.
- Add butter to the pan in which you fried garlic.
- Cook the vegetables on medium heat till they are a little soft.
- Mix the vegetables, eggs, and avocados along with mustard mayonnaise in a serving bowl. Season with salt and pepper. Garnish with chili flakes and crispy garlic.

Nutrition facts:

Per Serving: 1018 calories | 94 g fat | 22 g protein | 13 g carbs

Recipes PART 5
KETO SOUP

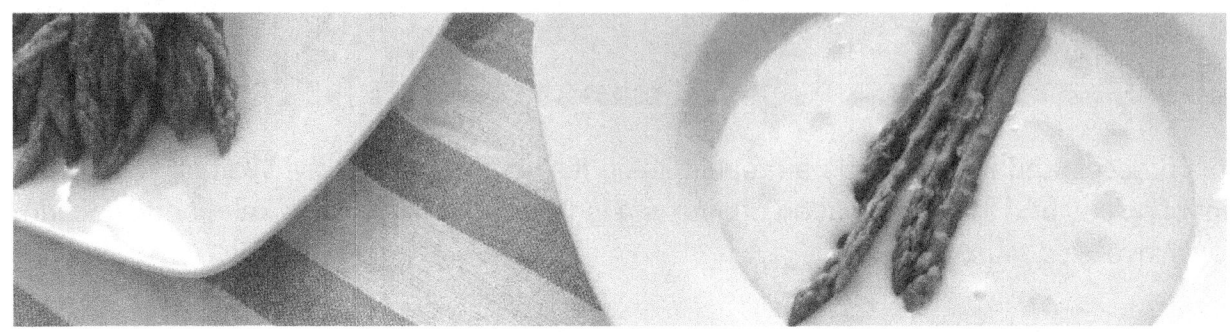

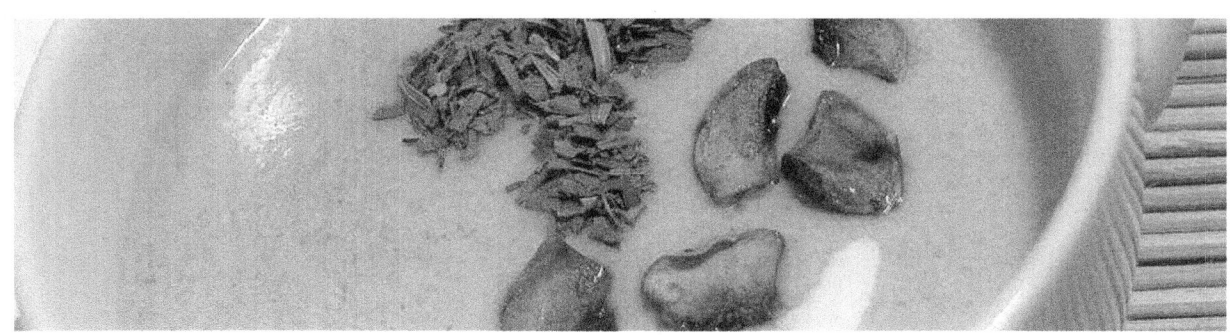

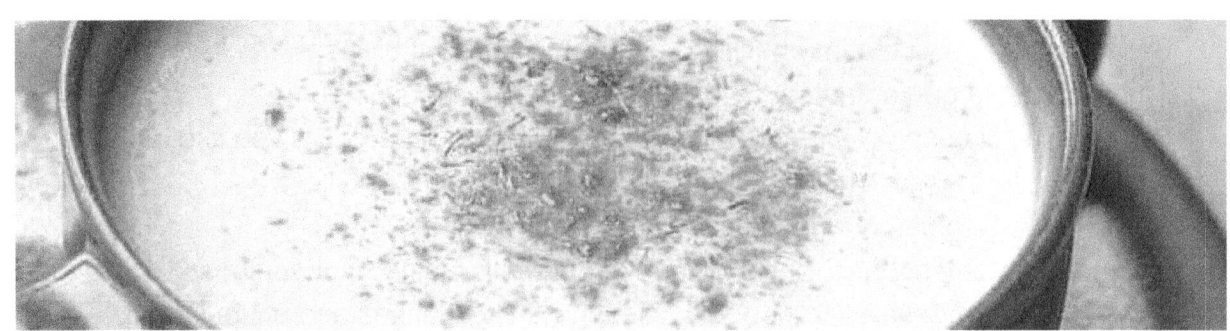

Chicken Enchilada Soup

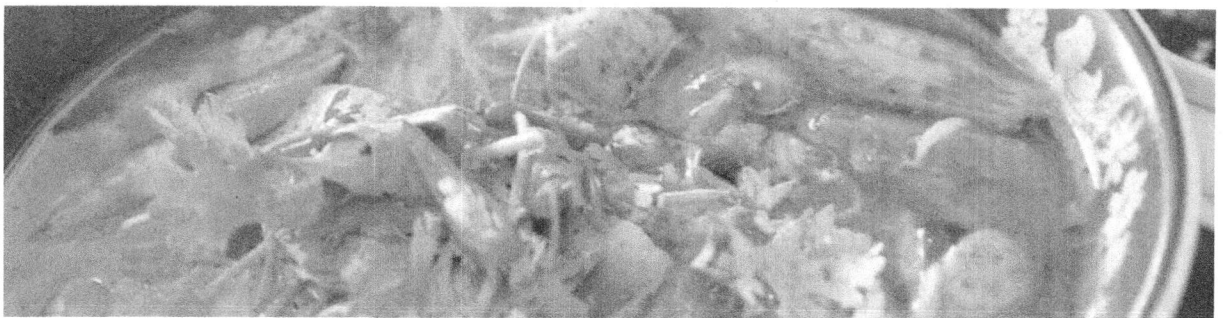

This warming soup is amazing for winters. It packs the punch from taco seasoning and the richness of sour cream, butter, and chicken broth. Besides, it's good for a large family.

Serving quantity: 8

Ingredients:

- 32 ounces boneless chicken breast
- 2 cups tomato puree
- 2 diced jalapenos
- ½ cup chopped onion
- 5 cups chicken broth
- ¼ cup butter
- ¾ cup sour cream
- ¾ tsp. salt
- 3 tbsp. taco seasoning

Directions:

Prep 15 min. | Cook 25 min. | Ready in 40 min.

- Put chicken, jalapenos, onion, tomato puree, butter, salt, and taco seasoning in an Instant Pot. Pour the chicken broth as well.
- Secure the lid and seal the vent.
- Set it to Soup function for 20 minutes.
- When the cooking time is over, leave it for 15 minutes to release the pressure naturally. When the soup is cooked, take out the chicken pieces with one cup of broth in a bowl. Shred the chicken with a fork and mix sour cream.
- Pour it back into the pot.
- Adjust seasonings according to your taste and serve hot.

Nutrition facts:

Per Serving: 302 calories | 17 g fat | 29 g protein | 6 g carbs

Zucchini Noodle Soup

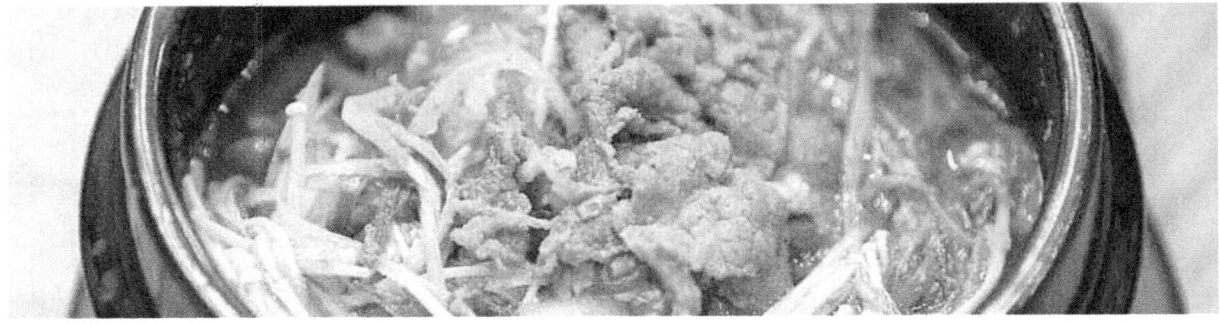

Replace the common noodles with zucchini noodles and you will have a healthy low-carb zucchini noodle soup. Serve this flavorful and nutritious soup with a squeeze of lime and enjoy it with your family.

Serving quantity: 8

Ingredients:

- 1 tbsp. coconut oil
- ¼ chopped onion
- 1 chopped jalapeno
- 2 minced garlic cloves
- 1 ½ tbsp. green curry paste
- 6 cups chicken broth
- 13 ounces coconut milk
- 16 ounces chicken breast, thinly sliced
- 1 thinly sliced red pepper
- 2 spiralized zucchinis
- 8 wedges of lime

Directions:

Prep 15 min. | Cook 15 min. | Ready in 30 min.

- Heat coconut oil in a large saucepan.
- Sauté onions for 5 minutes over medium heat.
- Add garlic, curry paste, and jalapenos and sauté for 1 minute.
- Pour coconut milk and chicken broth and mix well.
- Then add chicken, red pepper, and fish sauce. Let the chicken cook well.
- Then mix in the cilantro.
- Before serving, add noodles in the bowls and then pour the soup.
- Squeeze a wedge of lime in each bowl and serve.

Nutrition facts:

Per Serving: 260 calories | 16 g fat | 21 g protein | 6 g carbs

Garlic Chicken Soup

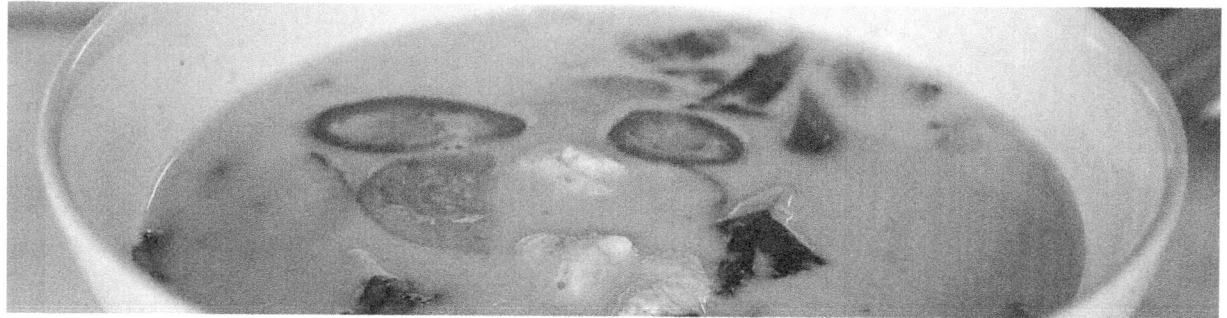

This soup is creamy because of heavy cream and cream cheese. It is also filled with amazing garlic flavor. Enjoy this hearty meal when you want to make something easy, filling, and yummy.

Serving quantity: 4

Ingredients:

- 2 tbsp. butter
- 2 cups shredded chicken
- 4 oz. cream cheese
- 2 tbsp. crushed garlic
- Salt and pepper, to taste
- 14 oz. chicken broth
- 1/4 cup heavy cream
- Paprika, lemon, and parsley (optional)

Directions:

Prep 10 min. | Cook 10 min. | Ready in 20 min.

- Add butter to a large saucepan over medium heat.
- Add shredded chicken, cream cheese, and garlic.
- After the cream cheese melts, add heavy cream and chicken broth. Mix well.
- Let it simmer for 5 minutes.
- Add salt and pepper according to your taste and the optional paprika, lemon, and parsley for a little extra punch if you want.

Nutrition facts:

Per Serving: 315 calories | 25 g fat | 18 g protein | 2 g carbs

Shrimp Chowder

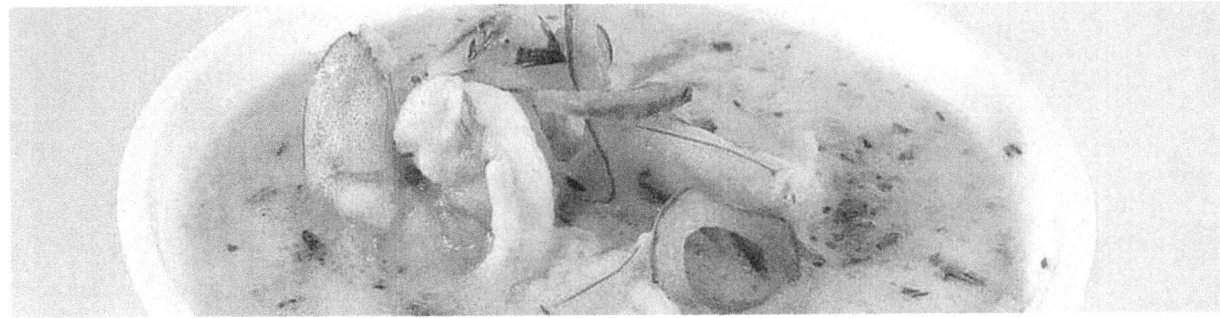

This is a rich, hearty, creamy, and flavorful soup perfect for cold weather. Made from shrimp, bacon, and chicken broth, this is exactly the thing for keto diet followers.

Serving quantity: 6

Ingredients:

- 16 ounces shrimp, peeled, deveined
- 6 slices chopped bacon
- 2 cups chicken broth
- 1 cup heavy whipping cream
- ½ cup onion, chopped
- 1 turnip, medium, cut into ½ inch cubes
- 2 cloves minced garlic
- ½ tsp. cajun seasoning
- salt and pepper, to taste
- chopped parsley, for garnish

Directions:

Prep 5 min. | Cook 25 min. | Ready in 30 min.

- Cook the bacon until crisp in a large pan.
- Drain the bacon in a lined plate and let the fat remain in the pan.
- Sauté onion and turnip in the same pan for 5 minutes till onion softens.
- Add garlic and cook for about a minute until fragrant.
- Add broth and let it simmer for about 10 minutes till the turnip becomes tender.
- Add shrimp and cream and stir for about 3 minutes till the shrimp cooks.
- Sprinkle seasoning, salt, and pepper.
- Add chopped parsley and serve.

Nutrition facts:

Per serving: 388 calories | 32 g fat | 17 g fat | 5 g carbs

White Chicken Chili Soup

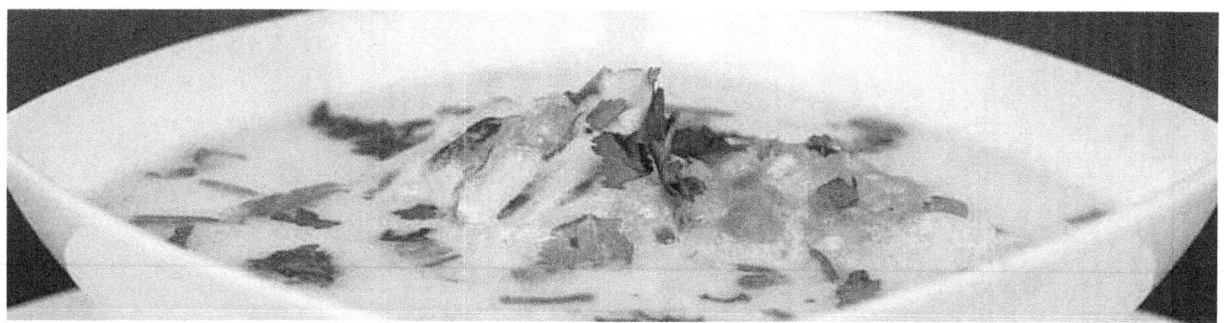

This creamy white soup is made in a slow cooker but the end result is totally worth your time and effort.

Serving quantity: 4

Ingredients:

- 32 ounces boneless and skinless chicken thighs
- 3 cups chicken broth
- 12 ounces cauliflower florets
- ¼ cup coconut oil
- ¼ cup chopped onion
- 2 minced garlic cloves
- 1 chopped jalapeno pepper
- 1 tsp. salt
- ½ tsp. black pepper
- 2 tsp. ground cumin
- chopped cilantro, for garnish

Directions:

Prep 10 min. | Cook 4 h | Ready in 4h 10 min.

- Put all ingredients in a slow cooker, except cilantro, and cook on high for 4 hours.
- When done, take out the chicken and shred it.
- Blend the soup and mix the shredded chicken back to the soup.
- Garnish with cilantro and serve.

Nutrition facts:

Per Serving: 408 calories | 24 g fat | 38 g protein | 7 g carbs

Creamy Asparagus Soup

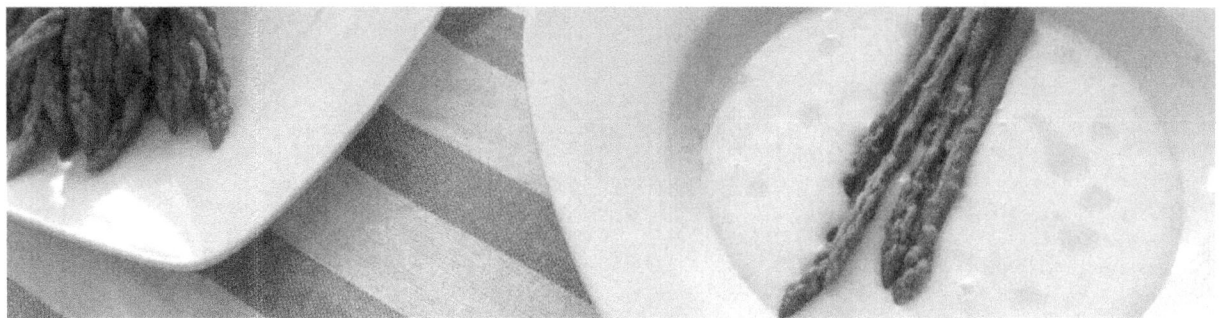

This light and creamy asparagus soup is keto and dairy-free. It's yummy, comforting, and only takes 30 minutes to cook.

Serving quantity: 4

Ingredients:

- 1 tbsp. avocado oil
- 8 ounces trimmed and chopped asparagus
- 1 chopped green onion
- 2 minced garlic cloves
- 2 cups chicken broth
- 1 ounce baby spinach
- 1 cup coconut cream
- salt and pepper
- 1 tbsp. lemon juice

Directions:

Prep 10 min. | Cook 20 min. | Ready in 30 min.

- Heat oil in a large saucepan over medium heat.
- Add asparagus, salt, and pepper and sauté for 4 minutes.
- Add onion and garlic and sauté for 1 minute.
- Then pour the broth and let it simmer for 10 minutes or until the asparagus becomes tender.
- Add spinach and cook for 2 minutes.
- Blend the soup and mix lemon juice and coconut cream.
- Adjust the seasoning and serve hot.

Nutrition facts:

Per Serving: 149 calories | 12 g fat | 4 g protein | 5 g carbs

Mushroom Soup

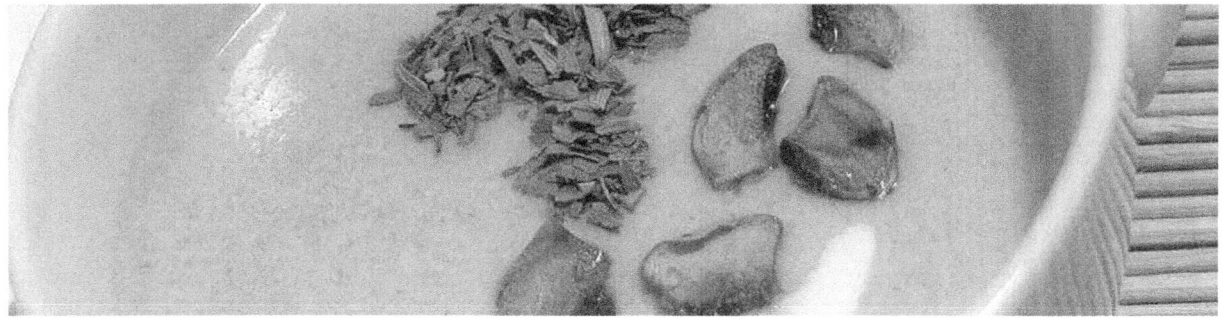

Mushrooms give such a nice flavor to any soup and this one tastes so good with butter and sage. Enjoy this creamy buttery mushroom soup with your family.

Serving quantity: 6

Ingredients:

- 16 ounces sliced mushrooms
- 2 tbsp. freshly chopped sage
- 6 tbsp. butter
- 4 cups chicken or vegetable broth
- ½ cup heavy cream
- salt and pepper, to taste

Directions:

Prep 10 min. | Cook 15 min. | Ready in 25 min.

- Heat butter in a large pot. Cook sage for 1 minute.
- Toss in the mushrooms and cook for 5 minutes or until tender.
- Add the broth and cook for 5 more minutes.
- Blend the soup.
- Pour it back in the pot and mix the cream.
- Serve hot.

Nutrition facts:

Per Serving: 208 calories | 18 g fat | 5 g protein | 5 g carbs

Cauliflower Soup

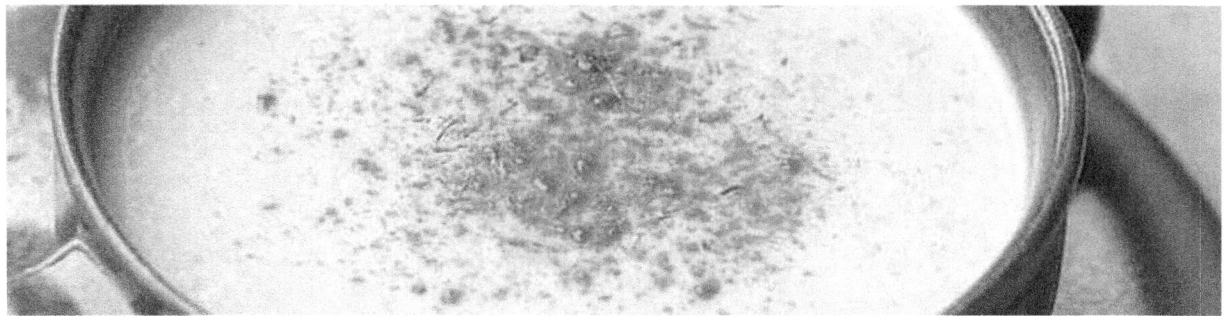

Make this soup in an Instant Pot, save some time and enjoy the rich flavors and texture of this delicious soup.

Serving quantity: 6

Ingredients:

- 1/4 cup chopped onion
- 2 minced garlic cloves
- 1 chopped celery stalk
- 6 chopped bacon slices
- salt and pepper
- 3 cups chicken broth
- 1 chopped cauliflower
- 2 cups shredded cheddar cheese
- 3/4 cup sour cream
- 1 green onion

Directions:

Prep 15 min. | Cook 25 min. | Ready in 40 min.

- Turn on the sauté function of your Instant Pot.
- Crip fry the bacon. Take it out and place it on a plate.
- Then sauté onion, garlic, and celery.
- Season with salt and pepper and cook for 5 minutes.
- Turn off sauté mode and add the broth.
- Toss in the cauliflower, close the lid, and manually set it on high for 5 minutes.
- When the time is up, let the pressure release naturally for 10 minutes.
- Open the vent to release the remaining pressure before opening the lid.
- Mix cream and 1 cup cheese. Blend well.
- Garnish with green onion, bacon, and the remaining cheese.

Nutrition facts:

Per Serving: 318 calories | 24 g fat | 15 g protein | 8 g carbs

Chicken Fajita Soup

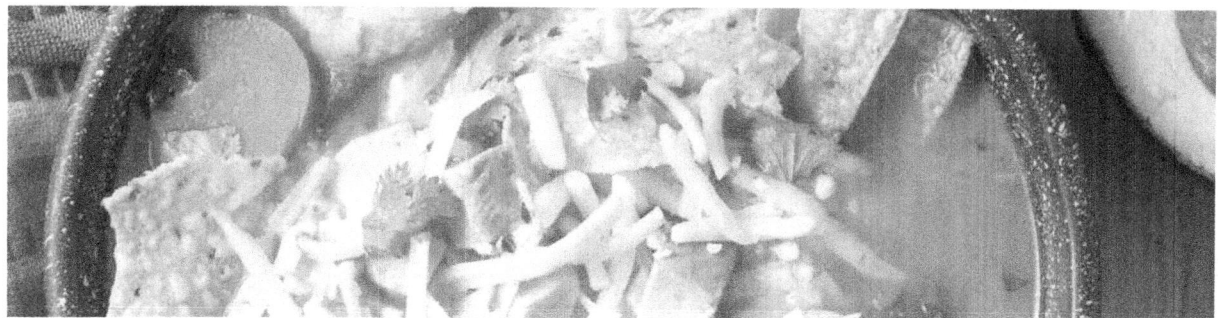

If you are looking forward to a heart-warming, a little spicy, and flavorful soup, then Chicken Fajita soup is what you should make to surprise the whole family. This low-carb soup is filled with healthy and tasty ingredients to make you feel good.

Serving quantity: 8

Ingredients:

- 40 ounces boneless and skinless chicken thighs
- 8 cups chicken broth
- ¼ cup chopped onion
- 2 chopped celery stalks
- ¼ cup sliced peppers
- 2 cups diced tomatoes
- ¼ cup diced green chilies
- 1 tsp. salt
- 1 tsp. black pepper
- 2 tsp. chili powder
- 1 tbsp. crushed garlic

Directions:

Prep 5 min. | Cook 25 min. | Ready in 30 min.

- Add all ingredients to a pressure cooker, seal, and cook for 25 minutes.
- Let the pressure release naturally.
- Take out the chicken, shred it and mix back in the pressure cooker.
- Serve with lemon wedges and chopped cilantro.

Nutrition facts:

Per Serving: 316 calories | 15 g fat | 35 g protein | 8 g carbs

Zucchini And Basil Soup

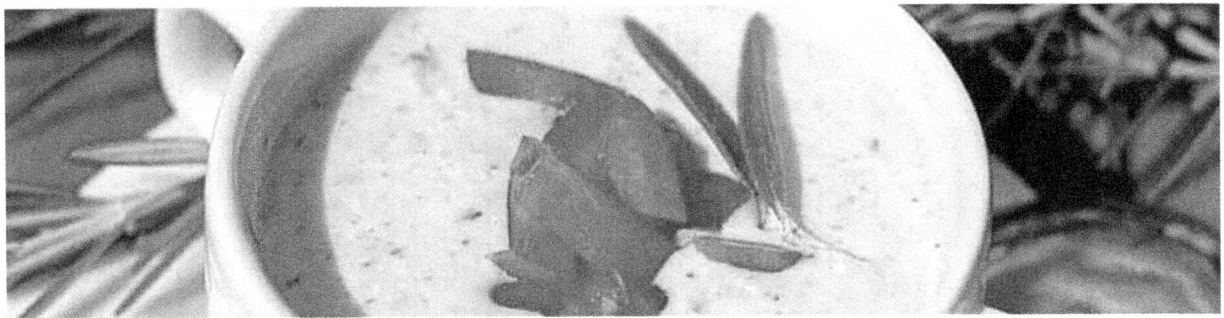

Low in carbs and full of healthy nutrients, you can make an excellent zucchini soup with a lovely touch of basil leaves to enhance the taste even more.

Serving quantity: 4

Ingredients:

- 1 tbsp. olive oil
- 2 garlic cloves
- 16 ounces zucchini, cut into cubes
- 2 cups chicken broth
- 1/2 tsp. salt
- 1/2 tsp. pepper
- 1/3 cup fresh basil leaves
- 1/2 cup whipping cream

Directions:

Prep 5 min. | Cook 30 min. | Ready in 35 min.

- Heat oil in a large saucepan over medium heat.
- Sauté garlic for 1 minute.
- Add salt, pepper, and zucchini and cook for 5 minutes.
- Add chicken broth and let it simmer on low heat for 10 minutes.
- Turn off the heat and add basil leaves.
- Blend the soup using an immersion blender or a food processor.
- Pour it back into the pot, adjust the seasoning to taste.
- Mix the cream, and serve hot.

Nutrition facts:

Per Serving: 171 calories | 14 g fat | 4 g protein | 6 g carbs

Recipes PART 6
KETO LUNCHES

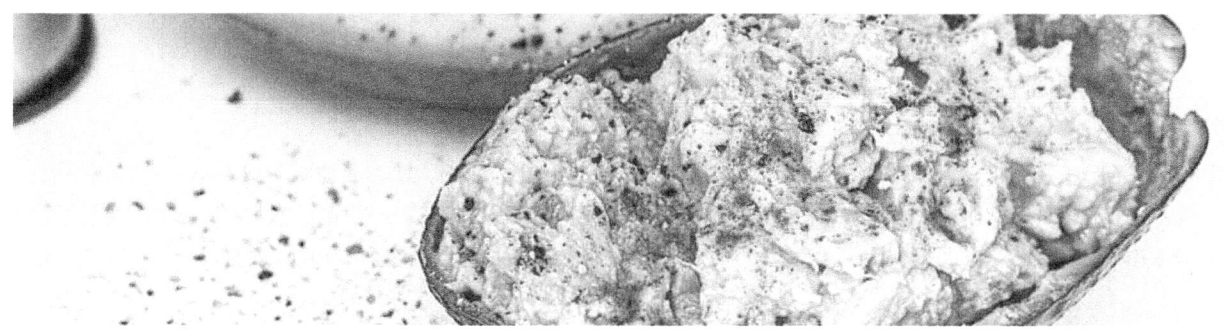

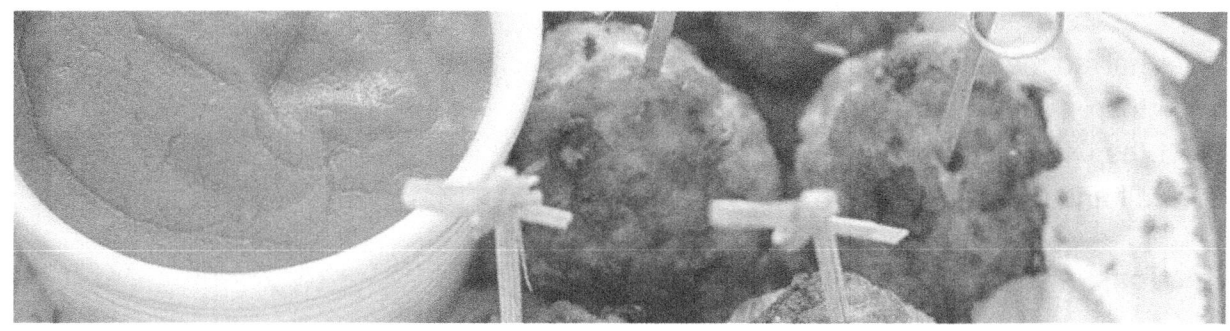

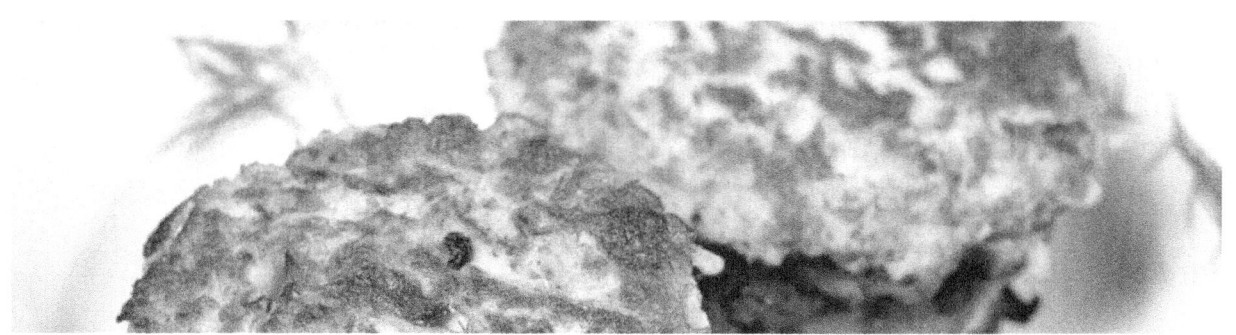

Salmon Avocado Devilled Egg

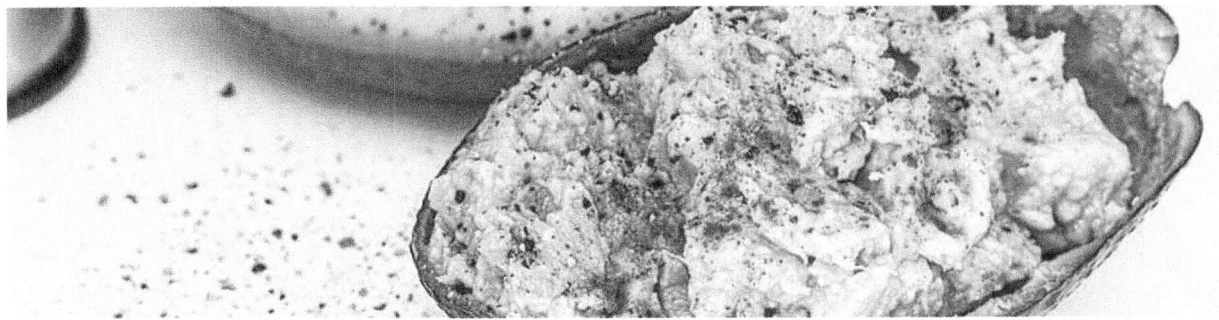

It's one of the easiest keto lunches to make, especially if you usually don't have much time to prepare lunch. The secret to this recipe is to choose ripe avocadoes and you can also substitute the sour cream with mayonnaise to add more richness to the dish.

Serving quantity: 1

Ingredients:

- 3 ounces salmon
- 1 halved medium avocado
- 4 tbsp. sour cream
- 1 tbsp. lemon juice
- Salt and pepper, to taste

Directions:

Prep 5 min. I Cook 5 min. I Ready in 10 min.

- Slice the avocado in half and remove the pit and discard it.
- In the empty spaces on the avocado slices, place the same amount of sour cream on top of each slice.
- Then, place smoked salmon on top.
- Sprinkle salt and pepper on it and squeeze the lemon to drizzle lemon juice on top.
- Garnish with parsley and serve

Nutrition facts:

Per Serving: 564 calories | 43 g fat I 21 g protein | 19 g carbs

Salmon With Pesto

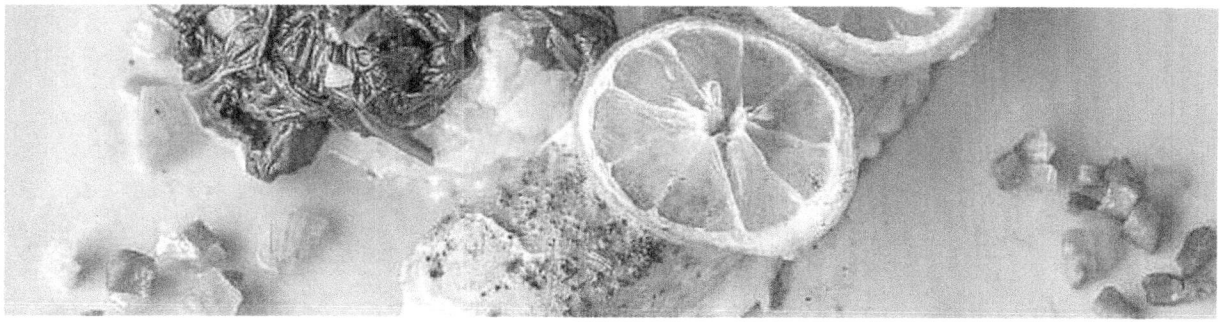

Beautiful pesto sauce lets the flavor of baked salmon shine through and you can enjoy this dinner without putting in too much effort. It's a win-win for a busy week night.

Serving quantity: 4

Ingredients:

Green Sauce:

- 4 tbsp. green pesto
- ½ cup Greek yoghurt
- 1 cup mayonnaise
- Salt and pepper, to taste

Salmon:

- 32 ounces salmon
- 4 tbsp. green pesto
- Salt and pepper, to taste

Directions:

Prep 5 min. | Cook 30 min. | Ready in 35 min.

- Grease a baking sheet and place salmon skin-side down.
- Rub salt, pepper, and pesto on top.
- Bake in the oven for 30 minutes at 400° F.
- Mix the ingredients of green sauce.
- Serve the salmon with green sauce and lemon wedges.

Nutrition facts:

Per Serving: 1044 calories | 88 g fat | 52 g protein | 3 g carbs

Chicken Jalapeno Fritters

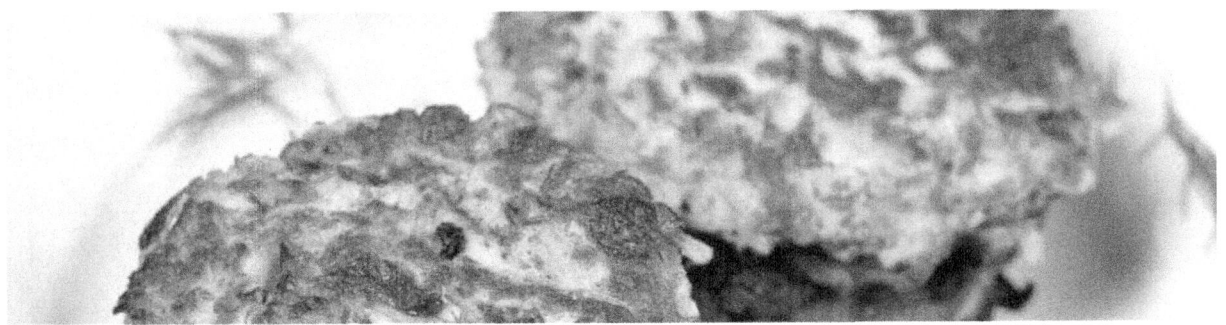

Chicken fritters are juicy, tender, and packed with flavor. The fritters become even better with jalapenos. You can use turkey instead of chicken and use coconut flour in place of almond flour since it won't affect your keto diet.

Serving quantity: 4

Ingredients:

- 2 eggs
- 24 ounces finely sliced skinless and boneless chicken breast
- 1 cup grated mozzarella cheese
- 3 seeded and thinly chopped jalapeno peppers
- 1/3 cup almond flour
- 1 sliced spring onion (reserve some for garnish)
- ¼ cup shredded parmesan cheese
- 2 tbsp. chopped parsley
- 1 tbsp. olive oil for frying
- salt and pepper, to taste
- ½ tsp. garlic powder

Directions:

Prep 10 min. I Cook 20 min. I Ready in 30 min.

In a large bowl, add all the ingredients except olive oil, starting with the sliced chicken. Mix everything well to combine and form the fritter mixture. On medium-low heat, heat up the oil in a large non-stick pan. Use a large spoon or an ice-cream scoop to scoop a portion of the fritter mixture onto the pan. Slightly flatten it to into the shape of a fritter. Place as many fritters as the pan can hold, without them sticking together, and fry the fritters in batches. Cook the fritters for 6 to 8 minutes or till both sides turn golden-brown on medium-low heat. When done, garnish with chopped spring onion and serve.

Nutrition facts:

Per Serving: 547 calories | 35 g fat | 49 g protein | 5 g carbs

Prosciutto Mozzarella Balls

A quick, easy yet fulfilling meal, the prosciutto mozzarella balls are a cheesy and flavorful treat that is low carb. By frying the prosciutto, it gets a smoky and salty taste that complements the mozzarella ball hidden inside it.

Serving quantity: 4

Ingredients:

- 8 ounces mozzarella balls
- 4 ounces sliced prosciutto
- Olive oil for frying

Directions:

Prep 5 min. | Cook 15 min. | Ready in 20 min.

- Take half of the prosciutto slices and layer them vertically on a cutting board.
- Layer the remaining prosciutto slices horizontally on top of the vertical layer.
- Put the mozzarella ball on the layered prosciutto slices upside down.
- Carefully but firmly, wrap the prosciutto slices around the mozzarella ball.
- If you are making the balls ahead of time, wrap the prosciutto mozzarella balls in cling film and place in the fridge till use.
- To fry the balls, heat up the olive oil in a pan or skillet.
- Cook till all the sides of the prosciutto turn crisp.
- Serve atop raw spinach leaves or with seasoned tomatoes.

Nutrition facts:

Per Serving: 268 calories | 20 g fat | 18 g protein | 2 g carbs

Green Beans And Bacon

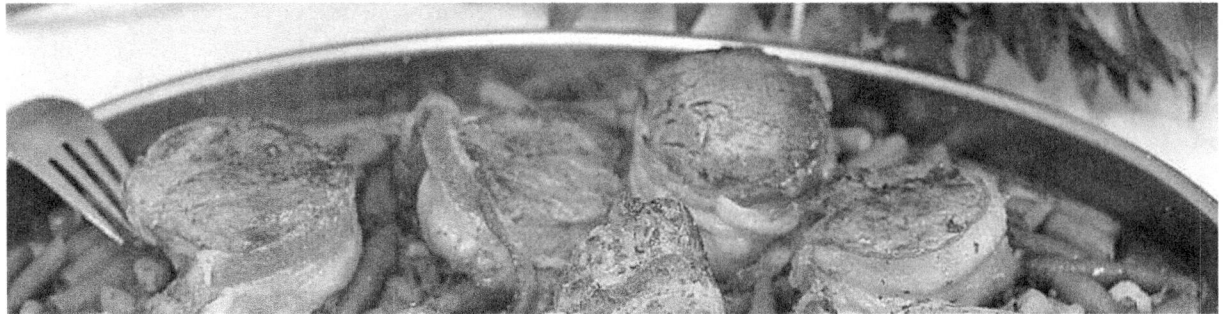

Certain vegetables make an excellent keto meal and green beans are amazing for you. This recipe is simple and very healthy.

Serving quantity: 6

Ingredients:

- 6 cups green beans, cut in half
- 5 slices diced bacon
- ¼ cup water
- 1 cup diced onion
- 1 tsp. salt
- 1 tsp. ground black pepper

Directions:

Prep 10 m | Cook 15 m | Ready in 25 m

- Turn on the sauté mode of Instant Pot.
- Add diced bacon and onion.
- Stir and add beans.
- Then add salt, pepper, and water.
- Put on high pressure for 4 minutes and then release pressure.
- Adjust salt and pepper to your taste.
- Dish out and serve!

Nutrition facts:

Per serving: 123 calories | 7 g fat | 4 g protein | 10 g carbs

Taco Pie

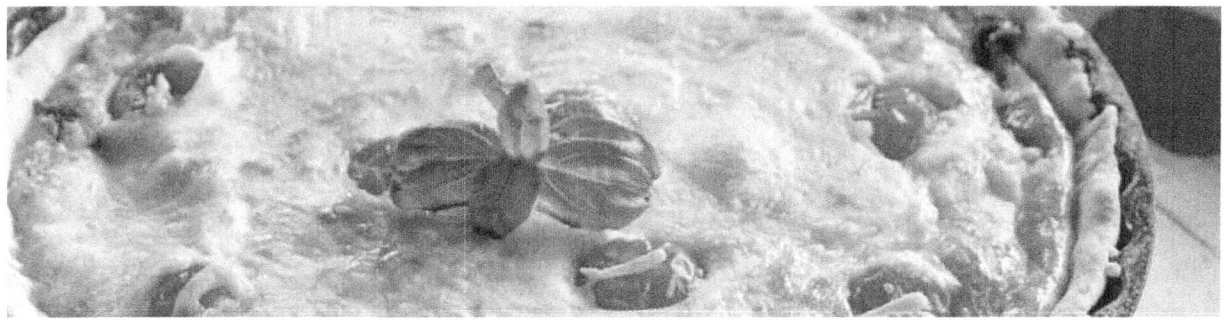

If you love some spice punch in your dinner, this easy taco pie is totally amazing. Packed with flavor and protein, add this pie to your weekly menu.

Serving quantity: 8

Ingredients:

- 16 ounces ground beef
- 3 tbsp. taco seasoning
- 6 eggs
- 2 garlic cloves, minced
- ½ tsp. salt
- ¼ tsp. pepper
- ½ cup heavy cream
- 1 cup shredded cheddar cheese

Directions:

Prep 15 min. | Cook 30 min. | Ready in 45 min.

- Preheat oven to 350° F and grease a 9-inch pie pan.
- Cook ground beef in a large pan over medium heat for 7 minutes.
- Add taco seasoning and cook over low heat for 5 minutes.
- Spread beef in the pie pan.
- Mix eggs, garlic, salt, pepper and cream in a large bowl and pour it over the beef.
- Sprinkle with cheese and bake for 30 minutes.
- Let it cool for 5 minutes, then slice up and serve.

Nutrition facts:

Per Serving: 367 calories | 28 g fat | 24 g protein | 2 g carbs

Chipotle Beef Chili

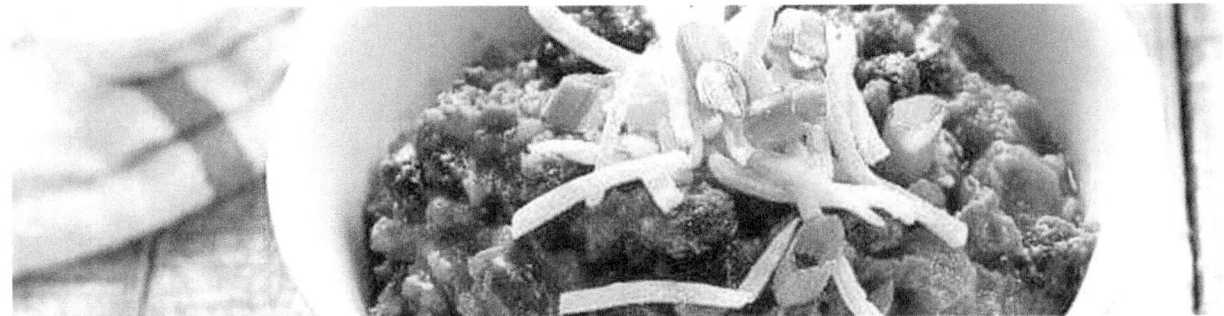

Ground beef chili is the best comfort food, not to mention a quick lunch dish. It takes only 10 minutes to simmer on the stove but you can also use an instant pot to lessen the time even further. It's best served when garnished with items like sour cream, sliced jalapeno, cheddar cheese, or cilantro.

Serving quantity: 6

Ingredients:

- 2 chopped celery ribs
- 1 tbsp. chili powder
- ½ tbsp. avocado oil
- 1 tsp. chipotle chili powder
- 32 ounces ground beef
- 1 tbsp. cumin
- 1 tsp. salt and pepper each
- 2 tsp. garlic powder
- 16 ounces beef bone broth
- 15 ounces no-salt tomato sauce

Directions:

Prep 5 min. I Cook 30 min. I Ready in 35 min.

- Over medium heat, heat up the avocado oil in a big pot and when heated, add in the chopped celery ribs. Sauté them till they soften or for 3 to 4 minutes.
- Transfer the sautéed celery to a bowl and place aside.
- Add in the beef and all the spices in the large pot and cook till the beef becomes brown and completely cooked. Adjust the heat to medium-low and pour in beef bone broth and tomato sauce. Then, cover the pot and let it simmer for 10 minutes and stir occasionally. Stir in the sautéed celery into the beef and mix well.
- Garnish with chopped spring onion or other toppings of your choice and serve.

Nutrition facts:

Per Serving: 386 calories I 23 g fat I 35 g protein I 7 g carbs

Keto Fried Chicken

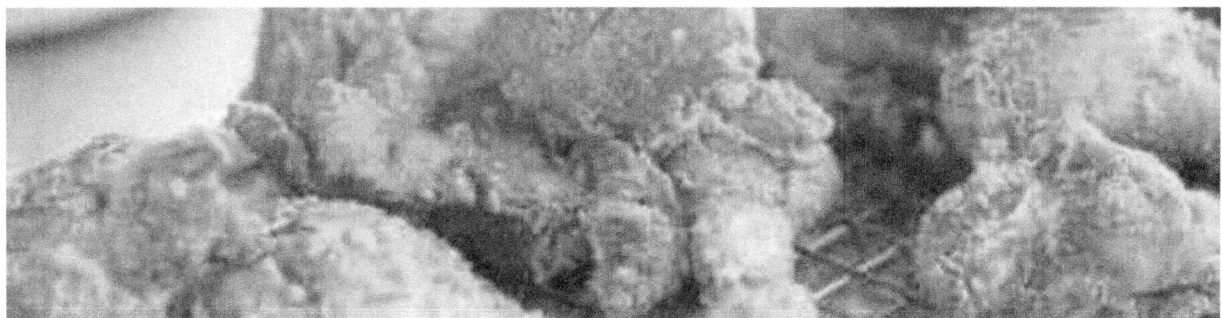

You can have fried chicken on keto if you substitute panko crumbs with whey protein powder. Using pickle juice as the brine or marinade will not only make your fried chicken keto-friendly, but it will also be healthier and more delicious.

Serving quantity: 4

Ingredients:

- 2 scoops unflavored 100% whey protein powder
- 24-ounce pickle jar
- ¼ cup shredded Parmesan cheese
- 1 tsp. paprika
- 8 medium-sized raw chicken breast tenders
- 2 tbsp. avocado oil
- Salt and pepper, to taste
- 2 eggs

Directions:

Prep 10 min. I Cook 20 min. I Ready in 30 min.

- Discard the pickles from the pickle jar. Then, place the chicken tenders inside a plastic bag or in a bowl. Add in the pickle juice to the plastic bag or bowl and mix with chicken if using a bowl. Put the chicken in the fridge for an hour at least to marinate it.
- In a plate, add the shredded Parmesan, salt and pepper, paprika, and the whey protein powder and mix well. In another plate, whisk the eggs to beat them.
- Over medium-high heat, preheat a skillet. Pour in the avocado oil and let it heat up while you coat the chicken. To coat or bread the chicken tenders, first dip them in the egg and then cover with the protein powder mixture.
- When the oil is hot, fry the tenders till they turn golden-brown and the inside is completely cooked. Serve right away.

Nutrition facts:

Per Serving: 345 calories I 15 g fat I 48 g protein I 2 g carbs

Mexican Ground Beef With Veggies

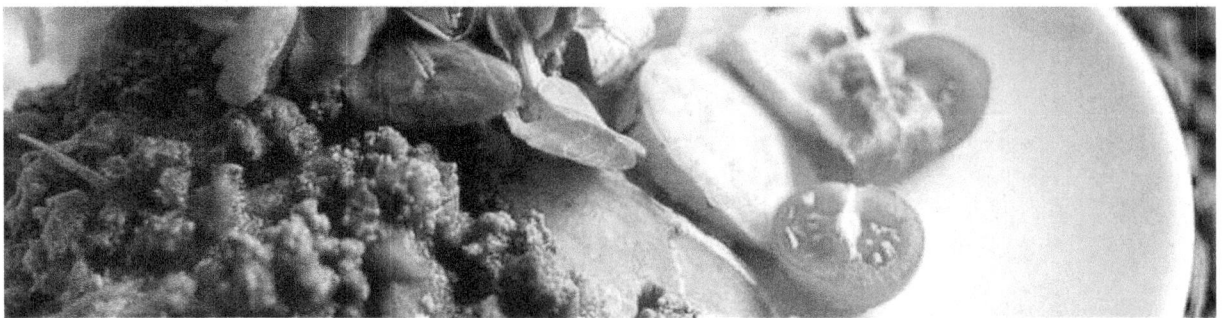

Serving quantity: 4

Ingredients:

- 16 ounces ground beef
- 1/3 cup green bell pepper
- ¼ cup diced onion
- 1 cup diced tomatoes
- 12 ounces cauliflower rice
- ½ cup chicken broth
- 3 tbsp. taco seasoning
- 1 cup shredded cheddar cheese

Directions:

Prep 10 min. | Cook 20 min. | Ready in 30 min.

- Cook ground beef in a large pan over medium heat for 5 minutes.
- Add bell pepper and onion and cook well.
- Mix the taco seasoning.
- Then add cauliflower rice, tomatoes, and chicken broth.
- Let it simmer for 10 minutes on low heat.
- Add the cheese and cover for 5 minutes.
- Serve with fresh vegetables and lemon.

Nutrition facts:

Per Serving: 510 calories | 35 g fat | 33 g protein | 13 g carbs

Bread Rolls

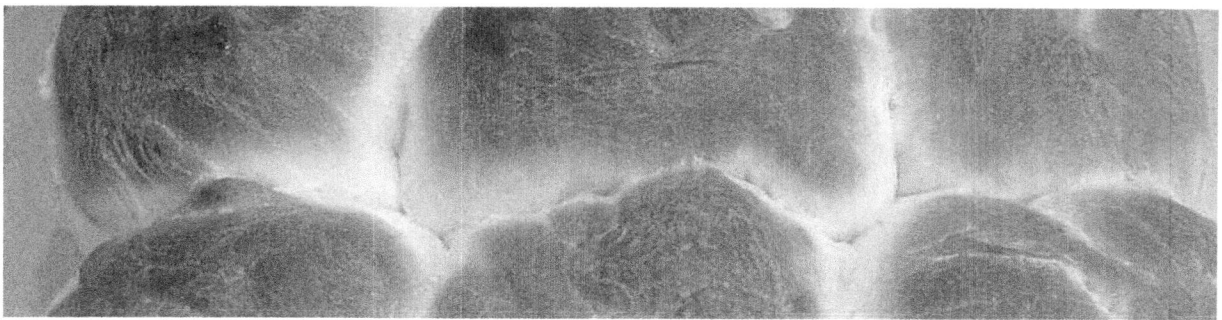

These keto dinner rolls are seriously life-changing. So fluffy and tasty and totally gluten-free! We use almond flour to make these. Eat them as a side dish for dinner.

Serving quantity: 12

Ingredients:

- 1 ⅓ cup almond flour
- 4 large eggs
- 3 cups mozzarella cheese, shredded
- 8 ounces block of cream cheese
- 1 tbsp. butter, unsalted

Directions:

Prep 35 min. | Cook 20 min. | Ready in 55 min.

- Preheat the oven at 400 °F.
- Melt and mix the cream cheese and mozzarella in a pan.
- Otherwise, melt them in the microwave for 30 seconds.
- Take a large bowl and add melted cheese, flour, eggs, baking powder and mix well.
- Refrigerate the mixture for 10 to 20 minutes.
- Roll them into 24 balls and refrigerate for another 10 minutes.
- Grease an iron skillet using butter.
- Place the balls in the skillet and bake for 20 to 25 minutes until cooked golden brown and fluffy.
- Serve them hot and fresh.

Nutrition facts:

Per serving: 251 calories | 19 g fat | 13 g protein | 5 g carbs

Chicken Paprika Meatballs

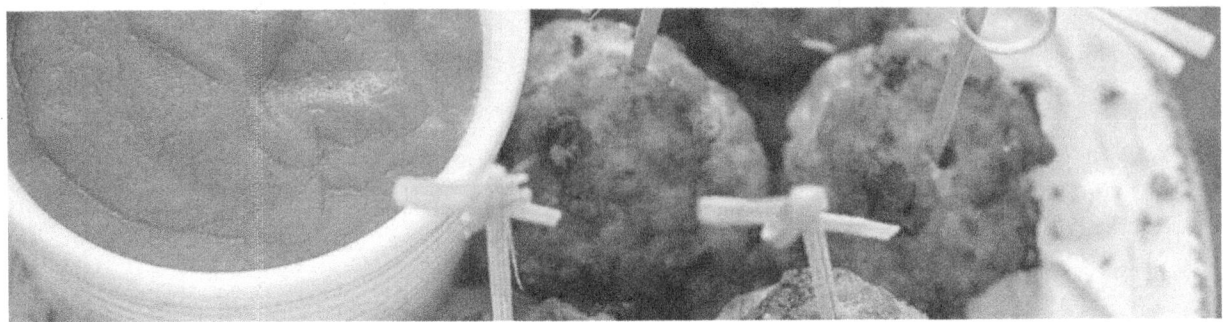

These low carb chicken meatballs are made with ground chicken and other everyday spices and herbs but they are made without any kind of breadcrumbs, which makes them keto-friendly. They taste cheesy and are gluten-free.

Serving quantity: 28

Ingredients:

- 16 ounces ground chicken
- 1 ½ tbsp. olive oil
- 1 tsp. onion powder
- ¾ cup shredded Parmesan cheese
- 1 egg
- 1 tsp. garlic powder
- ½ tsp. salt
- 1 tsp. smoked paprika
- ¼ cup freshly chopped parsley
- ½ tsp. cayenne powder

Directions:

Prep 10 min. I Cook 25 min. I Ready in 35 min.

- Preheat the oven at 400° F and place foil on a baking pan and spray non-stick spray on the foil.
- In a large bowl, add the cheese, ground meat, oil, egg, parsley, and all the spices; mix using your hands – knead to combine everything.
- Use a scooper or a large spoon and scoop a portion of the meatballs mixture onto your hands and make balls.
- Continue to make balls till mixture is finished – you should get 28 to 30 balls.
- Place the balls onto the baking pan.
- Bake the balls for 25 minutes and then take them out from the oven.
- Serve as is or with cauliflower rice.

Nutrition facts:

Per Serving: 58 calories I 4 g fat I 4 g protein I 1 g carbs

Lamb Chops

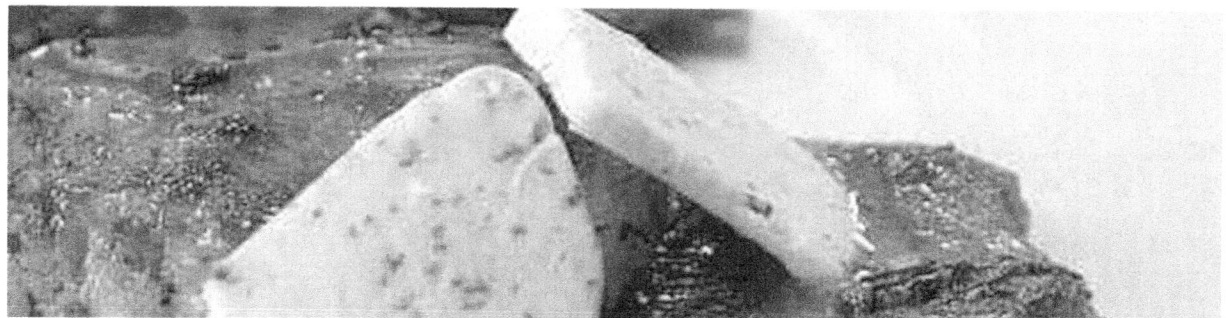

Totally keto-friendly with an air of elegance, this dish is simply delicious. The ingredients used are herb butter and lemon with the lamb chops.

Serving quantity: 4

Ingredients:

- 8 lamb chops
- 1 tbsp. olive oil
- 1 tbsp. butter
- Salt and pepper
- 4 ounces herb butter
- 1 lemon, cut into wedges

Directions:

Prep 5 min. | Cook 10 min. | Ready in 15 min.

- Let the lamb chops reach room temperature before cooking.
- Make cuts on fatty parts.
- Add salt and pepper to the chops.
- Either fry using butter or olive oil or grill after brushing oil.
- Cook for 10 minutes depending on the thickness of the chops.
- Dish out and serve with lemon and herb butter. Enjoy!

Nutrition facts:

Per serving: 761 calories | 62 g fat | 43 g protein | 2 g carbs

Low-Carb Curry Chicken

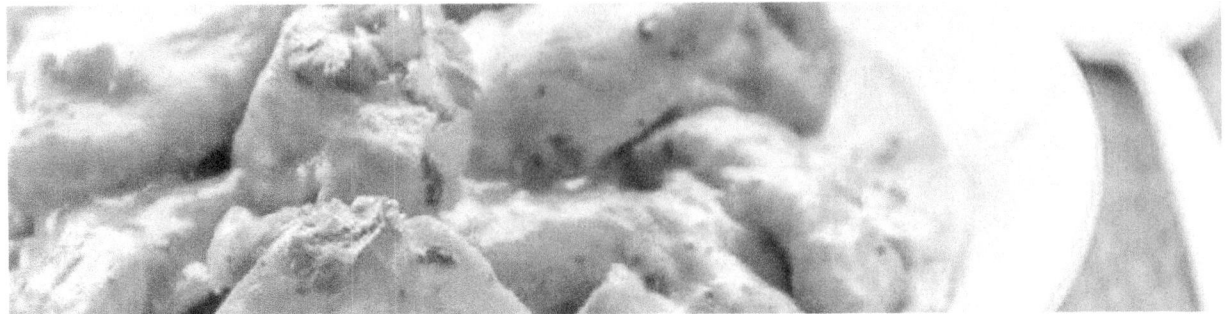

Chicken curry in keto diet is a delicious and fun meal. This coconut cream chicken curry is creamy, low-carb, and will be ready in only 30 minutes. You can serve it with cauliflower rice, zucchini noodles, or keto tortillas.

Serving quantity: 6

Ingredients:

- 16 ounces diced chicken breast
- 14.5 ounces drained, chopped tomatoes can
- 2 tbsp. olive oil
- 1 diced onion
- ¼ cup chicken broth
- 4 minced cloves of garlic
- 1 tsp. paprika
- ½ tsp. salt
- 1 ½ tbsp. curry powder
- 7 ounces coconut cream
- 1 tsp. ground ginger

Directions:

Prep 5 min. I Cook 25 min. I Ready in 30 min.

- Over medium heat, heat up 1 tbsp. of oil in a large pan.
- Stir in the chopped onion and sauté till it turns brown and translucent or for 7 to 10 minutes. Push the sautéed onion to one side and then adjust the heat to medium-high. Pour in 1 tbsp. of oil and place the chicken in one layer.
- Cook each side of the chicken for 1 to 2 minutes or till they turn golden-brown from the outside. Add in the chicken broth, chopped tomatoes, coconut cream, and all the spices to the pan and mix well. Taste and add more salt if needed. Let the mixture boil and then lower the heat. Cover the pan and simmer the curry for 15 to 20 minutes or till the chicken gets cooked completely from the inside and the sauce turns thick.

Nutrition facts:

Per Serving: 248 calories I 17 g fat I 14 g protein I 8 g carbs

Keto Cheesy Cauliflower

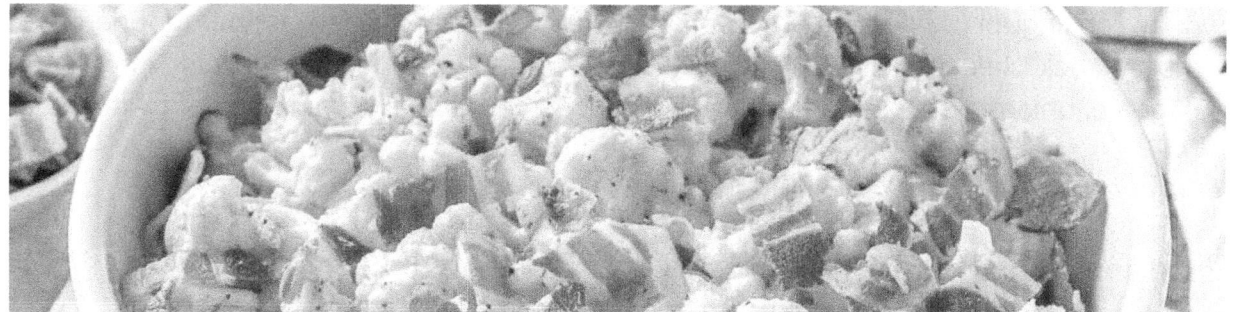

This is mac an' cheese keto style. Cauliflower is a perfect substitute for macaroni. Roasted cauliflower florets covered with a cheesy sauce will leave a creamy taste in your mouth and you can mix cooked, crumbled bacon to the dish to give it a nice crunch.

Serving quantity: 4

Ingredients:

- 1 head cauliflower chopped into small florets
- Sea salt and black pepper, to taste
- ¼ cup heavy cream
- 3 tbsp. butter
- ¼ cup unsweetened almond milk
- 1 cup grated cheddar cheese

Directions:

Prep 5 min. I Cook 20 min. I Ready in 25 min.

- Preheat the oven at 450° F. Use a foil or parchment paper to line a baking sheet pan.
- Melt 2 tbsp. butter in the microwave and toss the cauliflower with this melted butter in a large bowl.
- Sprinkle the florets with salt and pepper and toss again.
- Place the cauliflower florets on the baking sheet and arrange them.
- Bake or roast them till they become crisp but are still tender or for 10 to 15 minutes.
- In a microwave, heat up the heavy cream, milk, 1 tbsp. butter, and cheese till the mixture turns smooth and stir often.
- Do not burn or overheat the cheese mixture. Mix or toss the cauliflower with the cheese mixture and serve.

Nutrition facts:

Per Serving: 308 calories I 23 g fat I 11 g protein I 12 g carbs

Cheesy Beef Stuffed Peppers

If you're looking for a one-dish lunch recipe, then try these stuffed peppers topped with Monterey Jack cheese. This recipe uses classic stuffed pepper ingredients like ground beef, garlic, onion, tomatoes, and spices but it uses cauliflower rice instead of plain rice.

Serving quantity: 6

Ingredients:

- 16 ounces ground beef
- 1 tsp. dried oregano
- 2 tbsp. avocado oil
- 1 cup grated Monterey Jack cheese
- 1 14.5 ounces chopped tomatoes can
- 1 tbsp. tomato paste
- 1 tsp. paprika
- 1 chopped onion
- 1 tsp. salt
- 3 minced garlic cloves
- ¼ tsp. pepper
- 6 bell peppers, tops and cores removed
- 1 ½ cup cauliflower rice

Directions:

Prep 20 min. I Cook 1h I Ready in 1h 20 min.

- Preheat the oven at 400° F.
- Over medium-high heat, heat up the oil in a large 11 inch skillet.
- Add beef along with the spices to the skillet and cook for 5 to 7 minutes.
- Then, add in the garlic and onion and cook for 5 minutes.
- Stir in the tomato paste, cauliflower rice, and chopped tomatoes.
- Cook the mixture for 5 minutes.
- When done, divide the mixture between the 6 bell peppers and then top the mixture in each bell pepper with cheese.
- Clean or wipe the skillet and put the stuffed peppers in it.
- Cover the skillet with a lid and bake them in the oven for 30 minutes.
- The, take off the lid and bake again for 10 minutes or till the cheese becomes bubbly.
- Garnish with chopped parsley or spring onions and serve.

Nutrition facts:

Per Serving: 389 calories I 26 g fat I 21 g protein I 15 g carbs

Keto Bread Sandwich

This keto cloud bread sandwich is perfect to make if you're missing bread while on keto. It can be a little hard to make but it's a great substitute for regular bread.

Serving quantity: 4

Ingredients:

For the Cloud Bread:

- 4 ¼ ounces softened cream cheese
- ½ tsp. baking powder
- ½ tsp. ground psyllium husk powder
- 3 eggs
- ¼ tsp. cream of tartar

Sandwich Filling:

- 5 ounces cooked bacon
- 1 finely sliced large tomato
- 8 tbsp. mayonnaise
- 2 ounces lettuce

Directions:

Prep 15 min. I Cook 25 min. I Ready in 40 min.

- Preheat the oven at 300° F.
- Crack the eggs and separate the yolks from the whites.
- Mix in the cream of tartar and salt to the egg whites and whip with a hand mixer till it becomes very stiff.
- Add the cream cheese and psyllium husk powder to the egg yolks and mix together.
- Add the egg whites to the egg yolk mixture and gently fold the egg whites with the egg yolks.
- Do not overdo the mixing part otherwise the mixture won't remain whipped or cloudy.
- Line a baking sheet pan with parchment paper.
- Shape the cloud bread batter into 8 circles and bake them for 25 minutes or till they turn golden.
- Turn the cloud breads with their top part facing the plate and spread 1 tbsp. of mayonnaise on it and then top with bacon, lettuce, tomato, and a second cloud bread slice.
- Make four sandwiches in the same way. 1 tbsp. of mayonnaise is for each of the 8 cloud breads. Assemble and serve.

Nutrition facts:

Per Serving: 552 calories I 47 g fat I 20 g protein I 7 g carbs I

Tuna Steak

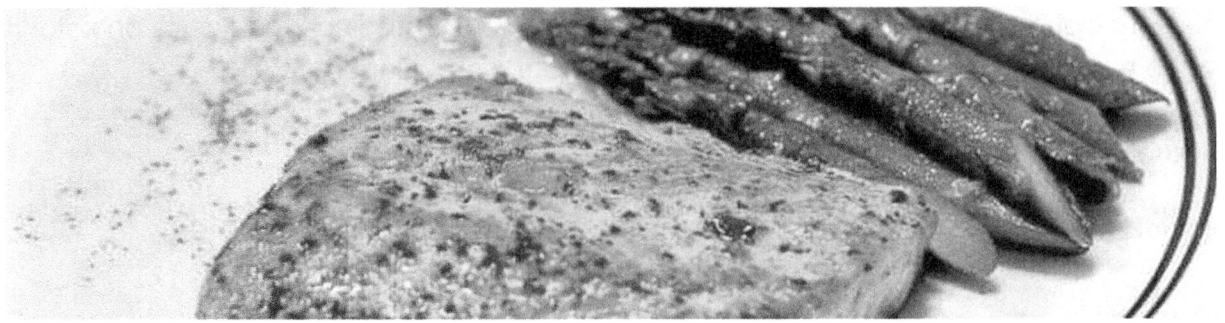

If you in the mood of having seafood for dinner, this recipe is your guide. You can get fresh or frozen tuna from the market and bake it in the oven.

Serving quantity: 2

Ingredients

- 2-6 ounces tuna steak (1 inch thick)
- 12 stalks fresh asparagus, large
- 1 lemon, fresh
- 6 tbsp. olive oil, extra virgin
- 1 tsp. dill weed, dried
- 1 tsp. garlic powder
- 1 tsp. salt & ½ tsp black pepper
- ⅓ cup parmesan cheese, grated

Directions:

Prep 10 min. | Cook 15 min. | Ready in 25 min.

- Preheat the oven at 400 °F. Put the tuna in a large bowl.
- Squeeze lemon and add salt, pepper, olive oil, and dill weed.
- Toss and turn gently till well mixed. Line the baking pan and set the steaks in them.
- Cover the top of the steaks with all the mixture using a spoon.
- Line another baking pan and take off the ends of asparagus stalks and spread them on the sheet. Lay out the onions cut in strips over asparagus.
- Add salt, pepper, parmesan, olive oil, and garlic powder. Roll them around to get it all coated. Put the pans in the oven. Check them after 10 minutes.
- Poke the asparagus with the fork to see if it is soft.
- Poke tuna with your finger to see if it is firm. Tuna takes about 10-12 minutes while asparagus takes about 5-10 minutes.
- When done, medium rare or well done, dish it out and serve.

Nutrition facts:

Per serving: 586 calories | 52 g fat | 17 g protein | 8 g carbohydrates

Salsa Chicken

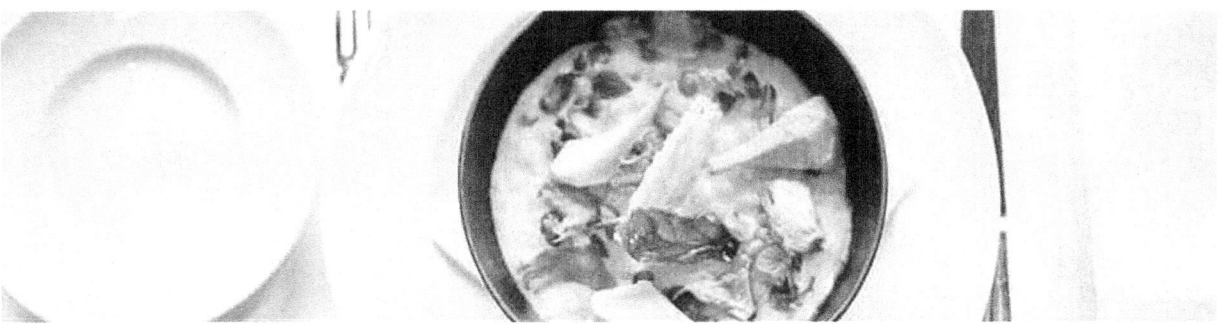

Salsa chicken is such a flavorful Mexican dish. This keto-friendly recipe will be your new favorite once you try it.

Serving quantity: 6

Ingredients:

- 32 ounces boneless chicken thighs
- 3 tbsp. taco seasoning
- 4 ounces cream cheese
- 1 cup salsa
- 1/4 cup chicken broth
- Salt and pepper, to taste

Directions:

Prep 5 min. | Cook 30 min. | Ready in 35 min.

- Put chicken thighs in an Instant Pot.
- Then season with salt, pepper, and taco seasoning.
- Add salsa, cream cheese, and broth.
- Close the lid and manually set it on High for 20 minutes.
- Let the pressure release naturally when the cooking time is over.
- Release any remaining pressure by opening the vent.
- Remove the lid and transfer the chicken to a separate plate.
- Blend the sauce for a smooth consistency.
- Shred the chicken and mix it with the sauce.

Nutrition facts:

Per Serving: 232 calories | 10 g fat | 30 g protein | 4 g carbs

Keto Pepperoni Pizza

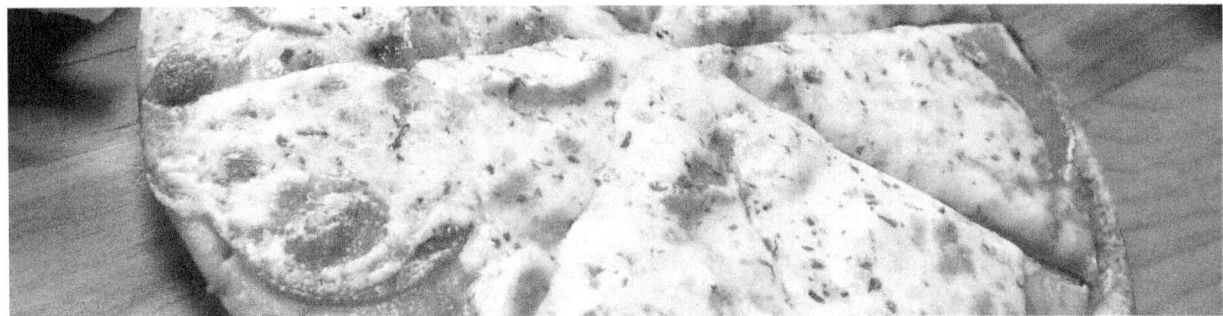

Miss pepperoni pizza? Here is the keto-friendly version of your favorite pizza. Make it at home and enjoy it without all the extra carbs and guilt.

Serving quantity: 2

Ingredients:

Crust:

- 4 eggs
- 6 ounces shredded mozzarella cheese

Toppings:

- 3 tbsp. tomato sauce, unsweetened
- 1 ounce pepperoni
- 5 ounces shredded cheese
- 1 tsp. dried oregano

Directions:

Prep 5 min. | Cook 25 min. | Ready in 30 min.

- Preheat oven to 400° F. Make crust in a bowl by mixing eggs and cheese.
- Spread the crust mixture on a lined baking sheet.
- Bake it for 15 minutes. Take out the crust and let it cool.
- Adjust the temperature to 450° F.
- Spread the sauce and top with pepperoni.
- Finish with cheese and dried oregano.
- Bake for 10 minutes.
- Drizzle a little olive oil and sprinkle pepper flakes before serving.

Nutrition facts:

Per Serving: 10475calories | 90 g fat | 53 g protein | 5 g carbs

Butter Chicken

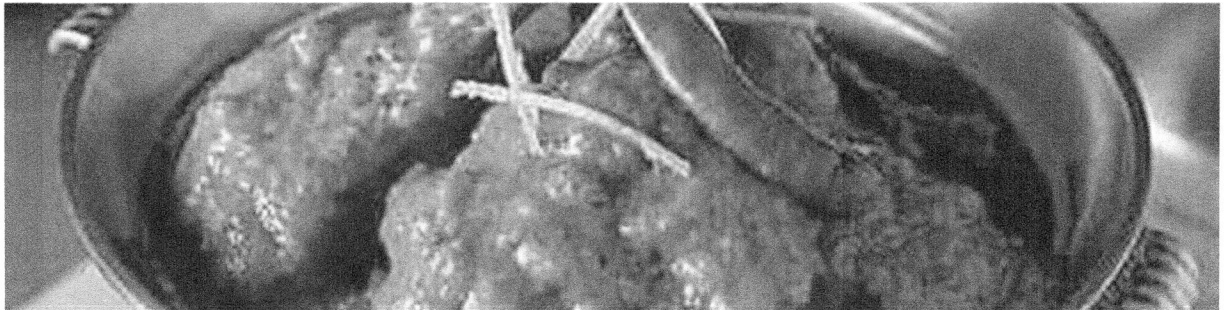

This low-carb chicken is cooked in butter and is extremely nutritious and delicious. It takes less time to prepare and the curry can be served with low carb rice or bread.

Serving quantity: 6

Ingredients:

- 24 ounces boneless chicken thighs
- 2 tbsp. avocado oil
- 2 tbsp. fresh sage, chopped
- 4 slices chopped prosciutto
- ½ cup butter
- salt and pepper

Directions:

Prep 5 min. | Cook 15 min. | Ready in 20 min.

- Remove the skin and cut chicken into 1 inch pieces.
- Season with salt and pepper.
- Heat a pan over medium heat and add avocado oil.
- Fry the chicken for 10 minutes till cooked and nicely browned from both sides.
- Take it out in a bowl and set aside.
- Melt the butter in a pan and add prosciutto and sage.
- Cook for about 4 minutes till the butter turns deep amber.
- Remove from heat and add and coat the chicken.
- Serve with cauliflower rice or zucchini noodles.

Nutrition facts:

Per Serving: 300 calories | 19 g fat | 28 g protein | 2 g carbs

Recipes PART 7
KETO DINNER

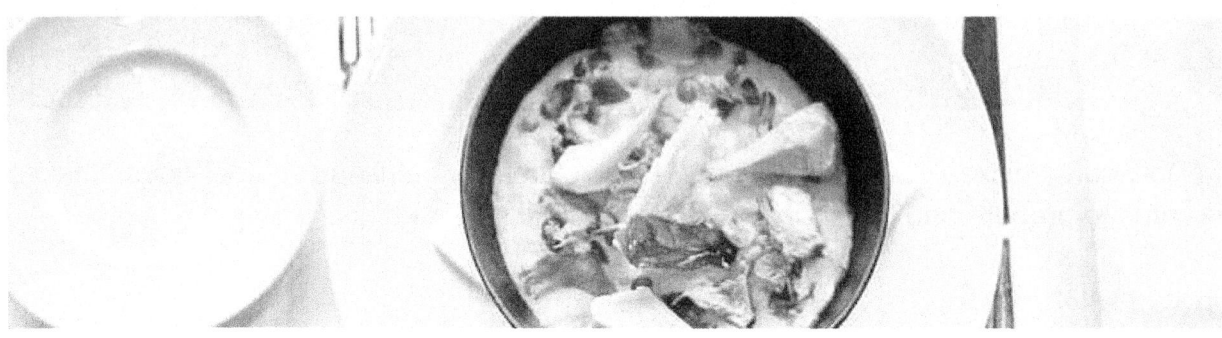

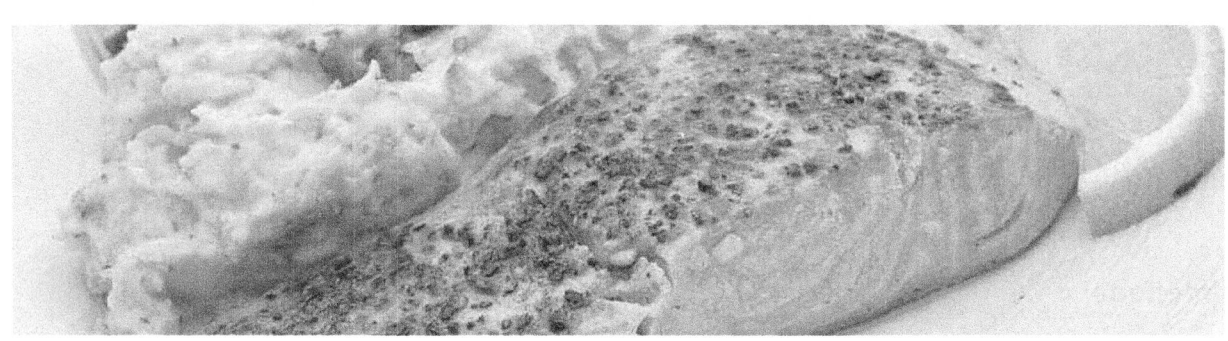

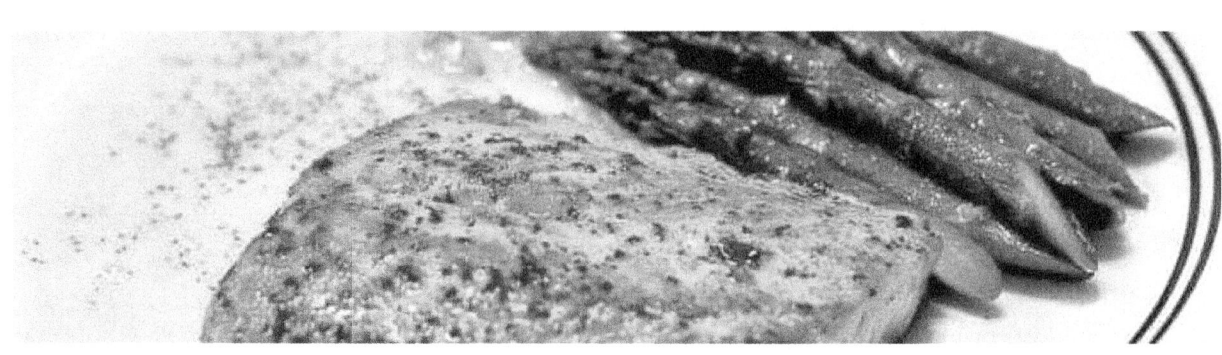

Skillet Lasagna

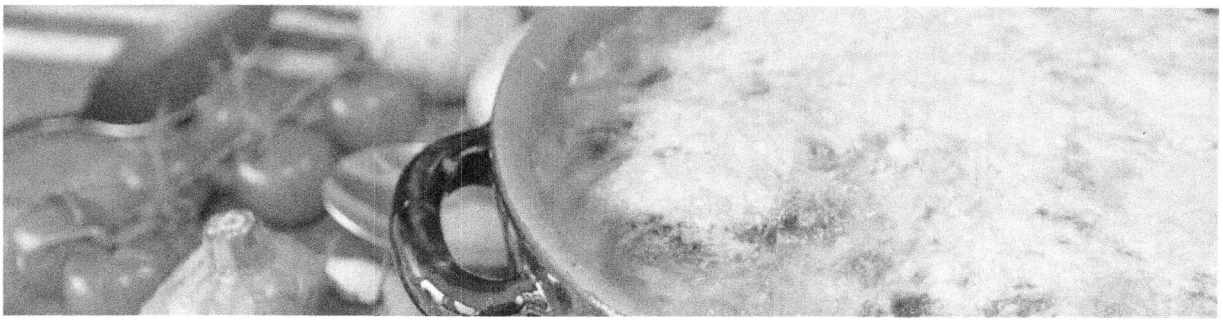

Cooking in one pan makes it easier to cook your dinner and it even reduces cooking time. This easy lasagna is rich, hearty, and low-carb; everything a keto dieter wishes for!

Serving quantity: 8

Ingredients:

- 2 zucchinis
- 2 tbsp. avocado oil
- 2 garlic cloves
- 1/2 tsp. red pepper flakes
- 1 tsp. italian seasoning
- 3/4 tsp. salt
- ½ tsp. pepper
- 24 ounces ground beef
- 1 cup tomato puree
- 1 cup ricotta
- ¼ cup grated parmesan
- 1½ cups shredded mozzarella cheese
- fresh basil for garnish

Directions:

Prep 10 min. | Cook 20 min. | Ready in 30 min.

- Slice zucchini into a quarter inch slices.
- Heat avocado oil in a large pan over medium heat.
- Add garlic and pepper flakes and sauté for 30 seconds.
- Add beef, salt, pepper, and Italian seasoning and cook for 8-10 minutes.
- Add zucchini and tomato puree and cook for 5 minutes.
- When zucchini and beef are cooked, add all the cheeses, cook on low heat until the cheese melts.
- Garnish with chopped basil and serve.

Nutrition facts:

Per Serving: 411 calories | 27 g fat | 33 g protein | 6 g carbs

Garlic Butter Salmon

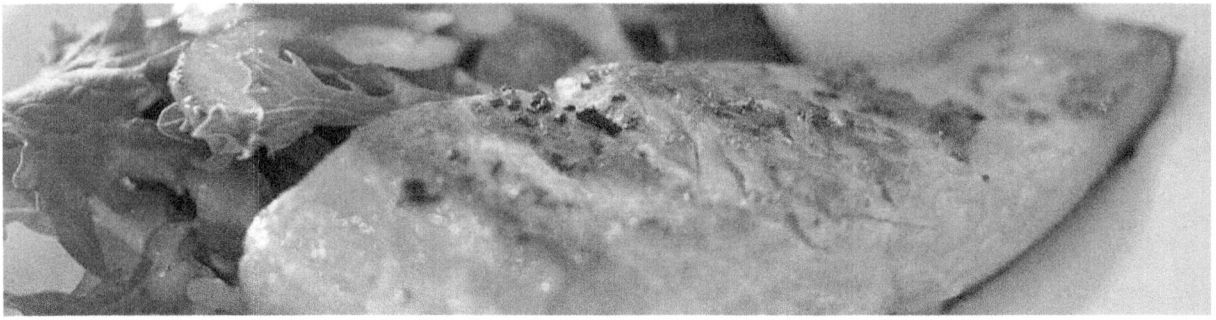

Cook salmon beautifully with garlic butter and love the natural taste of this amazing fish. The best part is that it only takes 30 minutes to cook this lovely dinner.

Serving quantity: 4

Ingredients:

- 24 ounces salmon fillet, cut into 4 equal pieces
- ¼ cup butter
- 3 garlic cloves, minced
- 2 tbsp. chopped parsley
- 16 ounces cauliflower florets
- salt and pepper, to taste
- 1 tsp. lemon zest
- lemon wedges for garnish

Directions:

Prep 8 min. | Cook 22 min. | Ready in 30 min.

- Preheat oven to 400° F, add 2 tbsp. of butter on a lined baking sheet and place it in the oven. Melt the rest of the butter in a small bowl.
- Mix lemon zest, garlic, and parsley in the butter.
- Add cauliflower florets in the baking pan when the butter melts.
- Season with salt and pepper and mix well.
- Put it back in the oven and bake for 10 minutes.
- In a large bowl, season the salmon fillets with salt, pepper, and mix in the garlic butter.
- Then place these coated fillets in the baking sheet and pour over garlic butter.
- Bake for 10 minutes and check with a fork if the fish is cooked.
- Bake 5 more minutes if it's undercooked.
- When the salmon is cooked, take out from the oven and serve with lemon wedges.

Nutrition facts:

Per Serving: 404 calories | 24 g fat | 37 g protein | 7 g carbs

Chicken Caprese

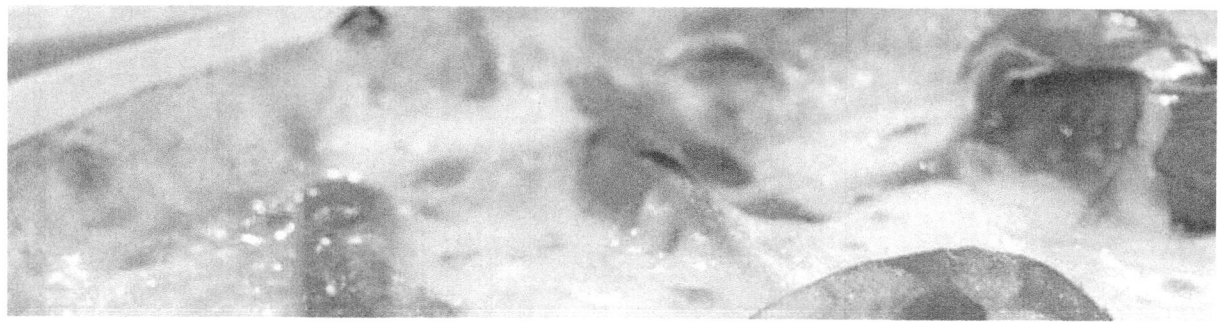

Here is a bit different take on Italian Caprese salad. This keto recipe is made with fresh vegetables, chicken, and cheese. It's easy to make and the whole family is going to love it.

Serving quantity: 4

Ingredients:

- 2 tbsp. avocado oil
- 5 boneless chicken thighs
- 6 ounces sliced mozzarella
- 1 tomato, sliced
- 1/4 cup chopped basil
- salt and pepper, to taste

Directions:

Prep 5 min. | Cook 35 min. | Ready in 40 min.

- Preheat oven to 375° F.
- Rub chicken with salt and pepper.
- Heat oil in a large pan and sear the chicken on both sides until it is golden brown.
- Place chicken in a single layer in a baking dish.
- Then layer the cheese and tomato slices.
- Bake for 25 minutes.
- Garnish with basil when it is cooked

Nutrition facts:

Per Serving: 333 calories | 19 g fat | 36 g protein | 2 g carbs

Lamb Kofta

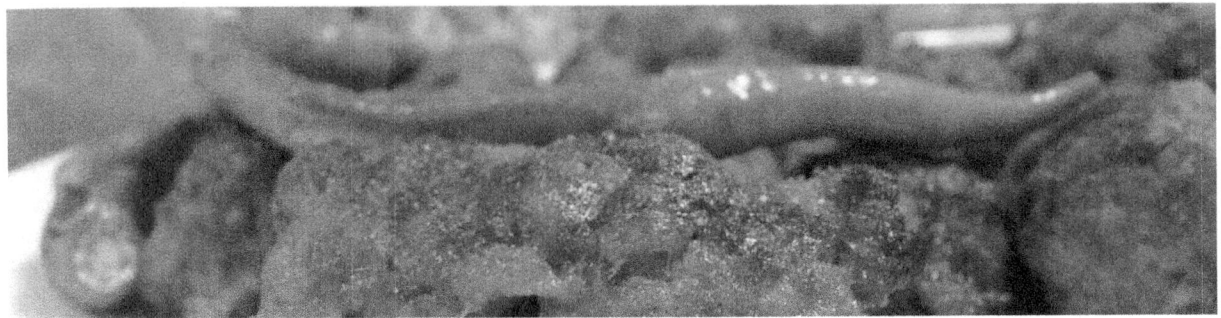

Lamb kofta is a delicious delicacy. It is keto-friendly and a dream come true for meat lovers.

Serving quantity: 6

Ingredients:

- 32 ounces ground lamb
- ¾ tsp. salt
- 1 tbsp. ground cumin
- ½ tsp. black pepper
- ½ tsp. cinnamon
- 1 tsp. paprika
- 2 tbsp. cilantro or parsley, freshly chopped
- 1 tbsp. coriander, grounded
- 2 tbsp. garlic, minced

Directions:

Prep 15 min. | Cook 12 min. | Ready in 27 min.

- Take a large bowl and combine all the ingredients well using your hands.
- Form them in ovals about 1-inch thick and 4 inches long. Make 12 of these.
- If you are using bamboo skewers, soak them in water for an hour.
- Put the koftas on a skewer if you want and air fry them for 10 to 12 minutes at 400°F. They are cooked when they are nicely browned.
- Alternatively, bake them at 375 °F or grill them over medium heat for 12 minutes.
- When done, let them rest for 5 minutes and serve.

Nutrition facts:

Per serving: 424 calories | 28 g fat | 38 g protein | 2 g carbs

Garlic Chicken

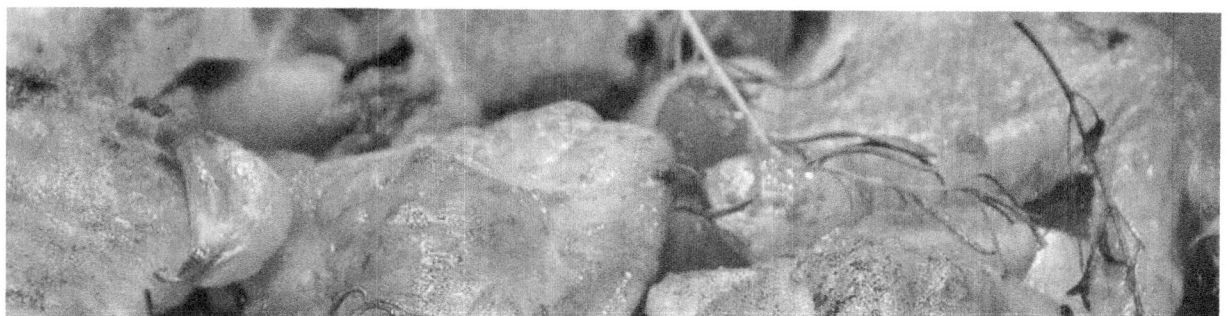

It is low-carb and has a fresh garlic and lemon taste. It doesn't take a lot of time and makes an excellent dinner for anyone craving something unique. The aroma is absolutely mouthwatering!

Serving quantity: 4

Ingredients:

- 32 ounces chicken drumsticks
- 7 sliced garlic cloves
- 2 ounces butter
- 2 tbsp. olive oil
- 1 lemon for juice
- ½ cup chopped parsley
- Salt, pepper

Directions:

Prep 15 min. | Cook 45 min. | Ready in 1 h

- Preheat the oven to 450 °F.
- Place the chicken pieces on a baking pan greased with butter and add salt and pepper to the chicken.
- Spray the lemon juice and olive oil over the chicken.
- Sprinkle the garlic and parsley as well.
- Bake for 30 to 40 minutes till the chicken becomes golden.
- Lower the flame at the end. It can take longer depending on the size of the drumsticks.
- Dish them out and serve with salad, cauliflower mash, or aioli.

Nutrition facts:

Per serving: 547 calories | 39 g fats | 42 g protein | 3 g carbs

Low-Carb Pasta

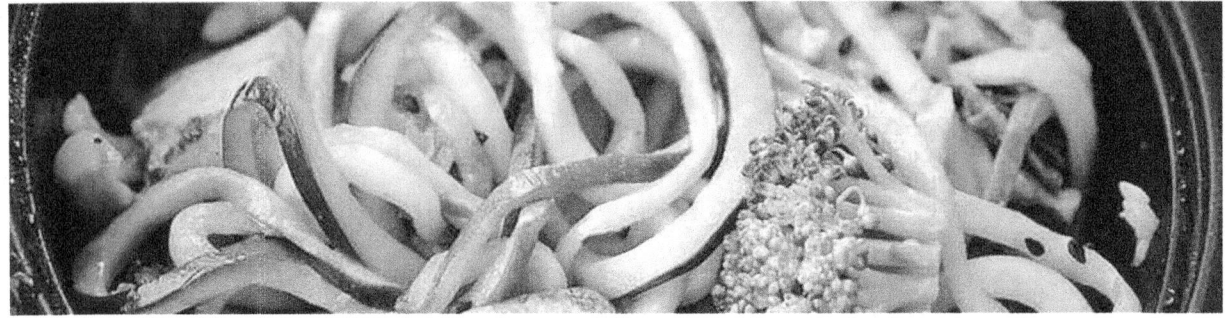

This dish is vegetarian and essentially plant-based. It is super healthy and delicious.

Serving quantity: 2

Ingredients:

- 4 zucchini squash, cut into noodles or use a spiralizer
- 7 asparagus stalks, cut into cubes
- 1 chopped garlic clove
- 1 tbsp. olive oil
- sea salt, pepper

Directions:

Prep 5 min. | Cook 25 min. | Ready in 30 min.

- Wash and prepare the vegetables.
- Use a spiralizer or cut to form zucchini noodles.
- Add olive oil to a skillet and heat over medium flame for 1 to 2 minutes.
- Add garlic and cook for 1 to 2 minutes.
- Add zucchini noodles and asparagus and cook for 10 to 15 minutes and stir every 3 to 4 minutes.
- Sprinkle salt, pepper, and herbs and continue cooking for 1 to 2 min.
- When done, dish out, serve, and enjoy!

Nutrition facts:

Per serving: 110 g calories | 7 g fat | 4 g protein | 7 g carbs

Butter Poached Shrimp

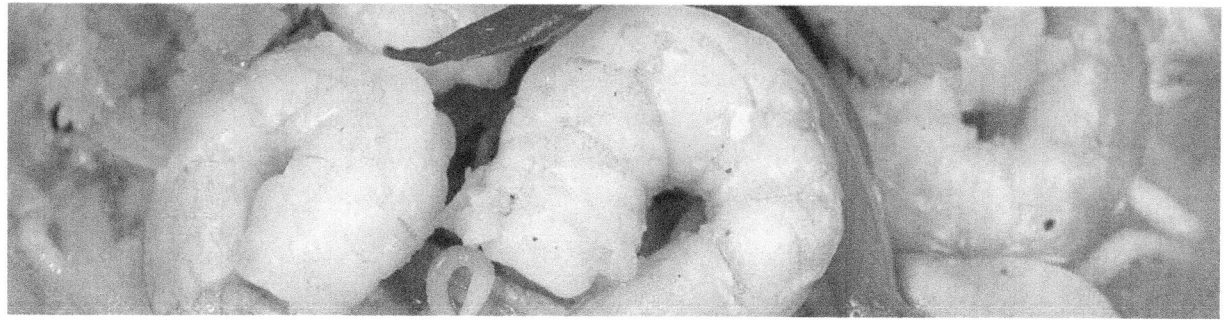

Keto dish cooked in less time? This is your champion. Tasty wild shrimp cooked in butter and served with zoodles or asparagus makes it a real deal for dinner.

Serving quantity: 4

Ingredients:

- 16 ounces shrimp, large, peeled, deveined
- 3 tbsp. water
- 1 cup ghee or butter
- 1 lemon zest
- 1 bay leaf
- 6 sprigs fresh oregano or ½ tsp. dried oregano
- salt, to taste
- basil for garnish

Directions:

Prep 10 min. | Cook 15 min. | Ready in 25 min.

- Boil water on high heat in a pan.
- Lower heat to medium and whisk butter or ghee until smooth.
- Add oregano, lemon zest, bay leaf, and shrimp and season everything with salt.
- Stir and spread it evenly.
- Cook for about 5 minutes on medium-low heat.
- Let the sauce come to a low simmer so that the shrimp is cooked well.
- Serve it on a plate with the garnish of fresh basil.

Nutrition facts:

Per serving: 309 calories | 27 g fat | 13 g protein | 1 g carbs

Mangolian Beef

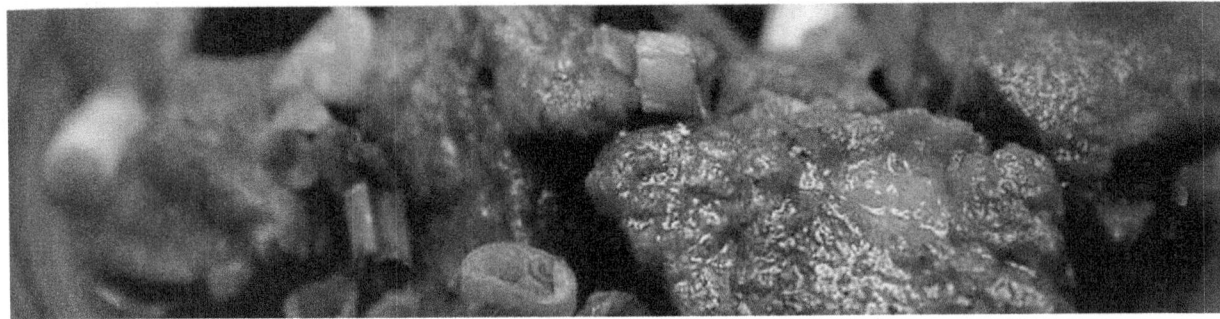

The beef is slow-cooked and highly tender, soaking all the spices and juices. Easy to prepare and served with cauliflower rice. It is a great family-style meal.

Serving quantity: 4

Ingredients:

- 88 ounces steak, flank, or sirloin
- 2 chopped green onions
- ¼ cup water
- stevia, to taste
- ¼ cup turmeric or soy sauce
- 2 cloves minced garlic
- ½ tsp. ground ginger
- 2 tbsp. sesame oil
- ¼ tsp. red pepper flakes
- ½ tsp. glucomannan powder or ¼ tsp. xanthan powder
- sesame seeds for garnish

Directions:

Prep 10 min. | Cook 6 h | Ready in 6 h 10 min.

- Thinly slice fresh beef and put it in the slow cooker.
- Whisk sesame oil, water, garlic, ginger, red pepper flakes, tamari, and brown sugar substitute in a bowl.
- Pour the mixture over the beef.
- Put the lid on the cooker and either slow cook for 4 to 6 hours or cook on high flame for 2 to 3 hours.
- When done, take some broth out and mix the glucomannan powder.
- Pour it back into the pot and mix until well coated.
- Spread sesame seeds and green onions over the beef and serve with cauliflower rice.

Nutrition facts:

Per serving: 388 calories | 25 g fat | 36 g protein | 2 g carbs

Salmon With Spinach

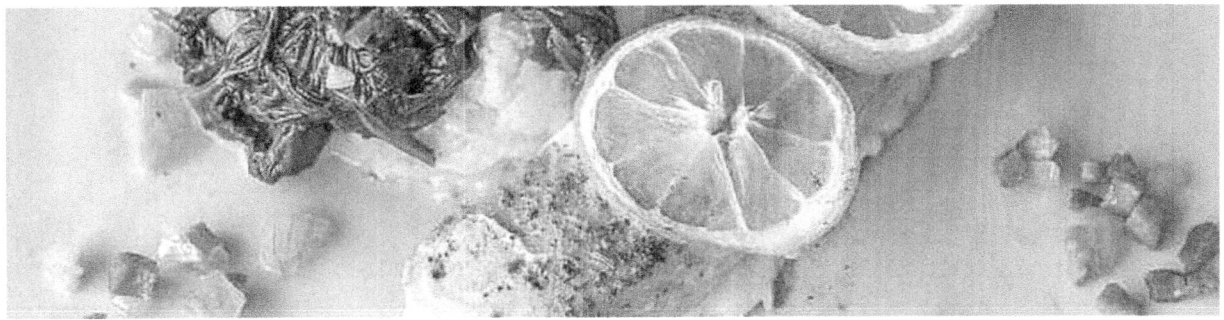

Salmon cooked with chili paste and served with spinach has a simple and elegant taste. It is so fresh, healthy, and tasty for anyone who likes fish. Totally keto-friendly!

Serving quantity: 4

Ingredients:

- 88 ounces salmon, cut into pieces
- 16 ounces fresh spinach
- 1 ounce grated parmesan cheese
- 2 ounces butter or olive oil
- ½ cup mayonnaise or sour cream
- 1 tbsp. chili paste
- salt and pepper

Directions:

Prep 5 min. | Cook 20 min. | Ready in 25 min.

- Set the oven at 400 °F.
- Use half the butter to grease a baking dish.
- Add salt and pepper to the salmon and place it on the baking dish, with the skin facing downwards.
- Mix mayonnaise, cheese, and chili paste separately and spread the mixture over the salmon.
- Put it in the oven and bake for 15 to 20 minutes till it changes color and flakes easily.
- Use the remaining butter to stir fry the spinach for about 2 minutes till wilts.
- Sprinkle it with salt and pepper to taste.
- Serve the oven-baked salmon with stir-fried spinach and enjoy!

Nutrition facts:

Per serving: 706 calories | 57 g fat | 41 g protein | 2 g carbs

Stuffed Avocado

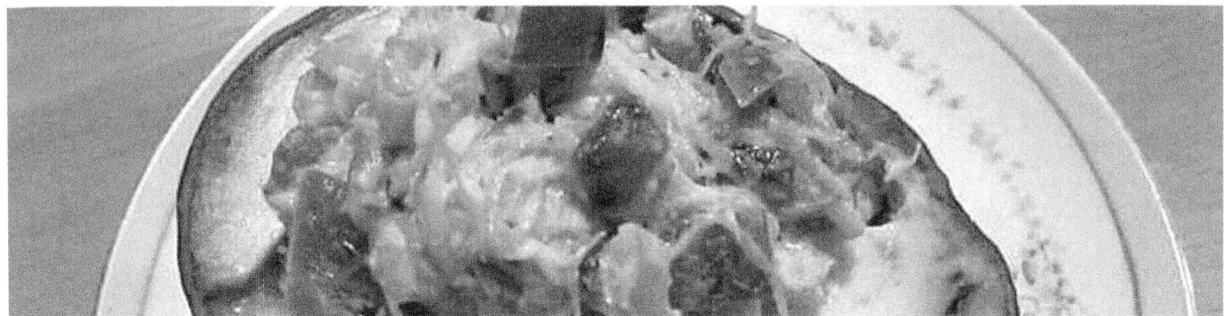

Stuffed vegetables and fruits have a lot of varieties and they are particularly easy to whip up on weeknights. What's more, it is very tasty as well.

Serving quantity: 8

Ingredients:

- 4 pitted and halved avocados
- 4 ounces shredded cheese, organic
- 2 cooked and shredded chicken breasts
- 4 ounces cream cheese
- ¼ tsp salt and pepper

Directions:

Prep 20 min. | Cook 10 min. | Ready in 30 min.

- Set the oven up to 400°F.
- Take a bowl and add half scooped out avocado, cream cheese, chicken, diced tomato, salt and pepper, and mix thoroughly.
- Scoop the mixture in avocado halves.
- Top with shredded cheese and place them on the lined baking sheet and put them in the oven.
- Bake for 8 to 10 minutes till the cheese melts and turns golden brown.
- Remove and serve.
- You can replace chicken with ground beef, tuna or crab as you like.

Nutrition facts:

Per serving: 265 calories | 21 g fat | 12 g protein 5 g carbs

Buttery Chicken With Broccoli

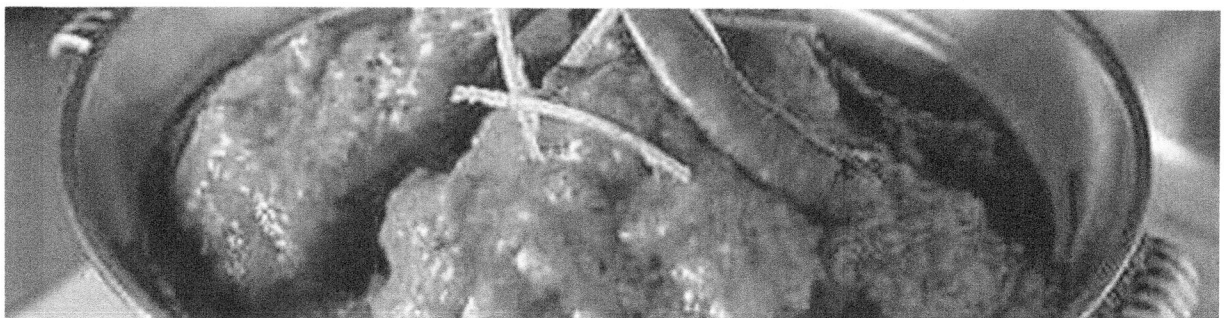

Simple but delicious keto recipe. You will be happy with it.

Serving quantity: 2

Ingredients:

- 9 ounces broccoli
- 10 ounces chicken
- 3 ounces butter
- salt and pepper, to taste

Directions:

Prep 5 min. | Cook 15 min. | Ready in 20 min.

- Wash and cut the broccoli.
- Heat half of the butter in a large frying pan and add chicken.
- Season the chicken with salt and pepper and cook it on both sides, 5 minutes each side.
- Make sure that it is cooked through.
- Add the rest of the butter and fry broccoli in the same pan.
- When everything is cooked, serve with fresh salad.

Nutrition facts:

Per Serving: 753 calories | 66 g fat | 29 g protein | 5 g carbs

Cheese Stuffed Meatballs

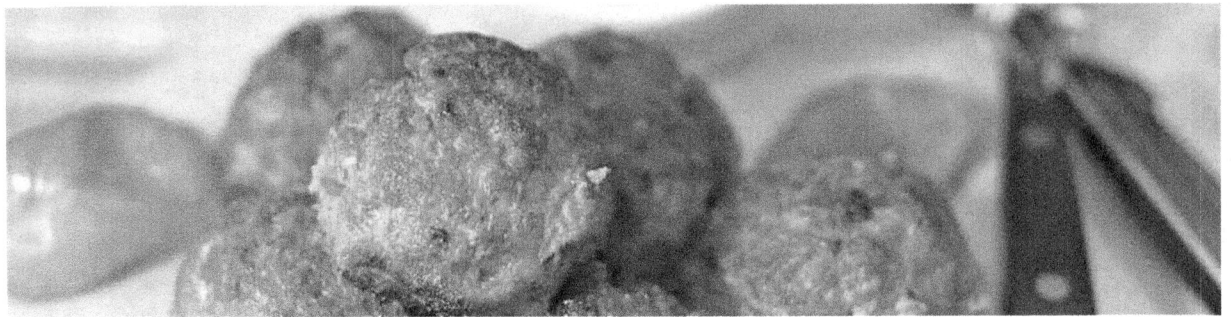

That oozing gooey cheese coming out of your meatball is what makes this dish a treat for you. It is so delicious that you would want to eat all of them by yourself.

Serving quantity: 4

Ingredients:

- 24 ounces ground beef
- 4 ounces mozzarella cheese
- ½ tsp. salt
- ¼ tsp. pepper
- 1 tbsp. dried basil
- 2 tbsp. cold water
- butter for frying

Directions:

Prep 15 min. | Cook 25 min. | Ready in 40 min.

- Add salt, pepper, basil, and cold water in the beef and mix well in a bowl.
- Make 10 flat patties.
- Cut mozzarella in 10 pieces and place one on each patty.
- Wrap the patties around the cheese and make balls.
- Fry on medium-low heat until they turn golden brown.
- Serve hot with lettuce wraps or fresh salad.

Nutrition facts:

Per Serving: 424 calories | 28 g fat | 39 g protein | 1 g carbs

Cabbage Casserole

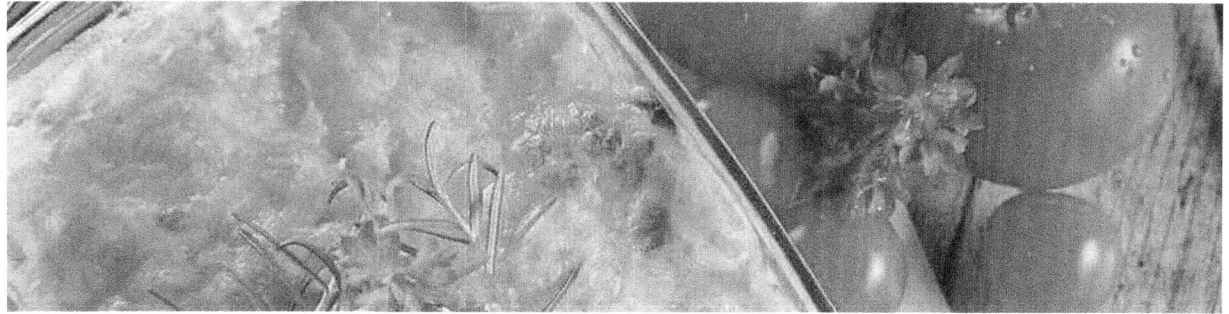

If you want to make a delicious dish out of something as humble as cabbage, try this cabbage casserole. Enjoy it with grilled meat of your choice.

Serving quantity: 6

Ingredients:

- 32 oz. green cabbage
- 1 onion
- 2 garlic cloves
- 1 cup heavy whipping
- 6 tbsp. sour cream
- 6 oz. cream cheese
- 4 oz. butter
- 6 oz. shredded cheese
- 1 tsp. salt
- ½ tsp. black pepper

Directions:

Prep 15 min | Cook 45 min | Ready in 1h

- Preheat oven to 400º F.
- Chop onion, cabbage, and garlic in a food processor.
- Melt butter in a large pan.
- Sauté chopped vegetables for 10 minutes.
- Add spices, cream cheese, cream, and sour cream.
- Mix well and let it cook for 10 minutes on low heat.
- Grease a baking dish and arrange the vegetable mixture in the dish.
- Sprinkle cheese and bake for 20 minutes.

Nutrition facts:

Per Serving: 629 calories | 57 g fat | 13 g protein | 11 g carbohydrates

Chicken Adobo

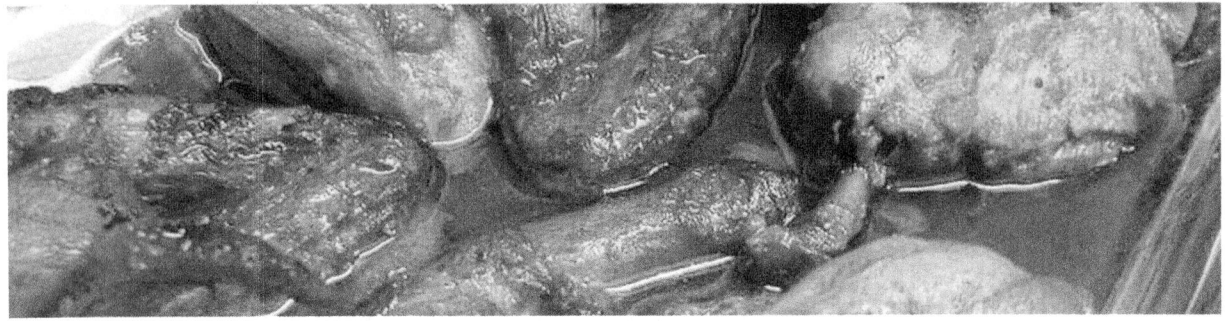

Chicken cooked in a pressure cooker takes little time and is extra tender. This recipe is from Philippines and is packed with a lot of flavors. It is keto-friendly as well. Serve with low carb cauliflower rice.

Serving quantity: 4

Ingredients:

- 36 ounces boneless chicken thighs
- 1 sliced onion
- 5 minced garlic cloves
- 3 bay leaves
- ½ cup soy sauce, low sodium
- ⅓ cup white vinegar
- ¼ tsp. cayenne, grounded
- salt and pepper
- 2 tbsp. olive oil
- 2 sliced scallions of green onions

Directions:

Prep 15 min. | Cook 35 min. | Ready in 50 min.

- Season chicken thighs with salt and pepper. Put the Instant Pot on sauté mode. Wait till it reads hot. When hot, add olive oil.
- Add half the thighs and cook on both sides for a few minutes.
- Take them out and repeat the process with the remaining chicken. Turn off this mode.
- Mix onion, garlic, vinegar, soy sauce, and cayenne in the pot.
- Add chicken and add bay leaf on top. Seal the lid and cook on high pressure for 10 minutes. Release the pressure and take off the lid.
- Let the sauce simmer for 15 minutes till it thickens.
- When done, sprinkle scallions and serve.

Nutrition facts:

Per serving: 376 calories | 21 g fat | 37 g protein | 7 g carbs

Keto Meatloaf

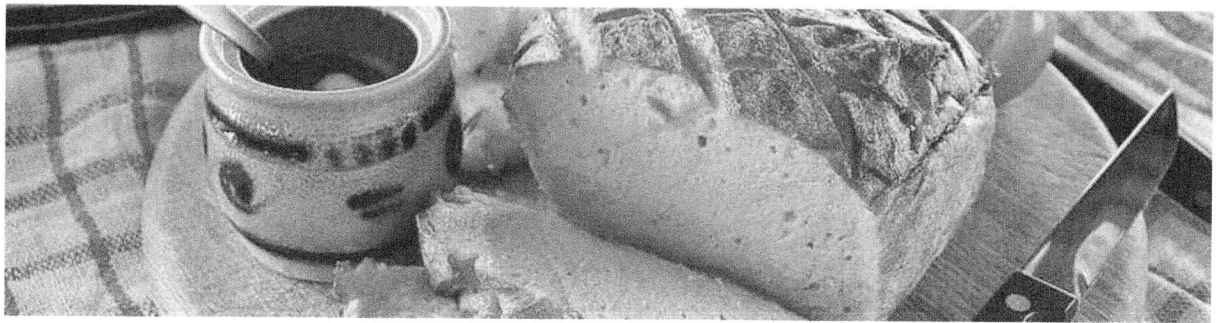

This keto meatloaf is a dinner recipe that can be eaten with whipped cauliflower. It has a wonderful aroma and needs to be put in the oven only. It can be served hot and fresh.

Serving quantity: 6

Ingredients:

- 16 ounces ground beef
- ½ cup cheddar cheese, shredded
- ½ cup sugar-free ketchup
- 1 red onion
- 4 garlic cloves
- 2 eggs
- ½ tsp. salt

Directions:

Prep 5 min. | Cook 50 min. | Ready in 55 min.

- Set the oven at 375 °F.
- Blend onion, garlic, and salt in a food processor till creamy but not pureed.
- Add cheese and eggs and blend in short intervals till well combined.
- Add beef in the mixture and combine.
- Transfer in a baking pan and put it in the oven to bake for 40 minutes.
- After 40 minutes, turn the heat up to 425°F.
- Remove it from the oven and add low-carb sugar-free ketchup and bake for 10 more minutes.
- When done, take it out and let it cool.
- Serve with whipped cauliflower.

Nutrition facts:

Per serving: 318 calories | 13 g fat | 40 g protein | 8 g carbs

Roasted Pork Belly

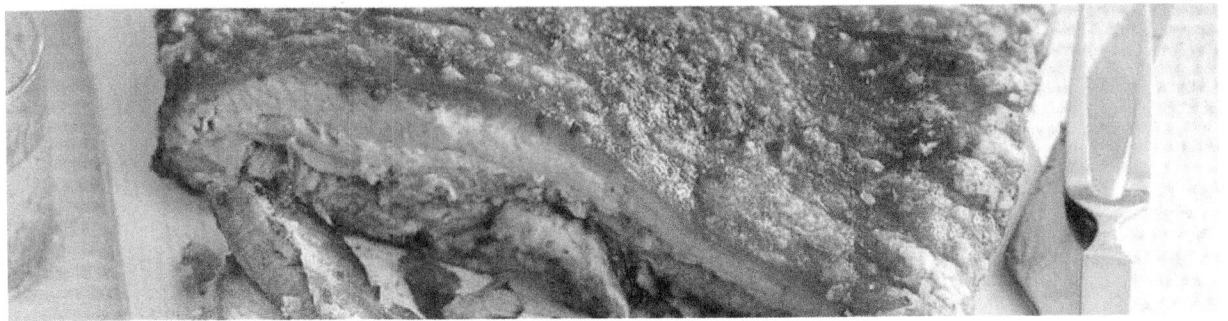

Pork belly has high-fat content which makes it perfect for a keto meal. With delicious fat juices and meat, dinner becomes a treat.

Serving quantity: 8

Ingredients:

- 32 ounces pork belly
- 2 tsp. olive oil
- 2 tsp. salt
- ½ tsp. pepper

Directions:

Prep 10 min. | Cook 1 h | Ready in 1 h 10 min.

- Set the oven at 450 °F.
- Score the skin of pork belly and use a paper towel to pat it dry.
- Marinate the belly with olive oil, salt, and pepper.
- Roast in a baking tray with skin side up for 25 to 30 minutes.
- Reduce the heat to 320 °F and roast for 1 hour or 1 hour 15 minutes.
- After removing from the oven, wrap it up in aluminum foil and let it rest for 20 minutes before serving.

Nutrition facts:

Per serving: 608 calories | 61 g fat | 10 g protein | 0 g carbs

Bacon Wrapped Chicken

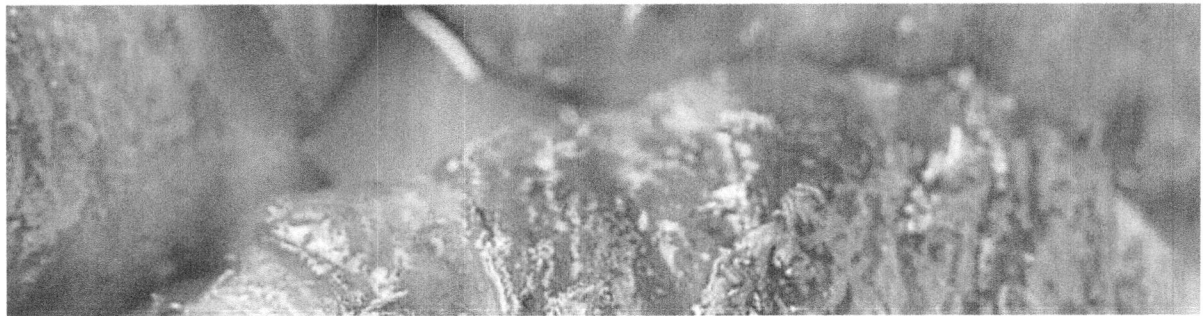

This one-pan dinner takes less time and is keto-friendly. It makes a nutritious meal because of vegetables baked along with meat. Any vegetables will do but the ones that are keto-friendly and can be cooked over high heat are most preferable.

Serving quantity: 6

Ingredients:

- 32 ounces chicken thighs, boneless and skinless
- 10 bacon slices
- 1 tsp. sea salt
- salt and pepper
- 1 tbsp. chili powder
- stevia, to taste
- 1 tsp. cumin powder
- 1 tsp. chipotle powder
- 1 tsp. onion powder
- ½ tsp. pepper
- ½ tsp. garlic powder

Directions:

Prep 7 min. | Cook 40 min. | Ready in 47 min.

- Preheat the oven to 375°F.
- Take a bowl and combine all spices in it.
- Roll chicken thighs in the spices and then wrap them with bacon.
- Line a sheet pan and place chicken over your choice of vegetables.
- Cook for 35 to 40 minutes until chicken is cooked and bacon is crispy.
- Take it out and serve.

Nutrition facts:

Per serving: 420 calories | 35 g fat | 22 g protein | 1 g carbs

Lamb With Kale

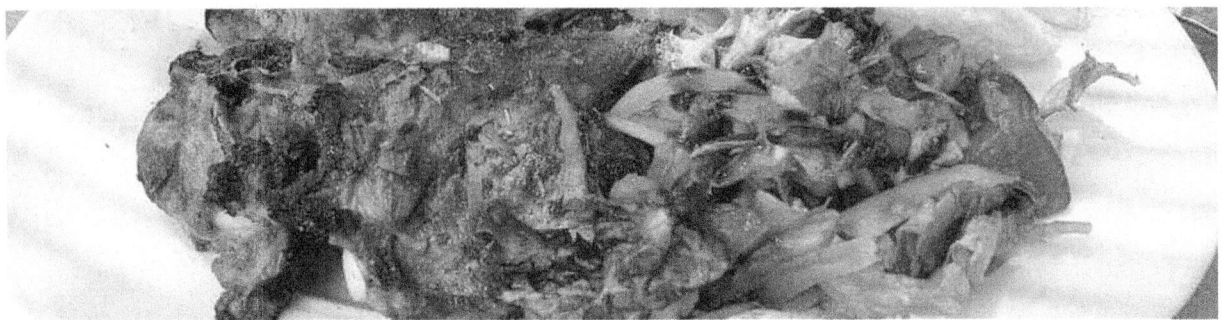

Lamb has such a nice flavor on its own but it gets even better when cooked with kale. Not only will you enjoy the juicy flavor of lamb, the kale will add some freshness to the dish.

Serving quantity: 4

Ingredients:

- 32 ounces lamb
- 1 bunch kale
- 1 tbsp. butter
- 1 tsp. sea salt
- 1 tsp. red pepper flakes
- 1 tsp. sesame seeds
- 3 tbsp. coconut oil

Directions:

Prep 5 min. | Cook 30 min. | Ready in 35 min.

- Fry meat in butter until it turns golden brown.
- Add salt and pepper flakes.
- Cover and cook for 25 minutes on low heat
- Add sesame seeds and kale and cook for 5 more minutes.
- Turn off the heat and let it cool for 5 minutes.
- Finally, add coconut oil and serve.

Nutrition facts:

Per Serving: 752 calories | 57 g fat | 42 g protein | 12 g carbs

Cauliflower And Broccoli Casserole

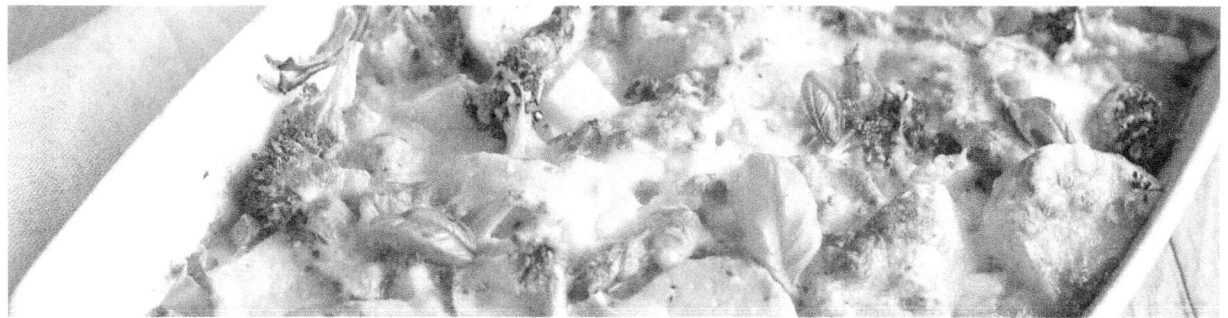

This filling family meal combines two low carb vegetables: cauliflower and broccoli. This combination tastes amazing!

Serving quantity: 6

Ingredients:

- 16 ounces broccoli florets
- 16 ounces cauliflower florets
- 7 ounces cream cheese
- 2 ounces butter
- 1 cup heavy whipping cream
- Salt and pepper
- 2 tsp. crushed garlic
- 8 ounces shredded cheese

Directions:

Prep 20 min. | Cook 40 min. | Ready in 1 h

- Preheat oven to 350 °F.
- Boil broccoli florets in a covered pot until it becomes tender.
- Strain broccoli and toss into a food processor.
- Add heavy whipping cream, cream cheese, butter, garlic, salt, and pepper.
- Make a smooth puree.
- Grease a baking dish and add cauliflower florets.
- Pour broccoli sauce and sprinkle the cheese.
- Bake for 40 minutes.

Nutrition facts:

Per Serving: 524 calories | 44 g fat | 17 g protein | 11 g carbs

Yakitori Chicken

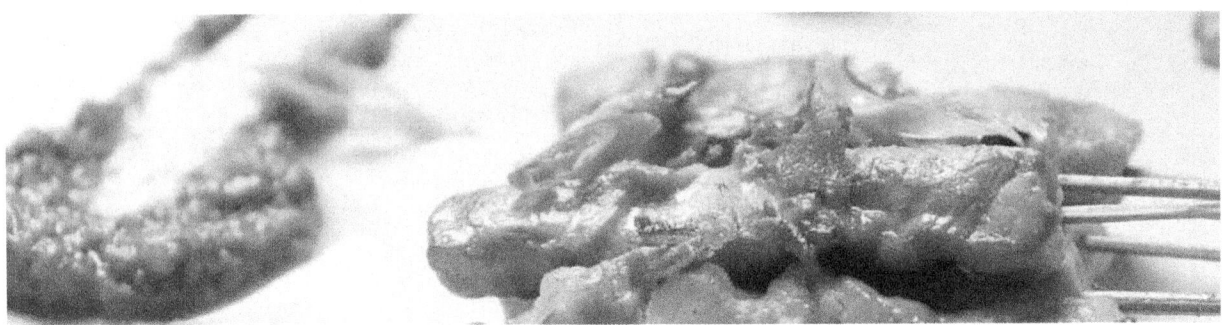

These are Japanese grilled chicken skewers and totally keto-friendly. What's yummier than grilled chicken anyway!

Serving quantity:

Ingredients:8

- 32 ounces boneless chicken thighs
- ¼ cup soy sauce or tamari
- ¼ cup water
- stevia, to taste
- 2 cloves minced garlic
- 1 chopped scallion
- 1 tbsp. sesame oil
- 2 tbsp. brochasweet
- ¼ tsp. xanthan gum
- 2 tsp. roasted sesame seeds
- 1 tsp. minced ginger
- ¼ tsp. hot pepper flakes

Directions:

Prep 15 min. | Cook 17 min. | Ready in 32 min.

- Add tamari, ginger, garlic, water, sweetener, brochasweet, sesame oil, hot pepper flakes in a saucepan, and boil over medium heat.
- Use ⅔ of the sauce to marinate chicken. Marinate it for 2 hours.
- Put the remaining sauce away to serve with the chicken.
- If you use bamboo skewers, soak them in water for 1 hour.
- Use either 8 large skewers or 12 small skewers.
- Heat the grill at medium-high flame and grease it.
- Thread the chicken on skewers and grill while brushing the marinating liquid.
- Grill for 5 to 6 minutes on each side and keep brushing the marinating liquid.
- When done, remove and serve them with the sauce.

Nutrition facts:

Per serving: 267 calories | 12 g fat | 36 g protein | 2 g carbs

REFERENCES

- Freeman JM, Kossoff EH, Hartman AL. The ketogenic diet: one decade later. Pediatrics. 2007 Mar;119(3):535–43. doi:10.1542/peds.2006-2447. PMID 17332207
- Martin-McGill KJ, Jackson CF, Bresnahan R, Levy RG, Cooper PN. Ketogenic diets for drug-resistant epilepsy. Cochrane Database Syst Rev. 2018 Nov 7;11:CD001903. doi:10.1002/14651858.CD001903.pub4. PMID 30403286
- Kossoff EH, Wang HS. Dietary therapies for epilepsy. Biomed J. 2013 Jan-Feb;36(1):2-8. doi:10.4103/2319-4170.107152 PMID 23515147
- Liu YM. Medium-chain triglyceride (MCT) ketogenic therapy. Epilepsia. 2008 Nov;49 Suppl 8:33–6. doi:10.1111/j.1528-1167.2008.01830.x. PMID 19049583
- Zupec-Kania BA, Spellman E. An overview of the ketogenic diet for pediatric epilepsy. Nutr Clin Pract. 2008 Dec–2009 Jan;23(6):589–96. doi:10.1177/0884533608326138. PMID 19033218
- Gano LB, Patel M, Rho JM. Ketogenic diets, mitochondria, and neurological diseases. J Lipid Res. 2014 Nov;55(11):2211-28. doi:10.1194/jlr.R048975. PMID 24847102.
- Stafstrom CE. An introduction to seizures and epilepsy. In: Stafstrom CE, Rho JM, editors. Epilepsy and the ketogenic diet. Totowa: Humana Press; 2004. ISBN 1-58829-295-9.
- de Boer HM, Mula M, Sander JW. The global burden and stigma of epilepsy. Epilepsy Behav. 2008 May;12(4):540–6. doi:10.1016/j.yebeh.2007.12.019. PMID 18280210
- Cai QY, Zhou ZJ, Luo R, Gan J, Li SP, Mu DZ, Wan CM. Safety and tolerability of the ketogenic diet used for the treatment of refractory childhood epilepsy: a systematic review of published prospective studies. World J Pediatr. 2017 Dec;13(6):528-536. doi:10.1007/s12519-017-0053-2. PMID 28702868.
- Wheless JW. History and origin of the ketogenic diet (PDF). In: Stafstrom CE, Rho JM, editors. Epilepsy and the ketogenic diet. Totowa: Humana Press; 2004. ISBN 1-58829-295-9.

ABOUT AUTHOR

"Du Bist Was Du Isst..." You Are What You Eat

Tasha Ryan is an authority in economics, finance management, and efficiency in the workplace. She is also an author of The Keto Diet for Beginners and other titles that centre around healthy diets and living, something she has been promoting for more than ten years. She lives with her husband, their daughter and their cat.

Unhappy with the weight she had steadily gained over the years, Tasha finally made a decision that she was going to lose at least some of it and began a thorough research into what might work best. Her journey ended when she discovered the ketogenic diet and immediately she knew that it was what she had been looking for.

With determination, lots of information, a range of tasty meals, and a willingness to try something different, Tasha managed to lose 40 pounds of excess weight and found that not only it made her look good but it also made her feel good, too.

With that momentum behind her, she began to understand that others may also benefit as she did. So, the author wrote her first book on the subject. She is following with a book in intermittent fasting and has more planned for the future.

Tasha's interest in healthy eating now occupies the entire ethos around the meals she prepares, cooking only healthy food for her family, who all love the variety of food that they can eat and the health benefits it brings. In her free time, she enjoys researching healthy living and dieting, creating amazing new recipes, and removing food addiction from the lives of her readers.

In the future, Tasha plans to share her experiences of losing weight, healing her body, and increasing efficiency to as many people as possible, improving their lives through simple recipes and great food.

Made in the USA
Coppell, TX
03 March 2022